Lecture Notes in Artificial Intelligence　　2101

Subseries of Lecture Notes in Computer S
Edited by J. G. Carbonell and J. Siekı

Lecture Notes in Computer Scieı
Edited by G. Goos, J. Hartmanis and J.

Springer
Berlin
Heidelberg
New York
Barcelona
Hong Kong
London
Milan
Paris
Singapore
Tokyo

Silvana Quaglini Pedro Barahona
Steen Andreassen (Eds.)

Artificial Intelligence in Medicine

8th Conference on Artificial Intelligence
in Medicine in Europe, AIME 2001
Cascais, Portugal, July 1-4, 2001, Proceedings

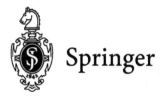 Springer

Series Editors

Jaime G. Carbonell,Carnegie Mellon University, Pittsburgh, PA, USA
Jörg Siekmann, University of Saarland, Saarbrücken, Germany

Volume Editors

Silvana Quaglini
University of Pavia
Department of Computer Science
Via Ferrata, 1, 27100 Pavia, Italy
E-mail: silvana.quaglini@unipv.it

Pedro Barahona
Departamento de Informática
Faculdade de Ciências e Tecnologia
Universidade Nova de Lisboa
2825-114 Caparica, Portugal
E-mail: pb@di.fct.unl.pt

Steen Andreassen
Aalborg University
Department of Medical Informatics and Image Analysis
Fredrik Bajersvej 7D, 9220 Alborg Øst, Denmark
E-mail: sa@miba.auc.dk

Cataloging-in-Publication Data applied for

Die Deutsche Bibliothek - CIP-Einheitsaufnahme

Artificial intelligence in medicine : proceedings / 8th Conference on AI in
Medicine in Europe, AIME 2001, Cascais, Portugal, July 1 - 4, 2001. Silvana
Quaglini ... (ed.). - Berlin ; Heidelberg ; New York ; Barcelona ; Hong Kong ;
London ; Milan ; Paris ; Singapore ; Tokyo : Springer, 2001
    (Lecture notes in computer science ; Vol. 2101 : Lecture notes in
    artificial intelligence)
    ISBN 3-540-42294-3

CR Subject Classification (1998): I.2, I.4, J.3, H.4, H.3

ISBN 3-540-42294-3 Springer-Verlag Berlin Heidelberg New York

Springer-Verlag Berlin Heidelberg New York
a member of BertelsmannSpringer Science+Business Media GmbH

http://www.springer.de

© Springer-Verlag Berlin Heidelberg 2001
Printed in Germany

Typesetting: Camera-ready by author, data conversion by PTP Berlin, Stefan Sossna
Printed on acid-free paper   SPIN 10839485   06/3142   5 4 3 2 1 0

Preface

The European Society for Artificial Intelligence in Medicine in Europe (AIME) was established in 1986 following a highly successful workshop held in Pavia, Italy, the year before. The aims of AIME are to foster fundamental and applied research in the application of Artificial Intelligence (AI) techniques to medical care and medical research, and to provide a forum for reporting significant results achieved at biennial conferences. In accordance with the latter aim, this volume contains the proceedings of AIME 2001, the eighth conference on Artificial Intelligence in Medicine in Europe, held in Cascais, Portugal, July 1–4, 2001. Previous conferences were held in Marseille (1987), London (1989), Maastricht (1991), Munich (1993), Pavia (1995), Grenoble (1997), and Aalborg (1999). This latter was a joint conference of AIME and ESMDM, the European Society for Medical Decision Making.

The call for papers of AIME 2001 required original contributions regarding the development of theory, techniques, and applications of AI in medicine. Contributions to theory included presentation or analysis of the properties of novel AI methodologies potentially useful in solving medical problems. Papers on techniques described the development or the extension of AI methods and their implementation, and discussed the assumptions and limitations of the proposed methods. Application papers described the implementation of AI systems to solve significant medical problems, and most of them presented an evaluation of the practical benefits of the system proposed.

The call resulted in 79 submissions, covering the areas of knowledge management, machine learning, data mining, decision support systems, temporal reasoning, case based reasoning, planning and scheduling, natural language processing, computer vision, image and signal interpretation, intelligent agents, telemedicine, careflow systems, and cognitive modeling.

All papers were carefully reviewed by at least two independent referees (77% by three referees), belonging to the Program Committee, supported by some additional reviewers. The review form addressed relevance of the paper content to AIME, originality and quality of the research, completeness, and organization of the paper. Eventually, 31 contributions were accepted for oral presentation, and 30 for poster presentation, with a "full paper" acceptance rate of about 39%. Thus, this volume contains 31 full papers and 30 short papers. In addition, the volume contains two keynote lectures written by the invited conference speakers. This year, keynote areas were the communication between agents within healthcare organizations and the sociotechnical approach to the design, implementation, and evaluation of knowledge-based systems. The choice of these areas stems from the recent debate within the medical community about the consequences of lack or default of co-operation among health care professionals. This is one of the main causes of poor care delivery. We think that AIME has the potentiality to take an active role in this debate, devoting efforts to the development of systems that take into account this medical community need. On the other hand, the 30 years history of AI in medicine shows that effective and efficient implementation of AI systems and, more generally, decision support systems in medicine, is often impaired by poor consideration of the real-word environment where such systems are intended to work.

We finish by thanking all those who contributed to the success of AIME 2001: the authors, the program committee members together with the additional reviewers, the local organizing committee members, the invited speakers Enrico Coiera from Australia and Jos Aarts from The Netherlands, the satellite workshops organizers, Peter Lucas (Bayesian Models in Medicine) and Stephen Rees (Computers in Anaesthesia and Intensive Care: Knowledge-Based Information Management), the tutorials' presenters Christoph Schommer (Application of Data Mining in Medicine), Jeremy Wyatt (Knowledge Management and AI in Medicine: What's the Link?), Gabriela Guimaraes (Unsupervised Neural Networks for Knowledge Discovery in Medicine), and Dan Steinberg (Multivariate Adaptive Regression Splines).

Last but not least we thank all the Institutions that sponsored the conference, namely IPE, Investimentos e Participações Empresariais, SA, Fundação para a Ciência e Tecnologia, and Fundação Calouste Gulbenkian.

April 2001

Silvana Quaglini
Pedro Barahona
Steen Andreassen

Organization

Scientific Program Chair: Silvana Quaglini (Italy)
Organizing Chair: Pedro Barahona (Portugal)
Tutorials and Workshops Chair: Steen Andreassen (Denmark)

Program Committee

Wil Van der Aalst (The Netherlands)
Stig K. Andersen (Denmark)
Steen Andreassen (Denmark)
Pedro Barahona (Portugal)
Robert Baud (Switzerland)
Riccardo Bellazzi (Italy)
Jan van Bemmel (The Netherlands)
Marc Berg (The Netherlands)
Enrico Coiera (Australia)
Carlo Combi (Italy)
Michel Dojat (France)
Rolf Engelbrecht (Germany)
John Fox (United Kingdom)
Douglas Fridsma (USA)
Catherine Garbay (France)
Barbara Heller (Germany)
Werner Horn (Austria)

Jim Hunter (United Kingdom)
Elpida Keravnou (Cyprus)
Cristiana Larizza (Italy)
Nada Lavrac, Ljubljana (Slovenia)
Johan van der Lei (The Netherlands)
Leonard Leibovici (Israel)
Silvia Miksch (Austria)
Marc Musen (USA)
Stelios Orfanoudakis (Greece)
Silvana Quaglini (Italy)
Alan Rector (United Kingdom)
Yuval Shahar (Israel)
Mario Stefanelli (Italy)
Mário Veloso (Portugal)
Jeremy Wyatt (United Kingdom)
Blaz Zupan (Slovenia)

Additional Reviewers

Ivano Azzini
Robert Kosara
Matjaž Kukar
Peter Lucas

Giovanni Magenes
Laura Maruster
Marko Robnik-Šikonja
Patrick Ruch

Andreas Seyfang
Ton Weijters
Xenophon Zabulis

Organizing Committee

Pedro Barahona
Mário Veloso

Joaquim Aparício
João Moura Pires

Gabriela Guimarães

Workshops

Bayesian Models in Medicine
    Co-chairs: Peter Lucas, University of Aberdeen, United Kingdom
    Linda van der Gaag, Utrecht University, The Netherlands
    Ameen Abu-Hanna, University of Amsterdam, The Netherlands

Computers in Anaesthesia and Intensive Care: Knowledge-Based Information
Management
    Chair: Stephen Rees, Aalborg University, Denmark
    Co-chairs: Silvia Miksch, Vienna University of Technology, Austria
    Michel Dojat, INSERM, France
    Jim Hunter, University of Aberdeen, United Kingdom

Tutorials

Application of Data Mining in Medicine
    Christoph Schommer, IBM German Development Laboratory, Germany
Knowledge Management and AI in Medicine: What's the Link ?
    Jeremy Wyatt, University College, London, United Kingdom
Unsupervised Neural Networks for Knowledge Discovery in Medicine
    Gabriela Guimarães, Universidade Nova de Lisboa, Portugal
Multivariate Adaptive Regression Splines
    Dan Steinberg, Salford Systems, San Diego, CA, USA

Table of Contents

Mediated Agent Interaction

Enrico Coiera

Centre for Health Informatics
University of New South Wales,
UNSW NSW 2055, Australia
ewc@pobox.com

Abstract. This paper presents a framework for agent communication and its mediation by technological systems. The goal of the framework is to provide quantitative mechanisms that will allow principled decisions to be made about the use and construction of mediating technological systems. Beginning with a simple model of interaction between agents, a model of communication influenced by bounded knowledge of others (or common ground) is developed. This leads to predictions that agent interactions generate equilibrium phenomena where optimal levels of grounding emerge over time between agents.

1   Introduction

Although computational and communication systems have had a largely independent development over the last century, there is no sharp demarcation between them either at a theoretical or technical level. Computational systems are as dependent on the transmission of data during calculation, as communication systems are dependent on the encoding and decoding of data for transmission. Indeed, a complex system like the World Wide Web clearly functions only because of the way that it marries communication and computation.

While there are bodies of work that either examine the human use of media, the transmission characteristics of media, or the computation of messages, we lack an integrated account of all three. At present we have strong models for several of the components of mediated interaction. Information theory models the process of message transmission across a channel. Computational theories model how an agent, given certain input, internal goals and resources, can construct or respond to a message. However, we have no adequate theoretical account that explains the behaviours that emerge when agents and channels combine to create a mediated interaction system.

This paper reviews the different bodies of communication research, identifies their specific deficiencies, and then outlines the scope for developing a new mediated communication theory. A framework for such a theory is then developed, based upon the notion of bounded mutual knowledge, or common ground, that is shared between communicating agents [1]. An examination of the costs of the grounding process then leads to the view that grounding is a kind of cost minimisation process, based upon

S. Quaglini, P. Barahona, and S. Andreassen (Eds.): AIME 2001, LNAI 2101, pp. 1–15, 2001.
© Springer-Verlag Berlin Heidelberg 2001

maximisation of agent utility, and results in cost-minimising equilibria developing between agents.

2   Three Views of Communication

Communication is the way we make our intentions known to the world, interact with others to achieve our goals, and the way that we learnt about our environment. Perhaps more than any other skill, the ability to hold conversation is the defining achievement of any intelligent agent. To do so requires knowledge of self and of other, and the ability to engage in a process of exploration whose bounds are imposed by mutual consent through interaction.

There are also physical bounds to communication, and these are provided both by the physical organs of agents, and by the communication channels they use to transmit messages. Communication channels are the intermediating links that agents use to converse, and the properties of channels also limit the forms a conversation can take. Sound, image and text all support very different conversational structures. Thus, communication is shaped both by the agents who wish to converse, and the mediating environment within which the conversation takes place.

Given its centrality in human society, communicative interaction has been looked at extensively over the centuries. Some have sought to develop technologies for communication or computation, whilst others have been motivated to understand and characterise the various forms of human interaction. Given these different intentions, we have communication theories that either emphasise the physical bounds to communication in technological systems, the knowledge bounds limiting rational agents, or the relativity of meaning arising out of the effects of context. It would be foolhardy to simplify these vast and complex bodies of work, but of necessity we can coarsely caricature three separate points of view:

- *Linguistic and social communication theories* (context centric) - Accounts of human communication have long been central to artists, musicians and writers, who have a profoundly different way of viewing communication to technologists. Fields like semiotics, communication theory [2], and philosophy have sought to emphasise how the context of communication profoundly alters the meaning that is drawn from a message. These ideas have coalesced into the notion of *post-modernism*, which emphasises the relativity of meaning for individual agents. More recently linguists have emphasised that language use, and the structures of conversations, are actively shaped within the context of a discussion [3]. Whilst providing a rich body of ideas, context centric theories are essentially qualitative, and do not provides us with quantitative mechanisms for making decisions about the design or management of communication technologies or computational processes.

- *Information theory* (channel centric) - In the classic information theoretic setting described by Shannon, a sender and a receiver exchange messages across a channel. The effect that different channels have in distorting the message is modelled statistically as the effect of noise. Information theory concerns itself with the most efficient way to encode a message given the space of all possible messages and the effects of noise on any given channel [4]. However, information theory says nothing about the meaning of a message, or how agents structure a message to suit a given context.

- *Computational theories* (model centric) - The communicative behaviours of agents can be partially accommodated in computational theories. The intentions and knowledge of each agent, as well as its decision procedures for constructing messages, can all be explicitly modelled as computable actions [5,6]. In particular, interacting agents can be modelled as Turing machines [7]. However, a Turing machine assumes messages are sent across a cost-free channel. Indeed, channels are usually not modelled at all in theoretical accounts of computation, but are left implicit. This assumption is often explicitly acknowledged as "cheap talk" in computationally inspired decision models like Game Theory [8].

Recently, there has been some movement between these three views. For example, context centric theorists have begun to realise that they must move away from highly-context dependent research to explore more general communication phenomena (e.g. [9]). At the other end of the spectrum, designers of interactive computer technologies have begun to admit the need for some understanding of the context of communication in the human-computer interaction. (e.g. [10]). In artificial intelligence circles, there has been a movement away from the model-centric view of computational intelligence towards one of *situated cognition* [11]. Here, the situation in which an agent interacts with the world in some way determines the behaviours that agents display [12]. Biological comparisons with the simple decision rules that drive organisms like ants are often used, pointing out the complex social behaviours that emerge through interaction with environmental structures.

The Scope and Role of a Mediated Communication Theory

Individually, the channel, context or model-centric views are limiting if we want to develop technologies that craft themselves around the meaning of conversations. If we wish to build communication systems optimised to the specific task needs of populations, that optimise their behaviour based upon the intent behind a conversation, or if we want to build autonomous software agents that have some scope for exploratory interaction with each other, then we need to close the gap between current theories. If successful, such a union of theories should allow us to answer two distinct classes of question:

- *Local communication decisions*: How should an agent communicate to maximise the outcome of an interaction? What combination of channels and media would be most favourable given the context of the interaction? Indeed, given a set of other agents to interact with, which ones are likely to be favourable choices, and what should be said to them to achieve the aim of the interaction? The resources available will always bound such choices for agents.
- *Global communication decisions*: Given an existing population of agents and communication technologies, what would the consequences be of introducing new communication technologies, or varying existing ones? Could the impact of the Web have been predicted in advance? Although we might find it hard to predict what individual agents might do in any given circumstance, we could make useful predictions about groups of agents. For example, given an

organisation with a set of information and communication problems, what mix of mediating technologies will provide the best solution?

The ultimate goal in answering such questions would be to identify quantitative mechanisms that allow principled decisions to be made about the use and construction of *mediated interaction systems*. By analogy, the periodic table arranged elements in a particular structure and lead to the identification of previously unknown elements. Similarly, one could hope that an interaction framework would provide coherence to our observations on the use of media, predict how different interaction settings will function, and where feasible, identify new forms of interaction and interaction technologies.

3   A General Setting for Communicative Interaction

Intuitively, an interaction occurs between two agents when one agent creates and then communicates a message to another. The intent of that act is to influence the receiving agent in some new way. A *mediated interaction* occurs when a communication channel intermediates between agents by bearing the messages between them. We will begin by developing a general model of what it means to have an interaction between two agents.

Definition 1: An **interaction** occurs between two independent agents A_1 and A_2 when A_1 constructs some message m, and passes it to A_2 across some communication channel c.

$$A_1 \xrightarrow[c]{m} A_2$$

The interaction between A_1 and A_2 occurs because A_1 has some intentions, and has decided to influence A_2 via the message, to satisfy its intention. We have thus placed our agents within a world in which they have choice over their own actions, and some ability to interact with the world to change it to suit their purposes.

In this model, agents are independent entities. Agents have no direct control over the behaviour of others (they can only attempt to influence behaviour through interaction), and they have no privileged knowledge of the internal state of other agents (they can only observe each other's behaviour in the world, and infer their internal state). Agents also operate with finite resources, and consequently need to minimise costs on resources and maximise the benefits of any action they contemplate.

The interaction between agents is dependent upon three things - the channel, the relationship between the agents, and the context within which they find themselves. We need to expand upon the simple interaction model presented above, to incorporate each of these elements. Of the three, most will be said about the effect of agent relationship upon communication.

Effects of Channel upon Interaction

Standard information theory describes how the outcome of an interaction is determined in part by the characteristics of the mediating channel c [4]. A message m is transmitted between the agents as a data stream D. The communication channel c is not neutral to D, but has a modifying effect upon it. Data may be affected by noise in the channel, for example. So, we note that when agent A_1 utters a data stream D_1, that it is then modified by c, to be received as D_2 by agent A_2 (Figure 1). Since the information theoretic aspects of channel noise on message transmission are standard results, they need not be described any further here, except to reinforce their importance in quantifying the overall characteristics of inter-agent interactions.

Effect of Agent Relationships upon Interaction

Agents have independent origins, independent resources and independent prior experiences, which modify their internal state over time. Thus, in this setting we are not permitted to look inside an agent and know what it knows, only to infer that from observable behaviour. Critically then, the private world models of the communicating agents M_1 and M_2 are not verifiably identical to any observer.

We can now refine our interaction setting to include this new element. An individual agent A_1 creates a data stream D_1, based upon its knowledge of the world M_1. A_2 receives D_2, and generates its own private interpretation of its meaning based upon D_2 (Figure 1).

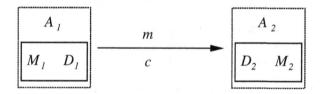

Fig. 1: The M-model of interaction (after McCarthy and Monk (1994)).

We next note that agents communicate more easily with other agents that have similar experiences, beliefs and knowledge. Intuitively we know that it takes greater effort to explain something in a conversation to someone with whom we share less common background. Conversely, individuals who are particularly close can communicate complicated ideas in terse shorthand.

Agents who share similar background knowledge can be termed *homophilus*, and dissimilar agents *heterophilus* [13]. The notion of homophily arose out of the analysis of social relationships between individuals of similar occupation and educational background. Homophilus individuals tended to have more effective communication amongst themselves, and the more individuals communicated, the more homophilus they became [14].

The degree of agent similarity is thus based upon the similarity of their knowledge about the world:

<u>Definition 2:</u> For interacting agents a and b with respective internal models M_a and M_b, with respect to a given message m, the degree of **homophily** between them $H_{a:b}$ is the ratio $f(M_a)/f(M_b)$, where $f(x)$ is some well-defined function on M_x.

This definition has the property that identical agents would have unit homophily. Further, one would expect that the cost of communicating between dissimilar agents is a function of the degree of homophily:

When $H_{a:b} = 1$ the interaction is *relationship neutral*. The agents are able to communicate with no effort diverted to managing misunderstandings, other than those caused by the effects of channel, such as noise.

When $H_{a:b} > 1$ the interaction is *relationship negative*. This means that agent a needs to explain part of a message to b, by transmitting background knowledge along with the principle message to permit b to fully understand. The negativity is associated with the fact that there is an extra cost imposed upon a.

When $H_{a:b} < 1$ the interaction is *relationship positive*. In this case, agent a needs to request background knowledge along with the principal message from b. The positivity is associated with the fact that there is an extra benefit for a, in that its knowledge will be expanded by interacting with b[1].

<u>Definition 3:</u> For interacting agents a and b with respective internal models M_a and M_b, with respect to a given message m, the **relationship distance** between the agents $D_{a:b}$ is $f(M_a) - f(M_b)$, where $f(x)$ is some well-defined function on M_x.

According to this definition, identical agents would have zero distance. Dissimilar agents have a finite distance and one would also expect that the cost of communicating between them is a function of that distance i.e.:

When $D_{a:b} = 0$ the interaction is *relationship neutral*.
When $D_{a:b} > 0$ the interaction is *relationship negative*.
When $D_{a:b} < 0$ the interaction is *relationship positive*.

Homophily and relationship distance are clearly closely related. For example, one natural interpretation of the two is to see both as a statistical estimates of a model i.e. $f(x)$ is a probability distribution function describing M_x. Further, from basic information theory, the information contained in an event is defined as the log of its probability i.e. $I_x = log\ p(x)$. We could then define:

$$H_{a:b} \quad = p(M_a)\,/\,p(M_b)$$
$$log\ H_{a:b} = log\ [p(M_a)\,/\,p(M_b)]$$
$$log\ H_{a:b} = log\ p(M_a) - log\ p(M_b)$$
$$= D_{a:b}$$
$$log\ H_{a:b} = D_{a:b} \tag{1}$$

---

[1] Receiving knowledge is not always 'positive' in any absolute sense. There are costs associated with receiving, processing, and maintaining knowledge, as we shall see later.

Thus $D_{a:b}$ can be interpreted as an information distance, directly derivable from $H_{a:b}$, which is some statistical representation of the content or behaviour of a given model. This definition brings with it all of the nice properties that come with information measures. However, it is worth emphasising that there are many possible interpretations of $f(x)$, not just this probabilistic one, with consequences for how one interprets the relationship between $H_{a:b}$ and $D_{a:b}$.

While distance or homophily can give us an indication of the likely costs and degree of success of an interaction, it may be necessary to actually examine the specifics of the knowledge that agents share. In linguistics, the shared knowledge between agents is called the common ground ([15, 3]), and we can try to operationalise that notion:

Definition 4: For interacting agents a and b with respective internal models M_a and M_b, the **common ground** $G_{a:b}$ between them is the intersection of their model spaces $M_{a,b}$.

Note that we are saying nothing at present about the way an individual concept might be represented internally within an agent. For knowledge to appear in the common ground, both agents have to be able to recognise that the other agent possesses knowledge that is functionally equivalent to their own for a given task and context.

Once common ground is known, we can begin to examine its effect upon message transmission. An idealised message can be thought of as containing two parts. The first is a model, and the second is data encoded according to that model [16]. Thus we can define a message from agent a to b as having the idealised form:

$$m_{a,b} = M_{a,b} + (D|M_a)$$

(2)

The model $M_{a,b}$ is that subset of agent a's overall knowledge that it has determined is needed to interpret the message data D. In information theory, this model would be the code used to encrypt data.

However, since some of the model $M_{a,b}$ is known or is assumed to be shared between agents, not all of it needs to be transmitted. The optimal model to be transmitted t will be:

$$t(M_{a,b}) = \{ x: x \, ?M_{a,b} \, ?x? \, M_{a,b} \}$$

(3)

and the actual message sent will be:

$$t(m_{a,b}) = t(M_{a,b}) + (D|M_a)$$

(4)

The effort required to transmit a particular message between two agents can be represented by the degree of message shortening that occurs because of the shared common ground between agents:

<u>Definition 5:</u> For interacting agents *a* and *b* with respective internal models M_a and M_b, the **grounding efficiency** for a message *m* sent from *a* to *b* is the ratio of the lengths of the actual message transmitted over the idealised message length determined by *a*:

$$G_E = \frac{t(m_{a\ b})}{m_{a\ b}}$$

$$= \frac{t(M_{a\ b}) + (D|M_a)}{M_{a\ b} + (D|M_a)}$$

(5)

Grounding efficiency thus gives us some measure of the resource requirements for an interaction between two agents, all else being equal. If the average grounding efficiency is calculated by summing over a number of interactions, it gives the efficiency likelihood of a future interaction, based upon past experience i.e.:

(6)

$$G_{E(av)} = \frac{1}{n} \sum_n \frac{t(m_{a\ b})}{m_{a\ b}}$$

One of the reasons agents create common ground is to optimise their interaction. By sharing ground, less needs to be said in any given message, making the interaction less costly. Consequently, the goal in grounding is to develop sufficient ground to accommodate the anticipated efficiency requirements of future interactions. One can identify three different classes of interaction, based upon grounding efficiency:

- When $G_E < 1$, the interaction is *ground positive* since some shortening of the message has occurred.
- When $G_E = 1$ the interaction is *ground neutral*. The message in this case is simply sent in its idealised form.
- When $G_E > 1$, the interaction is *ground negative*. This means that the message sent is longer than the idealised length.

The Effect of Context upon Interaction

The idea of the context within which an interaction occurs can be interpreted widely. Here it is understood to be the set of constraints upon communication imposed by the environment that is external to agents. Specifically, context imposes limits upon the physical resources available for communication. Examples of contextually constrained resources include time, bandwidth and money.

A channel forms part of the environment and limits the nature of any given communicative interaction. For example, when a channel mediates an interaction, we should be able to relate message-grounding requirements between agents to the transmission capacity of the channel that could successfully mediate their exchange:

<u>Definition 6:</u> For interacting agents *a* and *b*, a message *m* transmitted over a time *t* with a grounding efficiency of G_E, the **requisite channel capacity** *C* is:

$$C = \frac{m}{t} G_E$$

Recalling that average grounding efficiency is based upon the history of previous messages, making the channel capacity for the $n+1th$ message dependent upon the grounding history of the previous n messages:

$$C = \frac{m_{n+1}}{tn} \sum_{x=1}^{n} \frac{t(m_x)}{m_x}$$

(7)

With this equation, we connect together the triad of channel characteristics, context-specific message requirements and the nature of the relationship between communicating agents. It allows us to make three different types of inference:

- *Channel-centric inference*: For a given pair of agents and a message, we can specify channel capacity requirements.
- *Relationship-centric inference*: For a given agent, channel and time resource, we can say something about the common grounding that would help select an appropriate second agent to communicate with.
- *Task-centric inference*: Time can be considered a key task-limiting resource. For a pair of agents and a given channel, we can say something about the complexity of messages that can be exchanged between them over a given period of time.

The last of these suggests that we can generalise the previous equation further to incorporate other resources. Resource-specific versions of the equation can be crafted, substituting bandwidth for other bounded resources like time, monetary cost, utility of knowledge received etc. A general resource function, probably based upon utility, may be useful.

Grounding estimates lead to communication errors and inefficiencies

When agents create a message to suit a given context's needs, it must make guesses. For example, Equation 4 shows that a guess needs to be made about what model $t(m_{a,b})$ is to be transmitted in a message. This guess is based upon estimates ? of what model is needed to explain the data $?(M_{a,b})$, and what part of that model is already shared $?(M_{a,b})$. Thus grounding efficiency will always be a local measure when individual agents make it, since it is based upon local estimates of what needs to be transmitted:

$$t_a(M_{a,b}) = \{ \mathfrak{X}, x \ ? \ ?(M_{a,b}) \ ?x \ ? \ ?(M_{a,b}) \}$$

(8)

Consequently, errors occur in estimating both the common ground and the model needed for data interpretation. For example, an agent may end up explaining more of the model than is needed because it underestimates the common ground it shares with another agent, or conversely fails to explain enough. It may also simply lack the knowledge needed to interpret the data it sends. The possible error cases are summarised in Table 1.

Table 1: Communication errors based upon common ground estimates.

	$< ?_b (M_{a,b})$	$= ?_b (M_{a,b})$	$> ?_b (M_{a,b})$
$?_a (M_{a,b})$	*a confuses b:* *a* overestimates common ground with *b* - model message too short and *b* cant fully interpret	*a informs b:* *a's* estimate of common ground agrees with *b* - model message optimal	*a bores b:* *a* underestimates common ground with *b*- model message too long, telling *b* what it already knows

With the notion of common ground, we are thus able to move away from the rather abstract idea of homophily, and begin to explore more precisely how relationship as modelled by shared knowledge affects communication. It also begins to give structure to the different types of interaction that can occur between agents, and the errors, misunderstandings and inefficiencies that result.

4   The Costs of Grounding

One consequence of agents having independent world models is the behaviour of *grounding* where agents devote some portion of their total interactions to checking if they understand each other [17]. Grounding is the process in which agents specifically attempt to test the common language, knowledge and assumptions between them, and then attempt to modify deficiencies in their shared understanding to ensure the overall goal of an interaction succeeds.

We can think of grounding as a process for operationally testing and then ensuring M_1 and M_2 are sufficiently similar, within the context of a particular set of interactions, to guarantee a common interpretation of shared messages. Work in the psychological literature examines how people first establish, and then maintain, common ground whilst communicating [15].

Grounding is not a neutral process, but consumes some of the resources agents have available to communicate. These costs come in two varieties. Firstly, there are costs associated with interpreting the messages created in the process of grounding. Secondly, there are costs associated with maintaining the common ground itself, which we have characterised here as a common set of interpretive models of the world. These two costs have very different characteristics in relation to when they are incurred and how agents might choose to manage them, as we shall now see.

The Cost of Communicating Common Ground

If agents had identical models of the World, then the only costs of communication would arise out of transmitting across a noisy channel, and constructing and decoding messages according to shared protocols. However, when there is uncertainty about shared understanding, both sender and receiver incur extra costs during communication.

We can relate this grounding cost to the difference in the models between two communicating agents. For any given message, there may exist some additional background knowledge B that is possessed by the sending agent, and needed by the receiving agent to fully interpret its meaning. For example, if we tell someone to meet us at a certain location, but they do not know where it is, then we will also need to tell them additional information about its geographical situation and navigating a route there.

For a sending agent A_1, costs are incurred in inferring B based upon its best understanding of the other agent's knowledge and the progress of the conversation, and then communicating B.   There is clearly some monotonically increasing relationship between the cost of interaction for A_1 and the size of B. The more background knowledge we need to impart, the more effort it will require.

Equally A_2 bears reciprocal costs in receiving B in addition to the actual message. Again, there is an increasing set of costs associated with receiving, checking and testing B, as the size of B grows.

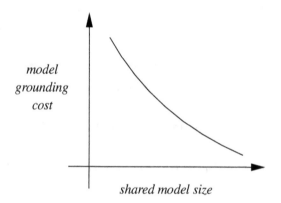

Fig. 2: The cost of grounding models decreases with the size of the shared model space between two agents.

So, for any two agents participating in an interaction, the cost of grounding rises with the difference in their models of the world. Conversely, and more directly, the cost of communication decreases as the degree of model sharing increases (Figure 2).

The Cost of Maintaining Common Ground

Agents interact in a dynamic world, and their knowledge of the world needs to be refreshed as the world changes around them. Thus the accuracy of any model possessed by an agent decays over time. For a model to retain its accuracy, it must be maintained at a rate commensurate with the rate of world change. It follows that there is an on-going requirement in any dynamic universe, for agents to update shared models.

Keeping knowledge up-to-date requires effort on the part of an agent, and this effort is related to the size of the up-date task. If we think of these shared models as formally represented structures, then we know that the maintenance and updating costs are exponential in shape, based on the costs of writing, de-bugging and updating software [18]. In fact, experience with software development shows that maintenance costs come not just from a need to keep up-to-date, but from the inherent flaws in the model building process. Our models are inherently flawed and 'de-bugging' costs rise with the size of a program. For the present argument, we only need note that many forces conspire to produce an increasing cost of model maintenance with model size. Consequently, the greater the size of the shared model of the world between two agents, the greater the need for updating and maintaining that model (Figure 3).

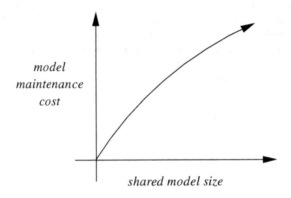

model maintenance cost

shared model size

Fig. 3: The cost of maintaining shared models increases with the size of the shared model space between agents.

Interactions are Shaped to Minimise Grounding Communication and Maintenance Costs

These two different costs associated with common ground give agents choices to either share mutual knowledge pre-emptively in anticipation of a communication, or just-in-time to satisfy the immediate needs of an interaction [1]. Since agents operate with finite resources, they will seek to minimise these costs on their resources. Firstly, agents have an incentive to minimise how much knowledge they share with each other, because maintaining and updating this shared body of knowledge is expensive. Intuitively we can think of the cost we incur 'keeping in touch' with people, and note that most people devote effort here commensurate with the value they place on the relationship and the amount of resource they have available for communication. In contrast, the less common ground agents share during a particular conversation, the more expensive that individual conversation will be, since additional knowledge will need to be communicated at the time. Intuitively, we can think of the effort one spends 'catching up' with an individual we haven't spoken with for some time, prior to getting to the point of a particular conversation. There are thus opposing incentives to minimise sharing of models prior to a conversation, and maximise the sharing during a conversation (Figure 4).

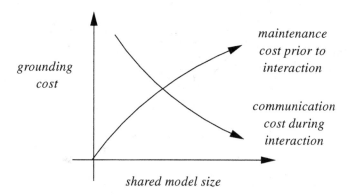

Fig. 4: Grounding costs at the time of a conversation decrease with shared models, but carry an ongoing up-date burden that increases with the size of the shared space between agents.

The total cost of grounding T is therefore the sum of costs during an individual set of interactions D and the model maintenance efforts prior to them P i.e. $T = D + P$. Interestingly, this line of reasoning predicts that the total interaction costs have a minimum at an intermediate level of model sharing, where the cost curves cross (Figure 5). Given a desire to minimise costs by individual agents, then it should also be predictable that they will seek to find such intermediate levels of model sharing since they are the most economical over a long sequence of interactions.

Fundamentally, every agent makes some assessment of the costs $C(x)$ and benefits $B(x)$ of a potential interaction x, and when the benefits exceed costs, elects to interact [19] i.e.:

if $B(x) > C(x)$ then do x else don't

What emerges then is a picture of a series of cost-benefit trade-offs being made by individual agents across individual interactions, and populations of interactions. The goal is to maximise the utility of any given interaction, through a maximisation of benefit, and minimisation of cost. The result of these choices is that agents try to choose a degree of shared common ground with other agents that minimises interaction costs, but is still sufficient to accomplish the goal associated with interactions. This leads to a hypothesis:

Hypothesis 1: The *law of the mediated centre* states that an interaction system of communicating agents will be driven to an intermediate level of model sharing over a series of interactions where the total costs of maintaining shared models and communicating models at interaction time are minimised. The mediated centre represents an interaction equilibrium point.

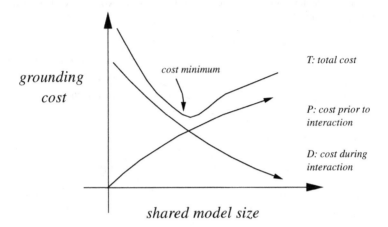

Fig. 5: Total grounding costs are based on costs during and prior to a conversation, and reach a minimum at an intermediate level of model sharing between agents.

Many factors modify decisions to model-share, in particular an individual agent's assessment of the duration of its relationship with another agent, and the costs of being caught short during an individual conversation. Thus, if an interaction with another agent is infrequent, then it may be cheaper to choose to ground only during individual interactions. If the agent is going to have a series of similar interactions, then it may be cheaper in the long run to establish a high level of shared common ground, and minimise grounding during individual interactions. Equally, if individual interactions are resource critical, for example being time-bound, then there may be little opportunity to ground at the time of an interaction. Consequently, even if interactions are infrequent, the cost of failure to communicate may make it important to establish prior common ground.

Similarly, there are costs associated with the channel chosen for an interaction. Some channels may allow rapid and high-quality transmission of a message, but be very expensive. Others may be slow but cheap, and in many circumstances sufficient for the task at hand. Channel costs are numerous and include:

- the actual price charged for using the channel
- the effect of noise on the transmitted message
- the effort involved in locating channel access
- the number of connection attempts required before another agent replies
- the opportunity costs involved in message delay due to the channels transmission characteristics like bandwidth and latency
- and similarly, the time it takes to transmit a message

5   Conclusion

In this paper, a framework for defining interactions between agents with only bounded mutual knowledge has been developed, extending upon earlier work [1]. The development of the theory to incorporate sequences of interactions between individual agents has lead to the notion of utility maximisation by agents, where they seek to optimise the degree of common ground between themselves.

The goal of developing such a mediated communication theory is to provide quantitative mechanisms for the design of interactions by individual computational agents, or for the design of interactions systems for use in complex organisations.

References

1.   E. Coiera, When Communication is better than Computation. *Journal American Medical Informatics Association.* 7, 277-286, 2000.
2.   P. Cobley (ed.), The Communication Theory Reader, Routledge, London, (1996).
3.   H. Clarke, Using Language, Cambridge University Press, Cambridge, (1996).
4.   J. C. A. van der Lubbe, *Information Theory*, Cambridge University Press, (1997).
5.   S. J. Russell, P. Norvig, *Artificial Intelligence - a modern approach*, Prentice Hall, Upper Saddle River, (1995).
6.   B. Moulin, B. Chaib-Draa, An overview of distributed artificial intelligence, in GMP O'Hare and NR Jennings (eds), Foundations of Distributed Artificial Intelligence, John Wiley and Sons, Inc., (1996).
7.   R. Herken (ed.), *The Universal Turing Machine - A half-century survey*, Oxford University Press, Oxford, (1988).
8.   H S. Bierman, L. Fernandez, Game Theory with economic applications, Addison-Wesley, Reading., Ma., (1995).
9.   C R. Berger, Chatauqua: Why are there so few communication theories?, Communication Monographs, 58, 101-113, (1991).
10.   B. Nardi (ed), Context in Consciousness - activity theory and human-computer interaction, MIT Press, Cambridge Ma., (1996).
11.   L. Suchman, *Plans and situated actions - the problem of human-machine communication*, Cambridge University Press, Cambridge, (1987).
12.   R Brooks, Intelligence without representation, Artificial Intelligence, 47,139-159, (1991).
13.   P. F. Lazarsfeld, R. K. Merton, Friendship as Social process: a substantive and methodological analysis, in M. Berger et al. (eds.), *Freedom and Control in Modern Society,* New York, Octagon (1964).
14.   E. M. Rogers, *Diffusion of Innovations*, 4th Ed., Free Press, New York, (1995).
15.   D Clarke, S. Brennan, Grounding in Communication, in L.B. Resnick J. Levine, & S.D. Behreno (Eds.), *Perspectives on socially shared cognition*, American Psychological Association, Washington, (1991).
16.   CS Wallace, DM Boulton, An infratio n measure for classification, Comp. J, 11, 185-195, (1968).
17.   J. C. McCarthy, A. F. Monk, Channels, conversation, co-operation and relevance: all you wanted to know about communication but were afraid to ask, *Collaborative Computing,*1:35-60 (1994).
18.   B. Littlewood, *Software Reliability: achievement and assessment*, Blackwell Scientific Publications, (1987).
19.   R.H. Frank, Microeconomics and behavior, 3rd Ed., McGraw Hill,New York, (1997).

On Articulation and Localization – Some Sociotechnical Issues of Design, Implementation, and Evaluation of Knowledge Based Systems

Jos Aarts

Department of Health Policy and Management
Erasmus University Rotterdam
P.O. Box 1738, 3000 DR Rotterdam, The Netherlands
E-mail: j.aarts@bmg.eur.nl

Abstract. The standard model of clinical work is a fixed sequence of tasks covering diagnosis and treatment of patients. Knowledge based systems have been designed according to this sequence. This ideal typical approach accounts for the relative modest success of knowledge based systems in healthcare practice. In reality however, clinical work is highly contingent, ad-hoc and idiosyncratic and therefore hard to fit into in a formal model. A physician is said to manage complex and diverse patient trajectories. Therefore the concept of a trajectory should not only relate to the course of the disease of a patient, but to all the organizational work during that course as well. We will highlight two aspects of this 'messy' view of clinical work and examine the consequences for the design, implementation and evaluation of knowledge based systems. *Articulation* refers to the fact that a lot of invisible work is being done in order to complete a visible task of a physician. A physician may see a patient, but before she can do that a lot of work has been done to assure that she actually sees the patient. *Localization* refers to the fact that clinical work is being adapted to local and situational circumstances. This is not primarily related to the variance in medical work as a result of uncertain knowledge about the true clinical state of a patient, but to the constant negotiating with colleagues, local opportunities and restraints and the possibilities of protocols and technologies. In short, the way how patient trajectories are being shaped by human and non-human elements. A knowledge based system that has the potential of adaptability to patient trajectories seems to offer new opportunities. Such an approach would place the user in the centerfold of the design, implementation and evaluation of such systems.

Introduction

The introduction of knowledge based systems in medicine has not been an easy task. To date not many systems are actively used in healthcare practice. Prominent examples are MYCIN that never made it to clinical practice because of the technological constraints of introducing computer systems into the clinic, and Internist1/QMR that eventually evolved into a teaching aid.

The most important arguments for introducing knowledge based systems in healthcare have been the following [1].

S. Quaglini, P. Barahona, and S. Andreassen (Eds.): AIME 2001, LNAI 2101, pp. 16–19, 2001.
© Springer-Verlag Berlin Heidelberg 2001

- Peer reviewed medical knowledge and the minds of the best practitioners have been captured in knowledge based systems and is made available to a wider group of users. Thus, it is hoped, variance in medical practice can be reduced.
- The knowledge base of medicine is increasing exponentially and no single human can even start to cope with it. Knowledge based systems can in principle encompass huge amounts of information and are therefore seen as means to relieve the information burden of the single practitioner.
- Humans are considered as flawed decision makers. Errors, biases, beliefs are part and parcel of the human decision making process. Knowledge based systems are seen to remedy this problem.

Researchers recognize that already the design of knowledge based systems is fraught with difficulties. Human experts are often blamed for these difficulties, because of the untrustworthy nature of human self-reporting. Often better modeling approaches and spending more time on eliciting expert knowledge are seen as a solution to overcome these difficulties. But Musen and Van der Lei state that the real problem in eliciting expert knowledge lies in the fact that the experts have so little insight into their own expertise [2]. In an ethnographic study of the maintenance of copying machines Suchman likewise relates that maintenance engineers tell what they think that they do instead what they really do [3].

Patient Trajectories

The standard view of clinical work is that of a cognitive process of the physician (or nurse). The physician sees the patient, assesses his condition, orders tests to ascertain a hypothesis or to decide more precisely a plan of treatment, initiates a treatment and evaluates her course of action. Knowledge based systems have been designed to support one or more tasks in this sequence. This paradigm of clinical work is so strong that most studies in medical informatics focus on individual physician behavior.

In reality a physician manages patient trajectories [4]. A patient trajectory includes the treatment of a patient's disease, the organizing of all the work done during the course of the treatment and the impact on those who are involved with that work and its organization. It follows that trajectories are highly contingent. People, protocols, technology, culture and organizational structure are all part of a patient trajectory. The study of the close relationship of the human and the non-human (technology, protocols, guidelines, organizational structure, etc.) is what is called the sociotechnical approach [5]. If a knowledge based system plays a role in supporting medical work it becomes part of that trajectory. Most trajectories are unproblematic and routine. Physicians know what needs to be done and how to organize that efficiently. This contradicts with the commonly held opinion that a physician has to cope with a growing amount of clinical knowledge. A patient trajectory can become problematic not only through the nature of the disease but also through the interactions with other elements of the trajectory. Managing a patient trajectory is not the same as managing a workflow. A workflow focuses fully on the tasks of one or several individuals and the questions how these tasks can be initiated and coordinated with help of (clinical) guidelines [6]. A workflow approach can be incorporated in a patient trajectory. An important aspect of modeling workflow is to model communication between the members.

If patient trajectories are being shaped by so many different elements, then it follows that a patient trajectory cannot be separated from its context and is localized by its nature. Elements of the trajectory should then be studied in this local context. Managing a patient trajectory is foremost a social phenomenon. In a more somber mood one can label clinical work as 'messy.'

On Articulation and Localization

Treating patients is very visible. But in order to manage a patient trajectory that centers around the treatment of a patient, a lot of work has to be done in order to complete medical tasks. Usually a physician has the largest view of the management of the disease of the patient, she knows what needs to be done and can rely on protocols that tell her what to do for a particular medical problem and what resources need to be mustered. Other people are needed to organize the job that the physician has requested. For example, nursing staff has to be available. Work schedules of nursing personnel have to be compliant with medical work. The order that a patient needs an X-ray means that a lot of work needs to be done in order to ensure that the job will be done. The patient needs to be prepared, a session needs to be scheduled, the patient needs to be transported, possible other planned activities needs to be rescheduled, people need to be telephoned, etc. Usually is this work highly invisible, but is the 'glue' that holds the patient trajectory together. Strauss calls it articulation work [4] (p. 151).

Managing patient trajectories is intricately connected with local and situational circumstances. Getting a medical job done is not primarily dependent on medical knowledge, but the result of a constant negotiation about what to do next. A physician will consult a colleague, be confronted with the financial constraint of his hospital, be angry about unavailability of nurses, etc. and these contingencies will determine to large part the clinical course of action. It is this what Strauss calls the messiness of patient trajectories. If knowledge based systems are to be used in healthcare practice they must become part and parcel of this messiness. Such a tool may become highly localized and function differently from what the designers originally envisaged [7] (p. 123).

Conclusions

I would like to draw some conclusions from the considerations above. A knowledge based system may be modeled on an analysis of the cognitive process of clinical decision making and based on universally agreed clinical knowledge, but in clinical practice it will become part of the negotiation process. I suggest that a knowledge based system can be successful if it contributes to coordination of work processes, i.e. if it becomes part of the 'glue' of a patient trajectory.

What does it mean for the design, implementation and evaluation of knowledge bases systems.

The design and implementation must be based on a careful analysis of clinical work practices. The analysis will not only rely on the modeling of cognitive clinical knowledge but also on a qualitative analysis of work practices by means of ethnography, document studies and non-structured interviews. Modeling and the design of formal tools are sides of the same coin, but, apart from linking data in a meaningful way, it needs to include the modeling of communication [8].

Like the design and implementation of any other technology it needs to be managed in close relation with its intended users. It has to be part of a social process. I will not elaborate on this issue, because it is treated elsewhere more extensively (see amongst others [9,10].

Evaluation should include the issue of localization. How adaptable a knowledge based system has to be, will depend on the extent that what is considered universally accepted knowledge, guidelines and protocols are subject of negotiations and how it will fit in a trajectory. It may be that the intended users will be different from what the designers expected.

References

1.   Shortliffe, E. H. (1987). "Computer programs to support clinical decision making." JAMA 258(1): 61-6.
2.   Musen, M. A. and J. van der Lei (1989). "Knowledge engineering for clinical consultation programs: modeling the application area." Methods Inf Med 28(1): 28-35.
3.   Suchman, L. A. (1987). Plans and situated actions, the problem of human machine communication. Cambridge, Cambridge University Press.
4.   Strauss, A. L., S. Fagerhaugh, et al. (1997). Social organization of medical work. New Brunswick, Transaction Publishers.
5.   Berg, M. (1999). "Patient care information systems and health care work: a sociotechnical approach." Int J Med Inf 55: 87-101.
6.   Quaglini, S., M. Stefanelli, et al. (2001). "Flexible guideline-based patient careflow systems." Artif Intell Med 22(1): 65-80
7.   Berg, M. (1997). Rationalizing medical work, decision support techniques and medical practices. Cambridge (MA), The MIT Press.
8.   Maij, E., V. E. van Reijswoud, et al. (2000). "A process view of medical practice by modeling communicative acts." Methods Inf Med 39(1): 56-62.
9.   Berg, M., C. Langenberg, et al. (1998). "Considerations for sociotechnical design: experiences with an electronic patient record in a clinical context." Int J Med Inf 52(1-3): 243-51.
10. Agre, P. E. (1995). Conceptions of the user in computer systems design. The social and interactional dimensions of human-computer interfaces. P. J. Thomas. Cambridge, Cambridge University Press: 67-106.

Prototype Selection and Feature Subset Selection by Estimation of Distribution Algorithms. A Case Study in the Survival of Cirrhotic Patients Treated with TIPS*

B. Sierra[1], E. Lazkano[1], I. Inza[1], M. Merino[2], P. Larrañaga[1], and J. Quiroga[3]

[1] Dept. of Computer Science and Artificial Intelligence, University of the Basque Country, P.O. Box 649, E-20080 Donostia, Spain
ccpsiarb@si.ehu.es
http://www.sc.ehu.es/isg
[2] Basque Health Service - Osakidetza, Comarca Gipuzkoa - Este, Avenida Navarra 14, E-20013 Donostia - San Sebastián, Spain
[3] Facultad de Medicina, University Clinic of Navarra, E-31080 Pamplona - Iruña, Spain

Abstract. The Transjugular Intrahepatic Portosystemic Shunt (TIPS) is an interventional treatment for cirrhotic patients with portal hypertension. In the light of our medical staff's experience, the consequences of TIPS are not homogeneous for all the patients and a subgroup dies in the first six months after TIPS placement. An investigation for predicting the conduct of cirrhotic patients treated with TIPS is carried out using a clinical database with 107 cases and 77 attributes. We have applied a new Estimation of Distribution Algorithms based approach in order to perform a Prototype and Feature Subset Selection to improve the classification accuracy obtained using all the variables and all the cases. Used paradigms are K-Nearest Neighbours, Artificial Neural Networks and Classification Trees.

Keywords: Machine Learning, Prototype Selection, Feature Subset Selection, Transjugular Intrahepatic Portosystemic Shunt, Estimation of Distribution Algorithm, Indications.

1 Introduction

Portal hypertension is a major complication of chronic liver disease. By definition, it is a pathological increase in the portal venous pressure which results in formation of porto-systemic collaterals that divert blood from the liver to the

* This work was supported by the Gipuzkoako Foru Aldundi Txit Gorena under OF097/1998 grant and by the PI 96/12 grant from the Eusko Jaurlaritza - Hezkuntza, Unibertsitate eta Ikerkuntza Saila.

S. Quaglini, P. Barahona, and S. Andreassen (Eds.): AIME 2001, LNAI 2101, pp. 20–29, 2001.

systemic circulation. This is caused by both an obstruction to outflow in the portal flow as well as an increased mesenteric flow. In the western world, cirrhosis of the liver accounts for approximately 90% of the patients.

Of the sequelae of portal hypertension (i.e. varices, encephalopathy, hypersplenism, ascites), bleeding from gastro-oesophageal varices is a significant cause of early mortality (approximately $30 - 50\%$ at the first bleed) [2].

The Transjugular Intrahepatic Portosystemic Shunt (TIPS) is an interventional treatment resulting in decompression of the portal system by creation of a side-to-side portosystemic anastomosis. Since its introduction over 10 years ago [17] and despite the large number of published studies, many questions remain unanswered. Currently, little is known about the effects of TIPS on the survival of the treated patients.

Our medical staff has found that a subgroup of patients dies in the first six months after a TIPS placement and the rest survive for longer periods. Actually there is no risk indicator to identify both subgroups of patients. We are equally interested in the detection of both subgroups, giving the same relevance to the reduction of both error types. The only published study [12] to identify a subgroup of patients who die within a period after a TIPS placement fixes the length of this period to three months. However, we think that our specific conditions really suggest lengthening this period to six months.

In this paper a new technique is presented that combines Prototype selection and Feature Subset Selection by an Estimation of Distribution Algorithm (EDA) approach. Although the application of the new EDA-inspired technique refers to the specific medical problem, the proposed approach is general and can be used for other tasks where supervised machine learning algorithms face a high number of irrelevant and/or redundant features.

Costs of medical tests are not considered in the construction of classification models and predictive accuracy maximization is the principal goal of our research. As the cost of the TIPS placement is not insignificant, our study is developed to help physicians, counsel patients and their families before deciding to proceed with elective TIPS.

The rest of the paper is organized as follows: the study database is described in section 2. Prototype Selection is introduced in section 3, while Feature Subset Selection (FSS) methods are described in section 4. Section 5 presents the Estimation of Distribution Algorithm, a new evolutionary computation paradigm. In section 6 the new approach used in this work is described, and experimental results are presented in section 7. Finally, the last section briefly summarizes the work and presents lines of future research in the field.

2   Patients. Study Database

The analysis includes 107 patients. The follow-up of these transplanted patients was censored on the day of the transplant. This censoring was done to remove the effect of transplantation when modeling the six-months survival of patients who undergo TIPS. If these patients were not censored, deaths due to surgical mortality related to transplantation might have influenced the selection of variables that are prognostic for the TIPS procedure. On the other hand, transplantation may prolong survival compared with patients who do not undergo TIPS. It is predictably found that survival in patients who undergo transplantation is significantly improved compared with those who do not undergo transplantation [12].

The database contains 77 clinical findings for each patient. These 77 attributes were measured before TIPS placement (see Table 1). A new binary variable is created, called *vital-status*, which reflects whether the patient died in the first 6 months after the placement of the TIPS or not: this variable reflects both classes of the problem. In the first 6 months after the placement of the TIPS, 33 patients died and 74 survived for a longer period, thus reflecting that the utility and consequences of the TIPS were not homogeneous for all the patients.

Table 1. Attributes of the study database.

History finding attributes:		
Age	Gender	Height
Weight	Etiology of cirrhosis	Indication of TIPS
Bleeding origin	Number of bleedings	Prophylactic therapy with popranolol
Previous sclerotherapy	Restriction of proteins	Number of hepatic encephalopathies
Type of hepatic encephalophaty	Ascites intensity	Number of paracenteses
Volume of paracenteses	Dose of furosemide	Dose of spironolactone
Spontaneous bacterial peritonitis	Kidney failure	Organic nephropathy
Diabetes mellitus		
Laboratory finding attributes:		
Hemoglobin	Hematocrit	White blood cell count
Serum sodium	Urine sodium	Serum potassium
Urine potassium	Plasma osmolarity	Urine osmolarity
Urea	Plasma creatinine	Urine creatinine
Creatinine clearance	Fractional sodium excretion	Diuresis
GOT	GPT	GGT
Alkaline phosphatase	Serum total bilirubin (mg/dl)	Serum conjugated bilirubin (mg/dl)
Serum albumin (g/dl)	Plateletes	Prothrombin time (%)
Parcial thrombin time	PRA	Proteins
FNG	Aldosterone	ADH
Dopamine	Norepineohrine	Epinephrine
Gamma-globulin		
CHILD score		
PUGH score		
Doppler sonography:		
Portal size	Portal flow velocity	Portal flow right
Portal flow left	Spleen lenght (cm)	
Endoscopy:		
Size of esophageal varices	Gastric varices	Portal gastropathy
Acute hemorrhage		
Hemodinamic parameters:		
Arterial pressure (mm Hg)	Heart rate (beats/min)	Cardiac output (l/min)
Free hepatic venous pressure	Wedged hepatic venous pressure	Hepatic venous pressure gradient (HVPG)
Central venous pressure	Portal pressure	Portosystemis venous pressure gradient
Angiography:		
Portal thrombosis		

3   Prototype Selection

Usually, three main approaches are used to develop Prototype Selection Algorithms:

1. Filtration of cases.
   These approaches are introduced in the firsts research works about prototype

selection, and use some kind of rule in order to incrementally determine which cases of the training database will be selected as prototypes and which of them discarded as part of the model. Some of the works keep wrong classified cases (Hart[4], Aha[1]), other approaches keep typical instances as prototypes (Zhang[22]) and some other algorithms select the correctly classified instances (Wilson[21]).

2. Stochastical search.

Among the stocastical search methods, some of them make use of Genetic Algorithms[7] to select prototypes. Cameron-Jones[3] offers an heuristic approach consisting on minimizing the lenght of the bit string that represents a group of well and wrong classified instances. These kind of algorithms have also been applied by Skalak[19].

3. Case weighing.

In these approaches a computation is done to weight the cases based on well classified or on more abstract concepts (Djouadi y Boucktache[6]).

3.1   Hart's Condensed Nearest Neighbor Algorithm

This algorithm constitutes the first formal proposal to built a condensation method (Condensed Nearest Neighbor, CNN, Hart[4]). The method defines the so called consistency concerned to the training set. It is said that a group of prototypes S is consistent with respect to another group D, if upon using S as the training set, it is possible to correctly classify the cases in D. It is desirable to obtain a condensed group of prototypes that is small and consistent. The corresponding algorithm is shown in Figure 1.

The operation mode of this method is very simple: it maintains in the training database those prototypes wrong classified taking as model the cases belonging to the S subset at each step. This is done under the presumption that wrong classified cases belong to the decision border. The CNN algorithm has a lineal order computational behavior in practice, obtaining quite reduced prototype subsets. It can not be assumed that the prototype subset obtained by applying this method is the minimal consistent group.

4   Feature Subset Selection

In supervised Machine Learning[13], the goal of a supervised learning algorithm is to induce a classifier that allows us to classify new examples $E* = \{e_{n+1}, ..., e_{n+m}\}$ that are only characterized by their n descriptive features. To generate this classifier we have a set of m samples $E = \{e_1, ..., e_m\}$, characterized by n descriptive features $X = \{X_1, ..., X_n\}$ and the class label $C = \{w_1, ..., w_m\}$ to which they belong ($w_i = 0$ or $w_i = 1$ in the two class problem we are working with). Machine Learning can be seen as a 'data-driven' process where, putting little emphasis on prior hypotheses than is the case with classical statistics,

Hart Condensation Algorithm

START
   As input, the algorithm should receive:
      The training database, D, containing N cases,
      $(\mathbf{x}_i, \theta_i), i = 1, ..., N,$

   Initialize the prototype set S to an empty set
   FOR each case belonging to D, $(\mathbf{x}_i, \theta_i)$ DO
      START
         IF the class given by the NN algorithm
         taking S as the training database is correct
         THEN
            Do not add the case to S
         ELSE
            Add the case to S
      END
   As output, the algorithm gives the set S containing the selected prototypes.
END

Fig. 1. Pseudo-code of the *Hart Condensation Algorithm*.

a 'general rule' is induced for classifying new examples using a learning algorithm. Many representations with different biases have been used to develop this 'classification rule'. Here, the Machine Learning community has formulated the following question: *"Are all of these d descriptive features useful for learning the 'classification rule'?"* Trying to respond to this question the Feature Subset Selection (FSS) approach appears, which can be reformulated as follows: *given a set of candidate features, select the best subset under some learning algorithm.*

This dimensionality reduction made by a FSS process can carry out several advantages for a classification system in a specific task:

   − a reduction in the cost of acquisition of the data,
   − improvement of the compressibility of the final classification model,
   − a faster induction of the final classification model,
   − an improvement in classification accuracy.

The attainment of higher classification accuracies is the usual objective of Machine Learning processes. It has been long proved that the classification accuracy of Machine Learning algorithms is not monotonic with respect to the addition of features. Irrelevant or redundant features, depending on the specific characteristics of the learning algorithm, may degrade the predictive accuracy of the classification model. In our work, FSS objective will be the maximization of the performance of the classification algorithm. In addition, with the reduction in the number of features, it is more likely that the final classifier is less complex and more understandable by humans.

Once the objective is fixed, FSS can be viewed as a search problem, with each state in the search space specifying a subset of the possible features of the task. Exhaustive evaluation of possible feature subsets is usually infeasible in practice because of the large amount of computational effort required. Many search techniques have been proposed to solve FSS problem when there is no knowledge about the nature of the task, carrying out an intelligent search in the space of possible solutions.

5   Estimation of Distribution Algorithms

Genetic Algorithms (GAs, see Holland [7]) are one of the best known techniques for solving optimization problems. Their use has reported promising results in many areas but there are still some problems where GAs fail. These problems, known as deceptive problems, have attracted the attention of many researchers and as a consequence there has been growing interest in adapting the GAs in order to overcome their weaknesses.

GAs are a population based method. A set of individuals (or candidate solutions) is generated, promising individuals are selected, and new individuals are generated using crossover and mutation operators.

An interesting adaptation of this is the Estimation of Distribution Algorithm (EDA) [14] (see Figure 3). In EDAs, there are neither crossover nor mutation operators, the new population is sampled from a probability distribution which is estimated from the selected individuals.

EDA
   $D_0 \leftarrow$ Generate N individuals (the initial population) randomly.
   Repeat for $l = 1, 2, \ldots$ until a stop criterion is met.
      $D_{l-1}^s \leftarrow$ Select $S \leq N$ individuals from D_{l-1} according to a selection method.
      $p_l(\mathbf{x}) = p(\mathbf{x}|D_{l-1}^s) \leftarrow$ Estimate the joint probability distribution of an individual being among the selected inviduals.
      $D_l \leftarrow$ Sample N individuals (the new population) from $p_l(\mathbf{x})$.

Fig. 2. Main scheme of the EDA approach.

In this way, a randomized, evolutionary, population-based search can be performed using probabilistic information to guide the search. In this way, both approaches (GAs and EDAS) do the same except that EDAs replaces genetic crossover and mutation operators by means of the following two steps:

1. a probabilistic model of selected promising solutions is induced,
2. new solutions are generated according to the induced model.

The main problem of EDA resides on how the probability distribution $p_l(\mathbf{x})$ is estimated. Obviously, the computation of 2^n probabilities (for a domain with n binary variables) is impractical. This has led to several approximations where the probability distribution is assumed to factorize according to a probability model (see Larrañaga et al. [11] or Pelikan et al. [15] for a review).

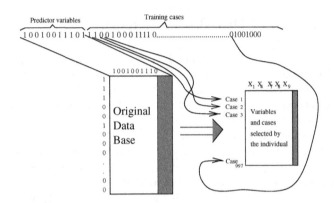

Among the first 10 bits, Xi=1 means that the i-th predictor variable is selected as part of the new training database. The next 1000 bits indicate which of the cases are selected

Fig. 3. Example of an individual codification.

6   New Approach

In the new approach used in this paper, a binary individual codification is used for the Prototype Seleftion and FSS[1]. Let n be the number of predictor variables in the initial training database, and let m be number of cases. We use a binary individual of $(n + m)$ bits length, where the first n bits indicate the selected predictor variables and the last m the selected cases. In both cases, a bit value of 1 indicates that selection is done and a value of 0 means rejection.

In other words, if the i-th bit $= 1$

$$\begin{cases} i \le n, \text{the} X_i \text{predictor variable is selected} \\ i > n, \text{ the } Case_{i-n} \text{is selected} \end{cases}$$

else the i-th bit value being 0 indicates no selection of the corresponding variable or case. Figure 3 shows a graphical example of the new approach.

---

[1] The variable corresponding to the class is not included

In other words, one individual $(x_1, \ldots, x_n, x_{n+1}, \ldots, x_{n+m})$ is represented by a binary string of lenght $n + m$, where, for $i = 1, \ldots, n$:

$$x_i = \begin{cases} 0 & \text{iff the } i\text{-th predictor variable is selected} \\ 1 & \text{in other case} \end{cases}$$

and for $i = n + 1, \ldots, n + m$:

$$x_i = \begin{cases} 0 & \text{iff the } i - n\text{-th case is selected} \\ 1 & \text{in other case} \end{cases}$$

7 Experimental Results

Three different classification algorithms have been used in the experimentation done, in order to show that the main Prototype Selection - Feature Subset Selection by Estimation of Distribution Algorithm (PS-FSS-EDA) approach could be used with most Machine Learning paradigms. The algorithms used are the 1-Nearest Neighbor (1-NN)[4] and a backpropagation (BP) based Artificial Neural Network[13] and C4.4 classification tree[16].

Validation is done by the Leave-One-Out (LOO) technique, which consists on classifying each case of the database by using the model obtained by the rest of the training cases. In other words, it is the Stone[20] X-Fold Cross-validation method in which the X equals the number of cases of the training database, 107 in our case. This validation technique is applied usually when the size of the database is minor than 1000.

Table 2. Well classified cases obtained using all the cases and all the variables, estimated by the Leave-One-Out validation technique

Classifier	Variables	Number of cases	Well classified	Percentage
1-NN	77	107	68	63.55
BP	77	107	73	68.22
C4.5	77	107	68	63.55

Table 2 shows the classification accuracy obtained by each of the classifiers used with the training database using all the 107 cases and all the 77 predictor variables, estimated by the LOO method.

The new proposed PS-FSS-EDA approach have been used with the same database. Obtained results estimated by the LOO technique are shown in the Table 3.

As it could be seen, accuracy results obtained by the three classifiers by applying PS-FSS-EDA paradigm outperform those obtained using all the cases and all the variables.

When the classification models are presented to the medical staff, they noted a large improvement in aplicability among the models induced with the aid of

Table 3. Well classified cases obtained by the PS-FSS-EDA approach, estimated by the Leave-One-Out validation technique

Classifier	Prototype average	Variable average	Well classified	Percentage
1-NN	5.12	37.38	83	77.53
BP	67.53	53.56	80	74.77
C4.5	?	?	76	71.03

FSS techniques and those that are constructed without FSS. Thus, by this dimensionality reduction, the confidence and acceptance in the models of our medical staff is increased. With the reduction in the number of needed measurements, an obvious reduction of the derived economic costs is achieved.

8   Summary and Future Work

A medical problem, the prediction of the survival of cirrhotic patients treated with TIPS, has been focused from a machine learning perspective, with the aim of obtaining a classification method for the indication or contraindication of TIPS in cirrhotic patients.

Although the new FSS EDA-inspired approach has been applied in this paper to the specific medical problem of TIPS indication, it has a general character and can be used for other kind of problems.

In the future, we plan to use a database with nearly 300 attributes to deal with the problem of survival in cirrhotic patients treated with TIPS, which also collects patients measurements one month after the placement of TIPS. We also plan to use more advanced probability estimation techniques, such as Bayesian networks [8], to study the relationships among the variables of the study database. We are also planning to use a classifier combination technique[18] in order to improve obtained results by using more than one classifier.

Acknowledgments. This work was supported by the PI 1999-40 grant from Gobierno Vasco - Departamento de Educación, Universidades e Investigación and the grant 9/UPV/EHU 00140.226-/2084/2000 from University of the Basque Country.

References

1. D. Aha, D. Kibler y M.K. Albert (1991): Instance-Based learning algorithms. *Machine Learning* **6**, 37-66.
2. P.C. Bornman, J.E.J. Krige and J. Terblanche, Management of oesophageal varices, *Lancet* 343 (1994) 1079-1084.
3. M. Cameron-Jones (1995): Instance selection by encoding length heuristic with random mutation hill climbing. *IEEE Proceedings of the eighth Australian Joint Conference on Artificial Intelligence*, World Scientific, 99-106.

4. B.V. Dasarathy (1991): *Nearest Neighbor (NN) Norms: NN Pattern Recognition Classification Techniques.* IEEE Computer Society Press
5. T.G. Diettrich, Approximate statistical tests for comparing supervised learning algorithms, *Neural Computation* 10 (1998) 1895-1924.
6. P. Djouadi, E. Boucktache (1997): A fast algorithm for the Nearest-Neighbor Classifier. *IEEE Transactions on Pattern Analysis and Machine Intelligence,* Vol. 19, No. 3, 277-281.
7. J. Holland, *Adaptation in Natural and Artificial Systems* (University of Michigan Press, 1975).
8. I. Inza, P. Larrañaga, B. Sierra, R. Etxeberria, J.A. Lozano and J.M. Peña, Representing the behaviour of supervised classification learning algorithms by Bayesian networks, *Pattern Recognition Letters,* 20 (11-13) (1999) 1201-1210.
9. I. Inza, P. Larrañaga, R. Etxeberria and B. Sierra (2000): "Feature subset selection by Bayesian network-based optimization", *Artificial Intelligence* **123**, 157-184.
10. R. Kohavi and G. John, Wrappers for feature subset selection, *Artificial Intelligence* 97 (1997) 273-324.
11. P. Larrañaga, R. Etxeberria, J.A. Lozano, B. Sierra, I. Inza, J.M. Peña, A review of the cooperation between evolutionary computation and probabilistic graphical models, in: Proceedings of the II Symposium on Artificial Intelligence CIMAF99, La Habana, Cuba, 1999, pp. 314-324.
12. M. Malinchoc, P.S. Kamath, F.D. Gordon, C.J. Peine, J. Rank and P.C.J. ter Borg, A model to Predict Poor Survival in Patients Undergoing Transjugular Intrahepatic Portosystemic Shunts, *Hepatology* 31 (2000) 864-871.
13. T. Mitchell (1997): *Machine Learning.* McGraw-Hill.
14. H. Müehlenbein and G. Paaß, From recombination of genes to the estimation of distributions. Binary parameters, in: *Lecture Notes in Computer Science 1411: Parallel Problem Solving from Nature – PPSN IV* (1996) 178-187.
15. M. Pelikan, D.E. Goldberg, F. Lobo, A Survey of Optimization by Building and Using Probabilistic Model, IlliGAL Report 99018, Urbana: University of Illinois at Urbana-Champaign, Illinois Genetic Algorithms Laboratory, 1999.
16. J.R. Quinlan (1993): "C4.5: Programs for Machine Learning", *Morgan Kaufmann Publishers, Inc.* Los Altos, California
17. M. Róssle, V. Siegerstetter, M. Huber and A. Ochs, The first decade of the transjugular intrahepatic portosystemic shunt (TIPS): state of the art, *Liver* 18 (1998) 73-89.
18. B. Sierra, N. Serrano, P. Larrañaga, E.J. Plasencia, I. Inza, J.J. Jiménez, J.M. De la Rosa and M.L. Mora (2001): Using Bayesian networks in the construction of a multi-classifier. A case study using Intensive Care Unit patient data. *Artificial Intelligence in Medicine.* In press.
19. D.B. Skalak (1994): Prototipe and feature selection by Sampling and Random Mutation Hill Climbing Algortithms. *Proceedings of the Eleventh International Conference on Machine Learning,* NJ. Morgan Kaufmann. 293-301.
20. M. Stone (1974): Cross-validation choice and assessment of statistical procedures. *Journal Royal of Statistical Society* **36**, 111-147.
21. D.L. Wilson (1972): Asymptotic properties of nearest neighbour rules using edited data. *IEEE Transactions on Systems, Man and Cybernetics,* Vol. 2, 408-421.
22. J. Zhang (1992): Selecting Typical instances in Instance-Based Learning. *Proceedings of the Ninth International Machine Learning Workshop,* Aberdeen, Escocia. Morgan-Kaufmann, San Mateo, Ca, 470-479.

Detection of Infectious Outbreaks in Hospitals through Incremental Clustering

Timothy Langford[1], Christophe Giraud-Carrier[1], and John Magee[2]

[1] Department of Computer Science, University of Bristol, Bristol, UK
{langford,cgc}@cs.bris.ac.uk
[2] Department of Medicine, Microbiology and Public Health Laboratory, Cardiff, UK
magee@cardiff.ac.uk

Abstract. This paper highlights the shortcomings of current systems of nosocomial infection control and shows how techniques borrowed from statistics and Artificial Intelligence, in particular clustering, can be used effectively to enhance these systems beyond confirmation and into the more important realms of detection and prediction. A tool called HIC and examined in collaboration with the Cardiff Public Health Laboratory is presented. Preliminary experiments with the system demonstrate promise. In particular, the system was able to uncover a previously undiscovered cross-infection incident.

1 Introduction

Nosocomial infections are estimated to affect 6-12% of hospitalised patients. These infections have significant effects on mortality, mean length of hospital stay and antibiotics usage, and result in many hundreds of thousand pounds annual cost to the National Health Services in the UK. Outbreaks, *i.e.,* multiple nosocomial infections caused by the same bacterial strain (*e.g.,* the infamous multi-resistant *Staphylococcus aureus* or MRSA), can result from many factors, including lapses in good practice, changes in procedure that introduce a new route of transmission, or the movement of patients between wards in the same hospital and between different hospitals.

Most detected outbreaks are limited to a single ward, a single medical/surgical team or a single treatment procedure. Detection and advice on treatment and control of infections (including nosocomial infections) are largely the responsibility of the local microbiology laboratory, run by the hospital or sometimes (in England and Wales) by the Public Health Laboratory Service. These laboratories receive specimens from the local hospitals and analyse them for bacteria. The bacteria are identified at the species level (there are about 4500 known species, of which about 500 cause human infection), and their susceptibility to a range of antibiotics (usually 3 to 12) appropriate to that species is assessed. These findings are then recorded and reported to the ward.

Outbreaks of nosocomial infection that are detected are typically first recognised by a laboratory worker, who, over a relatively short period, has handled several specimens yielding the same unusual species of bacterium, or a common species with an

S. Quaglini, P. Barahona, and S. Andreassen (Eds.): AIME 2001, LNAI 2101, pp. 30–39, 2001.

unusual pattern of antibiotic susceptibility. A possible cross-infection situation is recognised and records are searched for previous similar findings. This search often reveals that other closely similar or identical bacteria have been detected previously, and that all these infections are from either the same ward or same medical/surgical team. The cross-infection team then investigates the incident, and attempts to determine and rectify its cause. In a common alternative detection method, recent infections for a few species of particular interest are noted routinely on a board depicting the wards, and the board status is reviewed at each update, looking for anomalous concentrations of similar infections. Both methods are limited, labour-intensive and highly dependent on subjective interpretation.

Furthermore, modern hospitals may have more than 500 beds and laboratories may receive in excess of 100,000 specimens per annum. This means that clues to incidents are easily lost in the vast amount of data generated; no single member of the laboratory team sees all reports, and it is less likely that a single staff member will handle several specimens from an outbreak. In addition, the range of species that may be involved has increased markedly over the years. Outbreaks involving common species with „normal" susceptibility patterns are unlikely to be detected, and those outbreaks that are detected are often found late in their progress.

What is required is a systematic and ongoing search for structured anomalies in the report flow. Well established statistical techniques as well as recent advances in Artificial Intelligence, especially in the area of Data Mining, open up new possibilities for this kind of analyses in large bodies of data. This paper describes a procedure and software system, which support the automation of nosocomial infection detection through incremental clustering. The system, called HIC, has been trained and tested with data obtained from the Cardiff Public Health Laboratory (CPHL).

The paper is organised as follows. Section 2 outlines our case study with the Cardiff data. Section 3 shows how the raw data is transformed by HIC using clustering and sliding aggregation techniques to improve the design of detection and prediction mechanisms. Section 4 discusses the current implementation of outbreak detection based on thresholding the transformed data and reports on promising preliminary results obtained within the context of the Cardiff data. Finally, section 5 concludes the paper and highlights areas of future work.

2 The CPHL Data: A Characteristic Case Study

The CPHL currently holds about 7 years of historical diagnostic data, and new data is recorded daily. Each record or case corresponds to a particular sample collected on a given patient and is represented by a set of features as follows:

CASE_DATE : ORG_LOC : WARD : FIRM : SEX : AGE : HSP : LSN : <ANTIBIOGRAM>
where,

CASE_DATE	The date at which the specimen was submitted to the Laboratory
ORG_LOC	The anatomical origin of the case specimen (*e.g.*, urine, blood, faeces)
WARD	The infected patient's ward
FIRM	The patient's assigned medical team
SEX	The patient's sex

AGE	The patient's age
HPN	The Hospital Patient Number, a unique identifier for each patient
LSN	The Laboratory Specimen Number, a unique specimen identifier
<ANTIBIOGRAM>	The sample's antibiograms, including the species of organisms found and their antibiotic susceptibility patterns (see below)

The first 8 features define the context of the antibiograms. From the viewpoint of infection detection, the antibiograms can be regarded as the „core" data of each case since they provide information about bacteria found. Cases where no organism has been found constitute a good proportion of the recorded data, but these uninfected patients are not particularly relevant to detection of cross-infection.

Each antibiogram is represented as follows:

LSN : ORG_TYPE : ORG_ASP
where,
LSN	The corresponding case's LSN (see above)
ORG_TYPE	The type of the organism (*e.g.*, coliform, *Escherichia coli*, MRSA)
ORG_ASP	The antibiotic susceptibility pattern of the organism, *i.e.*, a list of the organism's resistance to a predefined set of 27 antibiotics, recorded as untested (no entry), sensitive (S), resistant (R) or intermediate (I)

The LSN feature serves only as a means to identify cases. The two other features carry the information that determines the type of organism. There are three main issues regarding the CPHL data that must be addressed by an automatic detection system. They are as follows.

- *Sparseness.* ORG_ASP has 4^{27} possible values. Although a reasonable amount of data is collected (bacteria from around 100 infections are identified and recorded each day), the fact that there are so many possibilities within each strain of bacterium means that the data is rather sparse. Hence, any direct attempt at clustering bacterial strains based on a symbolic comparison of their ORG_TYPE and ORG_ASP will lead to a large number of small clusters. This problem is further compounded by the fact that not all of the possible antibiotics are tested on every sample. Normally, only 6 to 12 tests are performed and recorded. The choice of tests performed reflects the organism species, the site and severity of the infection. In some cases, during a known outbreak, additional antibiotics may be tested to extend the possibility of identifying an outbreak-associated organism from an extended antibiogram pattern.

- *Test variation.* Two organisms with the same ORG_TYPE, but with different ORG_ASP should theoretically be regarded as distinct. However, test variations can cause small differences in the ORG_ASP between repeat analyses of the same organism. Similarity between ORG_ASPs can not require strict identity, but must account for „errors" in test reproducibility.

- *Time Dependency.* The sample data represents only one instance of the bacterium. The data contains no knowledge about how long the bacterium was present in the hospital environment before the data was obtained, or how long it remains in the hospital environment after it has been detected. Hence, the recorded data does not strictly provide an accurate representation of the actual frequencies of bacteria in the hospital environment. However, because each case has an associated date, the cases can be „trended" over time.

To accommodate the above characteristics and render the data more amenable to analysis, a number of transformations are applied, as detailed in the following section.

3 Data Transformation

This section deals with how the data can be utilised in a daily incremental way to allow a greater understanding of the distribution of infections in the hospital. The aim is to transform the data, using the concept of sliding aggregation, to make it more amenable to our selected data analysis methodology. Note that other methodologies may require different (or no) transformations.

3.1 Antibiograms Expansion

Antibiotic susceptibilities tend to follow rules. For example, a penicillin-sensitive *Staphylococcus aureus* will invariably also be sensitive to methicillin, and an ampicillin-sensitive *E. coli* is normally susceptible to co-amoxiclav and cephalosporin. Such rules can be used to fill in some of the missing susceptibility values based on recorded ones. In order to do so, the following meta-classes and corresponding classes of antibiotics were formed.

```
A PENICILLIN
    A PENICILLIN 0: PENICILLIN
    A PENICILLIN 1: AMPICILLIN, PIPERACILLIN
    A PENICILLIN 2: AUGMENTIN, (FLUCLOXACILLIN for Staph. aureus)
    A PENICILLIN 3: IMIPENEM
A QUINOLONE
    A QUINOLONE 0: NALIDIXIC ACID
    A QUINOLONE 1: CIPROFLOXACIN
A MACROLIDE
    A MACROLIDE 0: ERYTHROMYCIN
A TETRACYCLINE
    A TETRACYCLINE 0: TETRACYCLINE
A CEPHALOSPORIN
    A CEPHALOSPORIN 0: CEPHRADINE
    A CEPHALOSPORIN 1: CEFUROXIME
    A CEPHALOSPORIN 3: CEFTAZIDIME, CEFOTAXIME
AN AMINOGLYCOSIDE
    AN AMINOGLYCOSIDE 0: NEOMYCIN
    AN AMINOGLYCOSIDE 1: GENTAMICIN
    AN AMINOGLYCOSIDE 2: TOBRAMYCIN
A GLYCOPEPTIDE
    A GLYCOPEPTIDE 0: VANCOMYCIN
    A GLYCOPEPTIDE 1: TEICOPLANIN
UNGROUPED
    UNGROUPED: FUSIDIC ACID, TRIMETHOPRIM, NITROFURANTOIN, COLISTIN,
              CHLORAMPHENICOL, METRONIDAZOLE, RIFAMPICIN, MUPIROCIN
```

Within a meta-class (except for UNGROUPED), each class has an associated „level", where the higher the level the more potent the corresponding antibiotics with respect to bacterial tolerance. For example, within the A PENICILLIN meta-class, PENICILLIN, which belongs to the class A PENICILLIN 0, is a „weaker" antibiotic than FLUCOXACILLIN, which belongs to the class A PENICILLIN 2. With this classification, it is possible to design a simple set of rules expressing dependencies between antibiotic susceptibility and to use this to expand an ORG_ASP to explicitly reveal information that is implicit in the original patterns. For example, an original --SI--SRI... pattern may become R-SI--SRI... after expansion. A single (meta-)rule, instantiated as needed, is as follows.

IF A BACTERIUM IS RESISTANT TO AN ANTIBIOTIC IN GROUP G_LABEL N
THEN IT IS RESISTANT TO ALL ANTIBIOTICS IN GROUPS G_LABEL M FOR M N

Pattern expansion is attempted for all cases but only applied if the antibiotic in the original antibiogram is untested. If the antibiotic has been tested, the originally re-corded result takes precedence even if it contradicts the expansion rule's suggestion. By reducing sparseness, pattern expansion also facilitates clustering by improving the reliability of symbolic comparisons between patterns as discussed below.

3.2 Antibiograms Comparison

Clearly, the expansion rules discussed above limit the amount of symbolic mismatch between ORG_ASPs that should be treated as originating from the same organism. However, even then it is unrealistic to rely on exact symbolic matching. What is needed is a clustering mechanism based on some reasonable measure of similarity.

The similarity measure implemented in our system, combines a rather simple simi-larity coefficient with a user-defined threshold as follows. In order to be comparable, two antibiograms must have the same ORG_TYPE. If they do, the entries of their ORG_ASP patterns are compared in a pairwise fashion. Comparisons involving an I result or an empty entry in either pattern are ignored. The number of exact matches (*i.e.*, S-S or R-R) and the number of mismatches (*i.e.*, S-R or R-S) are used to com-pute the following similarity coefficient.

$$SimCoef = \frac{\# \, of \, matches}{\# \, of \, matches \ + \ \# \, of \, mismatches}$$

For example, the following two ECOLI antibiograms of length 15

```
ECOLI:   R  S  I  R  R  R      S  S  S  S  S  S  S
ECOLI:   S  S  S  R      R  S  S  R  S  I  R  I  S  S
```

give rise to 6 matches and 3 mismatches, and thus to a similarity coefficient of 0.67. A user-defined threshold can then be used to determine whether two organisms may be considered the same. For example, if the threshold is 0.6, the two ECOLIs above are deemed to be indistinguishable. Armed with SimCoef (and an associated threshold), it is possible to cluster antibiograms. This is accomplished in our system using a sliding aggregator as detailed in the following sections.

3.3 Sliding Aggregation

Sliding aggregation is a method that clusters data at two points in its operation in an incremental manner. Essentially, the mechanism is based on a period of time t, with a *sliding window* of n components (the fixed *window size*) in which the ordered data is placed. There must exist data for at least n time periods before the aggregator can be used. At the start, the leftmost compartment of the window contains data from the time period t_{-n+1} and the rightmost compartment of the window contains data for the time period t_0. The window then „slides along" the data, so that when data from a subsequent time period t_i (i 1) is added to the window, the oldest element (*i.e.*, t_{-n+i}) is removed from the window and all other elements occupy a new position directly to the left of their last position.

The operation of the sliding window can be used to implement a filter across any ordered set of data, although its performance is highly dependent on t, n, the size of the set of ordered elements and the ability to efficiently order the elements. With respect to the diagnostic data, it makes sense to set the time-period t to 1 day, hence each component of the window is the case data for the day it represents and incremental daily updates to the sliding window are possible. As the elements here are naturally ordered by time, the next critical choice is the value of the fixed window size n. The application domain suggests that n can be set to any value representative of the estimated time that organisms remain present in the hospital environment after detection. Currently, this is set to 35 days. (*i.e.*, $t=1$, $n=35$). Note that the use of the sliding window helps to compensate for the fact that the data represents investigated instances and does not account for the length of time that the bacteria remain in the hospital environment after detection (see section 2).

By clustering the case data within each component of the window with respect to their antibiograms, one may compare equivalent infections on a daily basis (section 3.3.1). Furthermore, one can also cluster daily clustered data within a window (section 3.3.2). By taking these results for each window on the data as a whole (*i.e.*, as the window slides or is updated with new data each day), the data can be transformed into a set of sequences for each bacterial type that is the aggregate of the data as the window slides along. The transformed data is more representative of the bacteria causing infections, more amenable to subsequent analysis, and can be readily presented for intuitive visual inspection by laboratory staff. Also, further transformations can be made readily. For example, one may consider an exponentially weighted modifier giving new data in the window a greater effect than older data.

3.4 Incremental Clustering

This section shows how antibiograms are clustered as data from the laboratory is added to the sliding aggregation system on a daily basis. For horizontal clustering, it is assumed that the aggregator window is full (*i.e.*, at least $n=35$ days' worth of data are available).

3.4.1   Vertical Clustering

Raw daily data is clustered using the above procedure and a threshold provided by the laboratory staff. Antibiograms of bacteria of the same organism type are compared to one another in turn until all have been compared. Each antibiogram has two frequency values associated with it: the „actual" frequency of the antibiogram and its „clustered" frequency. The actual frequency of an antibiogram is the number of times it occurs identically (*i.e.*, same ORG_TYPE and same ORG_ASP) in a day. The clustered frequency of an antibiogram is based on SimCoef (see section 3.1) and its associated threshold. Every time two antibiograms are considered sufficiently similar, their respective actual frequencies are added to each other's clustered frequencies. The following are two examples.

```
Organism: CNS          RRSS SR   S R    SS S
Actual Daily Frequency:    1
Clustered Daily Frequency: 7

Organism: MRSA         RRRS SR   S R    SS  S
Actual Daily Frequency:    12
Clustered Daily Frequency: 13
```

As vertical clustering is applied to all bacteria in the day's data, no information relating to the antibiograms' actual ORG_ASPs is lost, which is important to the subsequent horizontal clustering of the incremental process.

3.4.2   Horizontal Clustering

Clustered daily data make up the contents of the day's component in the sliding aggregator. Once the sliding aggregator has been updated, a further clustering operation is performed on the data. Here, the system tries to create the „highest clustered frequency" path through the sliding aggregator possible for each clustered antibiogram in the sequence. The output here is a sequence of both actual and clustered frequencies for each unique antibiogram within the window. This is achieved by beginning with the first cell and iteratively clustering each instance of the same organism/antibiogram type within it against all those in the next cell, then picking the first highest frequency antibiogram that satisfies the similarity measure. As progress through the window continues new previously unique antibiograms may be uncovered; for these new antibiograms a backward search through the aggregator window is performed before proceeding to ensure that each unique antibiogram in the window has its complete highest clustered frequency pattern enumerated. The following are two examples.

```
Organism: CNS          RRSS SR   S R    SS S
Actual Trended Frequencies:
    0:0:0:0:0:0:0:0:0:0:0:1:0:0:0:0:0:0:0:0:0:0:0:0:0:0:0:0:0:0:0:0
Clustered Trended Frequencies:
    0:0:0:0:0:0:0:0:0:0:0:7:2:1:2:1:6:4:2:3:2:0:5:2:6:4:6:4:2:1:1:1:5:5:1
Actual Trended Summation:        1
Clustered Trended Summation:     73
```

```
Organism: MRSA          RRRS SR    S R     SS S
Actual Trended Frequencies:
   2:6:4:3:2:2:1:0:9:12:3:4:2:1:0:4:3:4:7:3:1:1:4:4:2:4:2:0:0:9:4:6:0:6:6
Clustered Trended Frequencies:
   2:9:8:9:4:6:2:1:10:13:9:10:2:3:0:6:9:8:9:5:1:1:7:7:6:11:4:2:3:11:5:8:2:6:6
Actual Trended Summation:        121
Clustered Trended Summation:     205
```

At this point, the focus of the data has shifted from that of the original case data as a whole to that of the antibiogram. The system now has the opportunity to analyse the data with respect to particular organism/antibiogram type. Probability distributions over the other features in the cases can be calculated to provide a context to these infection levels. Also the summation of frequencies within the sliding aggregator can be obtained and used to construct higher-level sequences with respect to particular bacteria (filters, *e.g.*, exponential decay could also be applied to these).

4   Data Analysis – Detection

The data transformation methods of section 3 have been implemented in a software system, called HIC [5]. This section now details the detection mechanism used by HIC to uncover potential outbreaks and outlines a method to perform prediction.

Once a sequence of clustered frequencies has been obtained for each organism/antibiogram type, HIC can attempt to discover anomalous bunching of similar infections. The system could carry out this stage of the process in a variety of ways, either supervised or unsupervised. Currently, HIC relies on a rather simple thresholding method.

First, the stored „total" frequency for the organism/antibiogram is obtained. The expected frequency is then calculated from the date range over which the system data was collated and the size of the sliding aggregator window. This value can then be compared against the clustered value obtained from the sliding aggregator frequency total for the organism. The user defines a threshold, and if the sliding aggregator total is greater than the threshold times the expected frequency for the given organism, then this is noted as an anomaly and presented to the user for inspection. The following is a simple example.

```
Threshold = 1.8 (80%)
!! Possible Anomaly Detected !!
Sequence Frequency -  13
System Frequency -   7
Organism: KPNE       R    RS  SSSS S SSS  S
   0:0:0:0:0:0:0:0:0:0:0:0:1:0:0:0:0:0:0:0:0:0:0:0:0:0:0:1:0:0:0:0:0, sum = 2
   0:0:0:0:0:0:0:0:0:0:0:0:1:0:1:0:0:0:0:0:1:0:0:2:1:1:0:3:0:1:1:0:1, sum = 13
```

This is a fairly intuitive way of determining whether or not a specific organism has exhibited anomalous bunching. Yet, it has proved successful in detecting known outbreaks in the historical laboratory data. It is also suitable for unsupervised detection of anomalies in a data stream, with a default threshold that may be amenable to automatic adjustment by machine-learning methods in later versions of the system. It is also readily adapted to interactive supervised training of the system.

Details of the implementation of the HIC system are in [5]. The data provided by the Cardiff laboratory was used to train and test HIC. The experiment, which focused on detection, proved successful in highlighting a possible outbreak that remained undetected by the laboratory.

There is an ongoing infection problem with *Klebsiella* at the University Hospital of Wales. Briefly, there have been sporadic clusters of colonisation with a few cases of infection from 1995 to 1999. The strains involved were mostly identified to the species *Klebsiella aerogenes* and showed resistance to multiple antibiotics. The data downloaded as input for development of the cross-infection detection program included one of these clusters. This was not actually called as an outbreak, because small numbers of patients were involved, and the organisms were identified as multi-resistant *Klebsiella oxytoca*, rather than *Klebsiella aerogenes*. However, in retrospect, these organisms had closely similar antibiograms and biochemical patterns, and probably represented a cluster of nosocomial colonisation/infection. This cluster was strikingly obvious in the teaching set output from the detection program. There has not been sufficient time for fuller inspection of the output outside the *Klebsiella* group, where research interests engendered greater familiarity with the ongoing infection status. However, this result was promising, particularly as the cluster had not been recognised as such in the laboratory at the time the data was downloaded.

In another experiment extending HIC, automation was taken further as several methods of detecting outbreaks using thresholding techniques were tested [2]. The results have yet to be validated by the microbiologists.

5   Conclusion

This paper describes a system of automatic nosocomial infection detection and prediction, based on AI methods. The system uses clustering and sliding aggregation techniques to build sequences of data containing the actual and clustered frequencies centred on the organisms involved. This methodology is intended to transform the raw data into a form that takes into account the sparseness of the data, its instance based nature when gathered and the fact that values contained within it are subtly interchangeable. It maintains implicit information on the evolution of bacterial strains and their changing resistance to antibiotics over time. It also makes the data more amenable to subsequent analysis by, for example, Case-Based Reasoning, where it is possible to store higher-level aggregated sequences and feature-bound probability distributions of organisms that have previously led to outbreaks and to use them for the prediction of similar future outbreaks. Preliminary experiments with data from the Cardiff Public Health Laboratory on detection demonstrate promise, as in at least one situation, the system was able to detect a possible outbreak that had remained undetected by the laboratory.

The system's functionality could be extended as follows. Rather than using fixed, user-defined thresholds, the system must be capable of learning and adapting its thresholds for reporting anomalies on the basis of operator feedback based on „level of interest", „confirmed outbreak", „possible seasonal variation" and „antibiotic test variability". Other essential feedback items may be added in the light of development work. Changes in detection parameters should be checked automatically to see if these would have affected detection of previously confirmed outbreaks, or would have revealed previously undetected anomalies. Where an outbreak has occurred, but not been detected by the system, the operator should be able to specify the specimen numbers, species and susceptibility pattern involved. The system should then test modified parameters, optimising detection of the new and previously detected outbreaks, and reviewing the database. Previous parameters must be available for re-institution if the optimisation process fails, or if the new optimum is rejected by the user. It may be necessary to operate the system with several distinct threshold levels or interest profiles, particularly if other potential uses, such as detection of factors influencing frequencies of specific infections, are pursued.

Acknowledgements. The first author was supported in part by the MRC Health Services Research Collaboration and a British Council/JISTEC scholarship to IBM Tokyo Research Laboratory.

References

1. Althoff, K., Auriol, E., Barletta, R. and Manago, M.: A Review of Industrial Case-Based Reasoning Tools. AI Intelligence (1995)
2. Bouchoux, X.: HIC Dataset Report. Unpublished Manuscript, Advanced Topics in Machine Learning, University of Bristol, Department of Computer Science (1999)
3. Bull, M., Kundt, G. and Gierl, L.: Discovering of Health Risks and Case-based Forecasting of Epidemics in a Health Surveillance System. In Proceedings of the First European Conference on Principles and Practice of Knowledge Discovery in Databases (PKDD'97). LNAI, Vol. 1263, Springer (1997), 68-77
4. Kolodner, J.: Case-Based Reasoning. Morgan Kaufmann (1993)
5. Langford, T.: A Prototype System for Hospital Infection Control. Technical Report PR4-99-09, University of Bristol, Department of Computer Science (1999)
6. Leake, D. (Ed.): Case-Based Reasoning: Experiences, Lessons, and Future Directions. AAAI Press (1996)

Mining Data from a Knowledge Management Perspective: An Application to Outcome Prediction in Patients with Resectable Hepatocellular Carcinoma

Riccardo Bellazzi[1], Ivano Azzini[1], Gianna Toffolo[2], Stefano Bacchetti[3], and Mario Lise[3]

[1] Dipartimento di Informatica e Sistemistica, Università di Pavia, Pavia, Italy
{ric,ivano}@aim.unipv.it
[2] Dipartimento di Ingegneria Elettronica e Informatica, Università di Padova, Padova, Italy
toffolo@dei.unipd.it
[3] Dipartimento di Scienze Oncologiche e Chirurgiche, Sez. Clinica Chirurgica, Università di Padova, Padova, Italy, lisem@ux1.unipd.it

Abstract. This paper presents the use of data mining tools to derive a prognostic model of the outcome of resectable hepatocellular carcinoma. The main goal of the study was to summarize the experience gained over more than 20 years by a surgical team. To this end, two decision trees have been induced from data: a model M1 that contains a full set of prognostic rules derived from the data on the basis of the 20 available factors, and a model M2 that considers only the two most relevant factors. M1 will be used to explicit the knowledge embedded in the data (externalization), while the model M2 will be used to extract operational rules (socialization). The models performance has been compared with the one of a Naive Bayes classifier and have been validated by the expert physicians. The paper concludes that a knowledge management perspective improves the validity of data mining techniques in presence of small data sets, coming from severe pathologies with relative low incidence. In these cases, it is more crucial the quality of the extracted knowledge than the predictive accuracy gained.

1. Introduction

In almost all clinical institutions there is a growing interest in summarizing the experience collected over years on the diagnosis, treatment and prognosis of relevant diseases. Such interest is particularly high in case of severe pathologies with relatively low incidence; as a matter of fact, these problems are usually managed by the same experienced medical team over years. A summary may be useful to the team for performing self-assessment, or to the institution, in the light of preserving its intellectual asset when the team changes. The application of statistical or machine learning methods is a way to extract knowledge from the available data, or, in other words, to make available within the hospital institution the *implicit knowledge* that resides in the data

S. Quaglini, P. Barahona, and S. Andreassen (Eds.): AIME 2001, LNAI 2101, pp. 40–49, 2001.

(socialization) or to transform it in *explicit knowledge (externalization)*. Therefore, in this context, the goal of the application of modern data analysis methods is basically *institutional knowledge management (KM)* [1]. This fact is related with two important limitations in the exploitation of the results obtained:

1. The data are typically observational and collected retrospectively. They do not come from trials and they shouldn't be used for evidence-based purposes.
2. The data are the results of a local complex process. Their validity and the outcomes they show, in particular in presence of small data sets, may be limited to the institutional conditions in which they are collected.
3. The goal of the data analysis may be also related to a better comprehension of the information that is contained in the data, thus highlighting cases that do not confirm well-established knowledge or problems in the data collection procedures.

Unfortunately, this crucial point is usually neglected in the available literature. Medical literature shows often extreme attitudes with respect to the exploitation of this kind of data: the data may be neglected at all, since they are not collected from evidence-based studies, or they are claimed to support results that hold general validity. This is often the case when the problem under study do not allow for clinical trials, such as in low incidence surgically treatable cancers.

Rather curiously, also the machine learning community seem to have underestimated the relationships with the KM issues when arguing about the usefulness and comprehensibility of the representation of the extracted knowledge. Recently, a commentary of Pazzani [2] discussed the controversial opinions about the usefulness and understandability of representation formalisms, highlighting the need of cognitive psychology to support knowledge discovery. The consequence of this statement is that also the most effective Data Mining (DM) method for a certain problem (in presence of a similar performance) may be related with the particular KM issues to be faced with. Differences in the background of physicians and of the KM goal (externalization or socialization) can lead to different choices.

In this light, we have dealt with the problem of outcome prediction in patients with resectable hepatocellular carcinoma: this problem is fairly representative of a large class of prognostic problems that could be properly studied with a KM perspective. The work herein presented lies in the area of machine learning for outcome analysis; such area represents one of the most interesting directions for the application of DM in medicine [3].

2. The Medical Problem

Hepatocellular Carcinoma (HCC) is a severe disease with an yearly incidence of 3-5% in cirrhotic patients. HCC may lead to liver resection; such clinical decision depends both on the prognostic factors derived from the literature and on the physicians experience[4]. In the Institute of Clinica Chirurgica 2 of the University of Padova, more than one hundred patients underwent liver resection in the last twenty years. After this long time span, the need of quantitatively summarizing the experience gained was apparent. Such synthesis is also related to the identification of clinical or epidemiological factors that are able to predict the prognosis of resectable patients. The externalization of such knowledge may help to improve the indications for liver resection and the overall cost-effectiveness of the surgical procedures. The socialization of the knowledge may give some "day by day" prognostic rules that may be applied and progressively refined by a new clinical team. The overall data analysis procedure is useful to understand the quality of information contained in the data themselves.

Table I. Prognostic Factors

Prognostic Factors (Abbreviation)	Categories	Availability	# data
Gender (Sex)	M vs F	Pre	77
Age (Age)	Continuous	Pre	77
Cirrhosis (Tum)	0,1,2	Pre	77
Preoperative level of Albumin (Alb)	Continuous	Pre	75
Preoperative level of □-GT (GaGT)	Continuous	Pre	70
Preoperative level of GOT (GOT)	Continuous	Pre	74
Preoperative level of GPT (GPT)	Continuous	Pre	74
Preoperative level of LDH (LDH)	Continuous	Pre	66
Preoperative level of PT (PT)	Continuous	Pre	72
Preoperative level of α-fetoprotein (AFP)	Continuous	Pre	71
Child's class (Child)	A (1) vs B (0)	Pre	76
Number of nodules (Nod)	Integer	Pre	77
Diameter of largest nodule (Diam)	Continuous	Pre	77
Preoperative chemoembolization (Chemo)	Yes (1) vs No (0)	Pre	76
Intraoperative blood loss (Perd)	Continuous	Intra	73
Experience of the team (Exp)	Before (0) vs after '88 (1)	Intra	77
Type of hepatic resection (Res)	Anatom (0) vs non Anatom (1)	Intra	77
T classification (TNM)	T1-2 (0) vs T3-4 (1)	Post	72
Grading (Grad)	G1-2 (0) vs G3-4 (1)	Post	67

2.1 Data

From 1977 to 1999, 117 patients with HCC underwent liver resection at the Institute of Clinica Chirurgica 2 of the Università di Padova. Indications for surgery were made on the basis of clinical assessment and of a number of clinical exams and laboratory tests which are recognised to be prognostic factors for the HCC. The patients follow-up included α-fetoprotein (AFP) dosage every 3 months, abdomen US or CT scan of the liver every 6 months and chest X ray every 12 months. Tumor recurrence was defined as a lesion in the liver or in other organs, confirmed by percutaneous or open biopsy. From the clinical records, it was possible to derive a database of 90 patients that contained relevant clinical, surgical and pathological data. The outcomes were evaluated on the basis of a minimum follow up of 18 months, which leaded to reduce the number of cases to 77. Twenty prognostic factors, evaluated in the analysis were selected on the basis of the literature and of the physicians experience. Fifteen factors are pre-operative, while 5 are collected intra- or post-operatively. The list of factors is reported in Table I.

Recurrences occurred in 64 patients. Forty seven of these died of disease while 17 were alive with disease at the time of analysis. On the basis of these results, two categories of outcomes were considered: patients with early recurrence (<18 months) and late recurrence (>18 months) or no recurrent. The cut-off of 18 months was chosen since it represents the mean time of recurrence. The number of early recurrence patients was 39 and the number of late recurrence patients was 38.

3. Data Analysis

3.1 Prognostic Models for Liver Resection in HCC

In a related work, some of the authors of this paper studied the general problem of deriving a prognostic model for liver resection in HCC [5]. The approach followed was to test first classical survival models and in particular to extract the most relevant features through a multivariate score models based on the Cox's multivariate analysis for disease-free survival. This approach turned out to be unsuccessful for the prediction of early and late recurrent cases. Therefore, the data analysis was devoted to the application of methods capable of managing non-linearity and variable interactions, such as Naive Bayes classifier (NBc), Decision Trees, Feed-forward Neural Networks, Probabilistic Neural Networks and Support Vector machines. In this analysis, the NBc implementation described in [6] outperformed all the other methods. The NBc model was based on 8 factors only. Such factors were selected on the basis of a step-wise strategy and by exploiting the physicians experience. In the following we will refer to this model as the reference model, or model M0.

3.2 Building Models with a KM Perspective

Although the selected NBc showed a relatively low generalization error, it doesn't fulfill the main purposes of the analysis performed: it does not provide information on the relative importance of the different factors, and it is not able to derive any information on critical variable values. Therefore, we looked for the revision of the results obtained by better analyzing the problem characteristics and the physicians needs.

- As reported in Table I, the data set was not complete. Twenty-five patients had some missing data, and the factors with the highest percentages of missing data were LDH (14%) and Grad (13%). Moreover, a specific need of physicians was the chance of evaluating the quality of the knowledge derived (i.e. the prognostic model) also on other retrospective data, that might be made available by the collection of information from paper-based clinical records. Such data, by nature, are prone to contain missing values. This fact forces to use methods that are able to properly handle missing values.

- The first analysis performed by clinicians was devoted to look for a *scoring* model, that should be able *first* to select the most relevant factors and *second* to predict the outcome. Such capability should be preserved also by other methods.
- It is important, for KM purposes, to derive models useful both for externalization and for socialization. To this end, it might be crucial to provide users with both a relatively deep and understandable model for increasing explicit knowledge and a more simple, but relatively accurate model for supporting socialization.
- It is important to derive models whose predictions are justified by declarative statements. Since the data set is very small with respect to the dimensionality of the problem, it is crucial to be able to validate the extracted classifier and the knowledge contained in it.

For the reasons listed above, we devoted our study to revise and improve the results of induction decision trees (DT), since they seemed to accomplish for the three specific needs of the problem at hand. Moreover, the availability of easy to use software solutions makes easy and reproducible the performed analysis.

3.3 Model Selection

The basic goal of the DT induction process was to derive two different kind of models:

- Model 1 (M1): a DT able to express structured knowledge on the entire factor set. M1 should be used to reason about factors and data, and to accomplish for the task of externalization.
- Model 2 (M2): a DT with a minimum number of factors, that should be used to give a hint about patients prognosis during day by day clinical activity, i.e. for socialization.

The first direction that was looked for was related to improve feature selection. This step in model building is known to be critical, since partially or completely irrelevant/redundant to the target concept can affect the learning process. Moreover, some factors that are known to weakly affect the outcome may have an effect not measurable in small data sets. All these problems may be dramatically true for our classification problem, in which the outcome of the pathology is difficult to forecast. In particular, we have used a simple and integrated method based on the Information Gain (IG), described in [7]. In detail, we run the DT induction algorithm C5 with all (20) available factors: as is well known, C5 induces trees by selecting the splits that maximize IG. After training and pruning, a subset of factors are retained; such factors are considered to be the optimal ones with respect to IG. A new tree is then induced, with only the selected factors. After this procedure, only 8 factors were kept. The obtained DT was assumed to be our model M1. It is interesting to note that the derived features set was only partially overlapping with the ones used in M0. To obtain model M2 we applied the same procedure described above on the factor set used in M0, since we wanted to derive a model that was already accepted by physicians. We obtained a model with two features only.

The selected factors for the different models are reported in Table II.

Table II. Selected prognostic factors

Model	Factors
M0	**Pre**: GPT, Sex, LDH, Diam, Tum
	Intra: Res, Perd
	Post: Grad.
M1	**Pre**: GPT, GOT, AFP, Alb, Chemo
	Intra: Res, Perd
	Post: TNM.
M2	**Pre**: Diam
	Post: Perd

It is interesting to note that the model M2 founds its basis in the observation that the factor *Diam* is a statistical summary of the factors of model M1 (without *Perd*). In fact, we were able to derive a DT that is able to discriminate between the classes *Diam* ≥ 6 and *Diam* <6 on the basis of the factors: *Got, Gpt, AFP, Alb, Res, Chemo* and *TNM* with a generalization error, calculated after leave-one-out cross-validation, of 0.22.

4. Results

4.1 Models Prognostic Capabilities

For the DT induction we have exploited C5.0, the ID3 and C4.5 successor [8]. In particular, we have used See5 1.13[9]. NBc was implemented by using ROC 1.0, a software able to soundly derive Bayes classifiers in presence of missing data [10].

The prognostic capability of the selected models was investigated on the basis of the classical indexes for binary classifiers: Total accuracy = (TP+TN)/Total cases, Sensibility = TP/(TP+FN), Specificity = TN/(TN+FP), Positive Predictive Value = TP/(TP+FP) and Negative Predictive Value = TN/ (TN+FN), where TP is the number of True Positive classified cases, TN is the number of true negative cases, FP is the number of False Positive cases and finally FN is the number of False Negative cases. As positive cases we considered early recurrence patients. The indexes have been calculated by applying the leave-one-out method, in order to evaluate the generalization capability of the derived model; the generalization accuracy has been calculated as the average total accuracy of the prediction models obtained with the leave-one-out procedure. The leave one out approach is justified by the low number of cases available. Since the use of the derived model is foreseen both for externalization and socialization purposes, we also compared the models M2 and M3 through their Receiver Operating Characteristic (ROC) curves. The ROC curve is useful to depict the trade-off between hit rate (Sensitivity) and false alarm rate (1-Specificity). In particular, through the ROC curve it possible to understand if it is possible to increase the Specificity of the prognosis without affecting the Sensitivity too much, by changing one or more parameters of the classifier. In our case, we wanted to see whether and how we can influence the behavior of the classifier by changing the decisional threshold in favor of one or another class.

Tables III reports the performance indexes of the models M0, M1 and M2, respectively. It is straightforward to note that M1 is slightly better than M0; moreover, although only two factors are considered, M2 presents an increase of the generalization error with respect to M1 of only 8%. The rule base extracted from the training set for the model M1 is shown in Table IV.

Table III. Models results

Parameter	M0	M1	M2
Total accuracy	81.8% (63/77)	84.4% (65/77)	76.6% (59/77)
Sensibility	76.9% (30/39)	84.6% (33/39)	75.0% (30/40)
Specificity	86.8% (33/38)	84.4% (32/38)	78.3% (29/37)
Positive Predictive Value	85.7% (30/35)	84.6% (33/39)	74.4% (29/39)
Negative Predictive Value	78.6% (33/42)	84.4% (32/38)	78.9% (30/38)

Table IV. Rule set for model M1. In parentheses is reported the performance of the rule (n/m, where n is the number of cases covered by the rule and m the number of cases in which the rule fails).

R1: (12) GOT <= 34 and Perd <= 1600 and TNM = 0 Then class 0
R2: (10) Perd > 400 and Chemo =1 and TNM = 0 Then class 0
R3: (7) GPT > 150 and Alb > 3.2 and Chemo = 0 and TNM = 0 then class 0
R4: (4) GPT <= 57 and Chemo =1 and TNM = 0 Then class 0
R5: (4) AFP <= 28 and Res = 1 and TNM=1 Then class 1
R6: (7) Res = 0 and TNM =1 Then class 1
R7: (7) AFP > 28 and TNM = 1 Then class 1
R8: (56/22) GOT > 34 Then class 1
Default class: 0

The model M2 is translated into the simple rule set shown in Table V. The model M2 has been also tested on a validation set of 9 cases. For such cases it was only possible to derive from the clinical record the factor set used in M0. The total accuracy was 7/9, the sensibility was 3/5 and the specificity was 4/4. Rather interestingly, the same results were obtained with the model M0.

Table V. Rule set for model M2

R1: (2) Diam > 14 Then class 0
R2: (50/16) Diam <= 6 and Perd > 400 Then class 0
R3: (15/1) Diam > 6 and Diam <= 14 Then class 1
R4: (10/1) Perd <= 400 Then class 1
Default class: 1

Finally, the analysis of the ROC Curves (see Fig. 1), obtained by varying the misclassification cost, clearly depicts the difference in the robustness of the two models herein presented. In particular, the model M2 shows an average better performance, since its area under its ROC curve is closer to 1 than the one of M1.

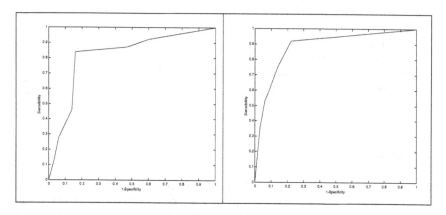

Fig. 1. ROC curves for the models M1 and M2.

4.2 Discussion

The derived model has been revised by a committee of expert physicians, working in the surgical team that was involved in the patients' treatment. The overall philosophy underlying the rules of the model M1 was considered acceptable by the experts. For example, *TNM* has been judged a good prognostic factor (in some sense related with *Grad*, used in M0) also on the basis of the clinical knowledge, and the role played by *GOT* in the derived rules confirmed a clinical hypothesis. However, some rules antecedents were considered to be not reliable; this problem was diagnosed to be related to the limited number of available data. For example, the presence in the rule R2 of the antecedent *Perd>400* was considered as a wrong precondition for the *late or no recurrence* class, since it is known that high values of *Perd* are related to early recurrence. Nevertheless, from an analysis of the data-base, it was possible to highlight that a certain number of early recurrent patients with high value of *Perd* were belonging to the *no or late recurrent* class. This problem also heavily affects the reliability of model M2. As a matter of fact, large values of *Diam* and high values of *Perd* are known to be prognostic indexes for early recurrence. Therefore, the derived rules R1 and R4 were considered unacceptable for socialization, while the rule R2 is interpreted as "although the Perd was high, the small value of Diam is a good prognosis for late recurrence". By analyzing the DT results, it was possible to note that the rules R1 and R4 are justified by a small number of supportive cases. Therefore, after having removed the cases that generate the rules R1 and R4, we induced a new DT on a reduced data set of 65 patients. Such rules are shown in Table VI; they showed an accuracy of 76% by applying leave-one-out cross validation. The new set of rules was judged to be coherent with the available knowledge and therefore useful for socialization. The data set covered by such rules is the 84% of the initial one.

Table VI. Rule set for model M2 with reduced data set

R1: (9) Diam > 7 Then class 1
R2: (14/3) Perd > 1600 Then class 1
R3: (42/10) Perd <= 1600 and Diam <= 7 Then class 0
Default class: 1

5. Conclusions

Medical literature is often reporting results of prognostic models built on small data sets, collected on severe pathologies with relatively low incidence. This fact is related to two basic needs emerging in such clinical applications: i) it is important to build models able to highlight what are the most important prognostic factors of the outcome; ii) it is crucial to be able to summarize the experience collected over years by the same clinical team and by the same institution in treating the pathology. Both of them are mainly KM tasks. More precisely, their solution resorting to DM techniques is plausible only within a KM perspective, without claiming that the results obtained hold general validity. This statement is justified by some simple theoretical considerations, based on computational learning theory and basic statistics [11,12]. For example, in the case of binary classifiers, we can compute the number of samples (n) of the training set needed to ensure that the true error will be no more than the estimated error plus a certain ε with reliability of δ. Under the simplified assumption that M prognostic factors are binary discretized, we obtain $n \geq 1/(2\varepsilon^2)(\ln |H| + \ln(1/\delta))$ [12], where $|H|$ is the hypothesis space. In the resectable hepatocellular carcinoma problem (with binary variables), if we suppose to exploit a learner that is able to reduce the dimension of $|H|$ from 2^{2^M} to 2^M, if we take $\delta=0.95$, we obtain $n \geq 6.95/\varepsilon^2$. Therefore, 69571 samples are needed to ensure $\varepsilon=0.01$, while with 77 samples, we only ensure $\varepsilon=0.3$. In this case, if a DM tool is able to obtain an error of 0.2, it is not possible to ensure that the true error would be less than 0.5. Finally, the dimension of the validation set needed to obtain an estimate of the error rate with a precision of 0.01 with 95% reliability is about 1000 samples. It is therefore apparent that accuracy (or any accuracy measure) cannot be considered as the only or the most important goal of this class of problems. The basic goal is on the contrary to provide to experts instruments for internal assessment and revision of the outcomes obtained, the operational procedures and the data collection. In other words, the basic goal is to provide quantitative means to transform the hospital clinics in a *learning organization*. This was the main goal of the work carried on in this paper. Rather interestingly, the only published paper on the application of DM techniques in the resectable hepatocellular carcinoma is an example of over-emphasis on the results obtained. In such paper, a Neural Network was applied in order to obtain the early prognosis of survival on a data base of 54 patients [13]. The authors showed the results of a successful validation on a unbalanced data set of 11 (10 survived and 1 died) new patients (100% accuracy). Such results were not obtained in our data set.

Finally, it is important to note that the work carried on in this paper has similar goals of the one presented in [14] on the use of confirmation rules, and in the work in [15] on the use of two stage models for guidelines development. As a future work, we plan to extend our work on hepatocellular carcinoma prognosis, by resorting to the technique proposed in [16], for taking into account censored data.

References

1. Nonaka I., Takeuchi H., The Knowledge-creating company, University Press, Oxford UK 1995.
2. Pazzani M.J., Knowledge discovery from data?, IEEE Intelligent Systems, 10-13, March-April 2000.
3. Kukar M., Besic N., Konomenko I., Auersperg M., Robnik-Sikonia M., Prognosing the survival time of the patients with the anaplastic thyroid carcinoma with machine learning, in: Intelligent Data Analysis in Medicine and Pharmacology, N. Lavrac, E. Keravnou, B.Zupan, 116-129, Kluwer, Boston, 1997.
4. Lise M., Bacchetti S., Da Pian P.P., Nitti D., Pilati P.L., Pigato P., Prognostic factors affecting long term outcome after liver resection for hepatocellular carcinoma, Cancer 82 (1998) 1028-1036.
5. Bacchetti S., Toffolo G., Volpato M., Da Pian P., Nitti D., Cobelli C., Lise M., Outcome prediction in patients with resectable hepatocellular carcinoma; comparison of a Multivariate score model and a Bayesian Model (submitted for publication).
6. Ramoni M., Sebastiani P., An introduction to the robust Bayesian classifier, KMI-TR-79, the Open University, UK, 1999.
7. Dash M., Liu H., Features Selection for Classification, Intelligent Data Analysis, 1997, http://www.elsevier.com/locate/ida.
8. Quinlan, J.R.: C4.5 Program for Machine Learning, Morgan Kaufmann, San Mateo CA (1994)
9. See5 Release 1.13, http://www.rulequest.com
10. Robust Bayesian Classifier (ROC), http://kmi.open.ac.uk/project/bkd
11. Duda R.O., Hart P.E., Pattern classification and scene analysis, Wiley, New York, 1973.
12. Mitchell T.M.: Machine Learning, McGraw-Hill, New York, 1997
13. Hamamoto I., Okada S., Hashimoto T., Wakabayashi H., Maeba T., Maeta H.: Prediction of the early prognosis of the hepatectomized patients with hepatocellular carcinoma with a neural network, Comput Biol Med 25 (1995) 49-59.
14. Gamberger D., Lavrac N., Jovanoski V., High confidence association rules for medical diagnosis, Proc. IDAMAP '99 workshop, 42-51., 1999.
15. Mani S., Shankle W.R., Dick M.B., Pazzani M.J.: Two stage Machine Learning model for guideline development, , Artif Intell Med, 16 (1999) 51-71.
16. Zupan B., Demsar J., Kattan M.W., Beck R.J., Bratko I: Machine Learning for survival analysis: a case of study on recurrence of prostate cancer, Artif Intell Med, 20 (2000) 59-75.

Discovering Associations in Clinical Data: Application to Search for Prognostic Factors in Hodgkin's Disease

N. Durand[1,3], B. Crémilleux[1], and M. Henry-Amar[2]

[1] GREYC, CNRS - UMR 6072
Université de Caen
F-14032 Caen Cédex France
{ndurand,cremilleux}@info.unicaen.fr
[2] GRECAN, EA 1772
Centre François Baclesse
F-14076 Caen Cédex 5 France
m.henry.amar@baclesse.fr
[3] present address: France Télécom R&D,
42 rue des coutures F-14066 Caen Cédex 4 France,
nicola.durand@rd.francetelecom.fr

Abstract. The production of suitable clusters to help physicians explore data and take decisions is a hard task. This paper addresses this question and proposes a new method to define clusters of patients which takes advantage of the power of association rules method. We present different notions of association and we specify the notion of frequent almost closed itemset which is the most appropriate for applications in the medical area. Applied to Hodgkin's disease to help establish prognostic groups, the first results bring out some parameters for which classical statistic methods confirm that they are interesting.

1 Introduction

Important medical data are collected during the treatment strategies of patients suffering from serious diseases like, for example, cancer. The use of relevant and efficient methods to explore such large data sets is not easy and we notice that these data are often under-used. Statistics are often used to validate suspected models and we are facing today to a new challenge: how may new models be discovered? By extracting from large amounts of data non trivial "nuggets" of information, Knowledge Discovery in Databases (KDD) is a semiautomatic way which may help the user for this work. Association rules are one of the most popular methods in KDD and the aim of this paper is to show their contribution to define a new method to gather patients who are similar from a certain point of view. These "clusters" of patients, in our context, may help to establish prognostic groups in Hodgkin's disease.

S. Quaglini, P. Barahona, and S. Andreassen (Eds.): AIME 2001, LNAI 2101, pp. 50–54, 2001.
© Springer-Verlag Berlin Heidelberg 2001

2   Associations and Clusters in Medical Area

2.1   Association Rules and Clusters

It is very common to try and structure a set of data in clusters in order to infer rules or other knowledge from them. In medicine, a cluster can group patients having similar and/or related features. The production of meaningful clusters in data mining is a hot topic. Similarity measures are often used. When data are complex and include categorical attributes, these measures are not easy to define [1]. Such situations are very usual in medical area. However, association rules method offers a background to produce clusters without requiring a similarity measure.

An association rule [2] is a statement of the form ``95% of patients that have gender = male and mediastinum = enlarged also get platelets $\in$ [100, 600[[1]``, 27% of patients in the database match this rule. This last number is called *support* of the rule, 95% is the *confidence* (i.e. the percentage of data that contain the consequent among those containing the antecedent). gender = male is an item and both antecedent and consequent are sets of items (or *itemsets*).

We claim that an itemset brings an intuitive way to define a cluster: it gathers patients who are similar according to items that are making up. According to the number of features and their frequencies in the patients data, the definition of a cluster can be more or less specific (and a cluster can collect a few or a large amount of patients). A sound idea is to use the itemsets generated during the process of mining the rules.

2.2   Method: Discovering Clusters of Patients

The search of clusters that we propose follows three main stages.

Frequent closed itemsets. The first stage provides all the frequent closed itemsets. The notion of frequency takes into account the "weight" of an itemset: if the frequency is not large enough, it means that the rule is not worth consideration. To generate clusters, for a given group of patients, we prefer to simply produce the sole and only itemset which is composed of the maximal number of items shared by the group: such an itemset is called *closed* itemset [3]. The idea is to catch the maximum amount of similarities among the data. We here propose to reuse this notion in a context of generation of clusters since a closed itemset catches the maximum amount of similarities among a set of data.

Almost closed itemsets. Nevertheless, in the medical area, it is well-known that data are particularly hard to explore: data are often noisy, missing values and redundancy often occur. From our point of view, one of the most difficult sides is the uncertainty intrinsically embbeded in the data. Physicians know that some examples escape from the rules and this fact makes difficult the use of data mining methods [4]. For association rules, we note that in practice, the "best"

---

[1] expressed in $10^{-9}/L$

rules that we are able to extract, are not characterized by a confidence level of 100%. To be efficient in a domain where there are always exceptions we relax the constraint of closure which is on the core of the closed itemsets [5] to allow for few exceptions in a cluster. From a technical point of view, this means that we mine the *almost* closed frequent itemsets. The number of exceptions is controlled by a parameter noted δ.

Constraints. The third stage of our method is the introduction of constraints. They are a way to take into account domain knowledge or expert know-how. A constraint can be about the domain or connected with the characteristics of the clusters (for instance, a cluster should contain a minimum number of items and patients). Only the clusters checking the constraints are kept. Moreover, it is also a pragmatic way to reduce the number of clusters.

Finally, let us note that it is hard to evaluate quantitatively the quality of the discovered clusters because, unlike classification, there is no predefined "correct value" that can be used to compute measures such as precision or recall.

3   Experiments

The used data set has been collected by the Lymphoma Group of the EORTC. It describes more than 4000 patients with early stage Hodgkin's disease (HD) treated with various protocols. Since protocols have changed with time, experiments where done on a selected subset (protocol H7, 816 patients, 1988-1993) [6]. Patients are divided in "favourable" (360 cases) and "unfavourable" (456 cases) prognostic groups described through 66 items. The data set contains 2825 missing values (five attributes concentrating 88% of the missing values).

In a first attempt, we searched for associations on all data (with a minimum support of 4% (i.e. 33 patients) and a maximum number of two exceptions by itemset). A large number of almost closed itemsets (850 417) were obtained and the selected clusters forming the "pseudo-partition" are difficult to interpret: in general, they contain a mixture of the prognostic groups or tend to be identified by the attributes corresponding to the definition of the prognostic groups.

Items belonging to the definition of the prognostic groups were then removed in order to better understand the role of the others (since experts were especially interested in biological data). 42 items remained. In order to distinguish subgroups of patients within each prognostic group, the data set was split according to the "favourable" and "unfavourable" values. We mined associations with the same parameters as before. From the "favourable" group, 4224 almost closed itemsets are extracted and 997 from the "unfavourable" group. Clusters were ranked on their treatment-failure associated rate. Are associated with a high risk of failure, in the "favourable" group, a low lymphocyte count, and in the "unfavourable" group, a low lymphocyte count and disease localized in the right supraclavicular region.

More investigation was made on the "unfavourable" group, after patients were separated according to the chemotherapy administrated: MOPP/ABV versus EBVP. For EBVP patients, a high level of white blood count (WBC) is associated with a high risk of failure while a low lymphocyte count is associated with a high risk of failure in MOPP/ABV patients. In order to confirm these observations, a classical survival analysis was performed that assesses the relevance of the WBC in EBVP patients only.

4   Conclusion

The production of meaningful clusters in data mining is a hot topic. We have presented a new approach to generate clusters of patients. This method is based on the search of closed itemsets and we have introduced the relaxation of the constraint of closure to be suitable in uncertain domains such as clinical data.

Applied to HD, using a clean database including patients with sufficient follow up, our method was able to discriminate few itemsets that may be prognostic. It was particular pertinent in the subgroup of patients experiencing the worse treatment failure free survival (i.e. EBVP patients of the "unfavourable" group). In the future, we will consider patients with early stage HD and unfavourable prognostic features together with patients with advanced stage disease and favourable prognostic features whose clinical outcome are similar thanks to the modern therapeutic strategies applied in order to highlight new itemsets potentially prognostic that could be used in clinical practice providing they are reproducible.

Considering the method to produce clusters, work has to be done to settle the best definition of an almost closed itemset in domains like medicine. Another way is to specify a proper strategy to obtain a clustering of the data.

Acknowledgements. The authors thank Artur Bykowski and Jean-François Boulicaut for stimulating discussions and the use of `min-ex` software.

References

[1] G. Das and H. Mannila.   Context-based similarity measures for categorical databases. In *proceedings of the Fourth European Conference on Principles and Practice of Knowledge Discovery in Databases, PKDD 00*, number 1910 in Lecture notes in artificial intelligence, pages 201–210, Lyon, F, 2000. Springer-Verlag.

[2] R. Agrawal, H. Mannila, R. Srikant, H. Toivonen, and A. I. Verkamo. *Fast discovery of association rules*, chapter 12. Advances in Knowledge Discovery and Data Mining. AAAI/MIT Press, 1996.

[3] N. Pasquier, Y. Bastide, R. Taouil, and L. Lakhal. Efficient mining of association rules using closed itemset lattices. *Information Systems*, 24(1):25–46, Elsevier, 1999.

[4] B. Crémilleux and C. Robert. A theoretical framework for decision trees in uncertain domains: Application to medical data sets. In E. Keravnou, C. Garbay, R. Baud, and J. Wyatt, editors, *6th Conference on Artificial Intelligence In Medicine Europe (AIME 97)*, volume 1211 of *Lecture notes in artificial intelligence*, pages 145–156, Grenoble (France), 1997. Springer-Verlag.

[5] J. F. Boulicaut and A. Bykowski. Frequent closures as a concise representation for binary data mining. In *proceedings of the Fourth Pacific-Asia Conference on Knowledge Discovery and Data Mining, PAKDD 00*, volume 1805 of *Lecture notes in artificial intelligence*, pages 62–73, Kyoto (Japan), 2000. Springer-Verlag.

[6] E. M. Noordijk, P. Carde, A. M. Mandard, W. A M. Mellink, M. Monconduit, H. Eghbali, U. Tirelli, J. Thomas, R. Somers, N. Dupouy, and M. Henry-Amar. Preliminary results of the EORTC-GPMC controlled clinical trial H7 in early stage Hodgkin's disease. *Ann. Oncol.*, 5 (Suppl. 2):S107–S112, 1994.

Visualisation of Multidimensional Data for Medical Decision Support

A. Rosemary Tate[1,2], Joshua Underwood[2], Christophe Ladroue[1],
Rosemary Luckin[2], and John R. Griffiths[1]

[1] CRC Biomedical MR Research Group, St George's Hospital Medical School,
University of London, Cranmer Terrace, London, UK.
[2] School of Cognitive and Computing Sciences, University of Sussex, Falmer,
Brighton, UK.

Abstract. Medical decision support tools are not widely used by clinicians, perhaps because most do not explain the decisions. We describe
an approach for case-based systems using automated pattern recognition techniques. Multivariate methods estimate the degree of similarity
between a new case and those in the database, and graphical displays
allow users to combine this information with their own expertise. The
approach is demonstrated by an example, the SpectraVisualizer, which
allows radiologists to interpret magnetic resonance spectra. The variables in the overview are derived directly from the signals obtained from
the scanner. Spectra with similar classification profiles can be linked to
clinical history, images and expert commentary.

1 Introduction

Medical decision support tools have had a long and chequered history. Early
systems, frequently aimed at automating diagnosis, were often perceived to be
in direct competition with the clinician [1]. Perhaps as a consequence few systems
supporting diagnosis are in use today [2]. Another major cause of non-acceptance
of diagnostic systems may be the lack of transparency and failure to provide
explanations of how system decisions are reached. We propose an approach for
case-based decision support which, instead of providing set answers, uses pattern
recognition techniques to help the users make their decisions by allowing them
to compare their data with known cases, and also "prototypical" cases, and to
estimate the degree of similarity between them.

2 The Framework

Most medical decisions will be based on balancing evidence obtained from a
number of different sources, for example, symptoms, patient data, family history, blood tests, scans etc. When there are only a few such variables these
can be displayed as univariate plots and graphs. However, with many features
this becomes more difficult and more sophisticated "multivariate" visualisation

S. Quaglini, P. Barahona, and S. Andreassen (Eds.): AIME 2001, LNAI 2101, pp. 55–58, 2001.
© Springer-Verlag Berlin Heidelberg 2001

techniques are required. The main idea of our approach is to provide linked interactive displays, which allow the user to compare cases with each other and also with prototypes or typical data from each class. Statistical classification methods are used to generate relevant similarity measures and additional tools are provided to help focus the user's attention on the most significant features for any particular classification problem. The main requirement for the proposed system is (ideally) a large computerised database of labelled cases, which can be used to train the system and provide comparisons for new data.

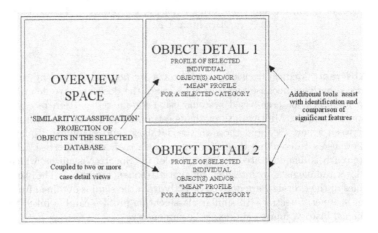

Fig. 1. Framework for a decision support system. The overview space on the left displays a 2-D projection of the cases in the database. The "detail" views on the right allow profiles of individual objects to be displayed.

The framework, depicted in Figure 1 consists of a number of "co-ordinated visualisations" [3] or "views" on the data. The main view is the 'overview' which shows database cases in a scatter plot; distance between cases is inversely proportional to their similarity. This view allows the identification of groups, subgroups and similar cases in the data set. Clicking on any case provides access to detail views which show the profiles of the individual object(s); these can include statistically generated typical objects for each group. Users can introduce new cases and these are automatically positioned appropriately in the overview.

There are various techniques for "projecting" multivariate data onto two or three dimensional scatter plots. Many of these are "unsupervised" methods, which aim to preserve the the original structure of data as much as possible e.g principal component analysis. However, where the aim is decision support, (rather than data exploration) supervised methods which take into account the label (e.g. diagnosis or prognosis) of the examples to find a suitable projection are generally more appropriate. For example, Linear Discriminant Analysis (LDA) [4], where the objective is to find linear combinations of the variables which best separate the classes. The way that the details are displayed will depend very much on the individual objects, and also the particular application. An example is described below.

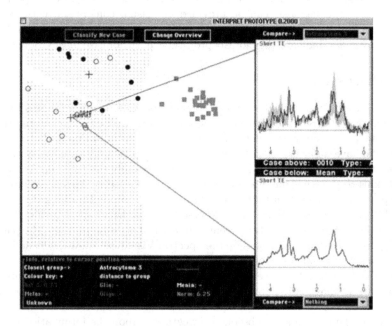

Fig. 2. User interface for Spectra Visualizer prototype. The overview (left) shows a 2-D scatterplot of spectra from low and high grade astrocytomas (filled and open circles) and normal brain (squares). The detail views (right) show spectral profiles for the two selected cases, together with a statistical profile (mean +/- one standard deviation) of the high grades (top right)

3   Example: The Spectral Visualizer

This system aims to enable radiologists to use data from Magnetic Resonance Spectroscopy (MRS) in the diagnosis of brain tumours. Support is provided via two-dimensional "overviews" generated by LDA of the MRS data. Any case in an overview can be selected and spectra, MR images and clinical information compared with the corresponding data for any other case.

At the top-level the entire dataset is classified into three groups, normal brain, malignant and benign tumours. Users can view how a case classifies at this top level and then apply their clinical expertise to select a suitable lower level overview showing a limited number of more specific candidate diagnoses. Spectra from tumours of the same type tend to cluster together in overviews and classification of a spectrum can therefore be read visually in terms of its membership of the disease clusters. System classifications may be used to add weight to the user's tentative diagnosis, perhaps suggested by initial inspection of the images, or to prompt consideration of alternative diagnostic hypotheses. Evidence for a diagnosis can be provided via visual comparison with spectra from similar cases and statistically "disease typical" spectra; boundaries drawn in the overview indicate the closest 'prototypical' mean case at any point.

4   Discussion

The approach to medical system development presented here addresses two important issues. Firstly, the role of the system and the nature of the information it presents, and secondly the method adopted for the visualisation of that information. We have described a design model that recognises the need for systems to adopt the role of enabling medical practitioners to apply their existing knowledge and skills to the problem of a new case requiring diagnosis. This is preferable to the provision of a system that attempts to actually present a diagnosis.

The second issue that we have addressed reflects the manner in which we propose that patient data can be presented to clinical decision-makers. The pattern recognition techniques adopted by the Spectral Visualizer allow the visualisation of an abstraction of the complete underlying data set. This abstraction enables the decision-maker to concentrate attention upon the most salient features for their current diagnostic pursuit. The provision of different perspectives or viewpoints upon the visualisation of this data abstraction supports a decomposition of the problem space and subsequent integration upon the formulation of a diagnostic hypothesis. The empirical validation of the framework presented in this paper is ongoing and the results to date offer much support for its potential.

Acknowledgements. Financial support has been provided by the EU (INTERPRET IST-199-10310). We also thank Dr. Carles Arús and physicians from participating hospitals and the British Council, Royal Society and Cancer Research Campaign.

References

1. J. Fox. Computers, decision making and clinical effectiveness. In Jo Lenagham, editor, *Rethinking Information Technology in Health.* Institute of Public Policy Research, 1998.
2. E. Coiera. Question the assumptions. In P. Barahona and J. P. Christensen, editors, *Knowledge and Decisions in Health Telematics – The Next Decade*, pages 61–66. IOS Press, Amsterdam, 1994.
3. C. North and B. Shneiderman. Snap together visualization: Can users construct and operate coordinated visualizations? *International Journal of Human-Computer Studies*, 53:695–714, 2000.
4. W. J. Krzanowski. *Principles of Multivariate Analysis.* Clarendon Press, Oxford, 1988.

A Clustering-Based Constructive Induction Method and Its Application to *Rheumatoid Arthritis*

José A. Sanandrés[1], Víctor Maojo[1], José Crespo[1], and Agustín Gómez[2]

[1] Medical Informatics Group. Artificial Intelligence Laboratory.
School of Computer Science. Universidad Politécnica de Madrid. Spain
{sanandre,vmaojo,jcrespo}@infomed.dia.fi.upm.es
[2] Clinical Epidemiology Research Unit. Hospital 12 de Octubre. Madrid

Abstract. We present a hybrid constructive model of induction. As a benchmark we used a database of rheumatoid arthritis patients. Combining Machine Learning and Clustering algorithms we obtained clinical prediction rules. Our model creates new features thru clustering methods, improving traditional ML methods.

Keywords. machine learning; inductive learning; constructive induction; clustering; rheumatoid arthritis

1 Introduction

We present a new method of constructive induction of machine learning (ML) applied to a medical domain, rheumatoid arthritis (RA). We have studied the relationship among attributes evaluated at the beginning of the disease and attributes that measure the long-term health status in patients.

ML algorithms analyze medical databases to extract knowledge, that can be used to help the physician in medical diagnosis and prognosis problems by improving objectivity and reliability [6].

We combined various ML and clustering algorithms and we applied them to medical records from a local hospital. One of our goals is to increase accuracy and comprehensibility of the results by our methods.

2 Model

ML methods reviews [7] show that there is not an optimal method for all domains [2]. The performance of a method is related to the domain properties.

A ML system can use only one representation language (homogeneous system) or more (hybrid system). Homogeneous systems may have problems when there are subspaces with different properties [11]. In a hybrid system the searching procedure selects the best representation language for each subspace.

S. Quaglini, P. Barahona, and S. Andreassen (Eds.): AIME 2001, LNAI 2101, pp. 59–62, 2001.

Stochastic Dependencies (SD) There is a stochastic dependency in an example set E among a set of numeric attributes $NA_1, NA_2, \ldots, NA_m$ when it holds: $\begin{array}{l} \exists f(NA_1, NA_2, \ldots, NA_m) \to \Re \\ \forall e_j \in E, f(NA_1, NA_2, \ldots, NA_m) > 0 \end{array}$

Functional Dependencies (FD) There is a functional dependency in an example set E among a set of numeric attributes $NA_1, NA_2, \ldots, NA_m$ when it holds: $\begin{array}{l} \exists g(NA_1, NA_2, \ldots, NA_m) \to \Re \\ \forall e_j \in E, g(NA_1, NA_2, \ldots, NA_m) = 0 \end{array}$

SDs, corresponding to regions in the space, can be found by using unsupervised clustering methods [3]. FDs can be obtained using statistical regression methods. We have chosen SDs, because functional dependencies can be considered as a particular case of the former type.

Inductive transformation generates new features from dependencies. The set of features representing the dependencies is evaluated for each example, and the values for the new features are added to the example definition. The set of transformed examples, containing the original and new features, is given to the ML algorithm.

3   Data

This is a retrospective cohort epidemiological study, carried out at the 12 de Octubre Hospital in Madrid, Spain . The database contains information about 374 patients diagnosed with RA.

Medical experts in RA chose 21 predictive variables. These variables were evaluated in the first year after the first. The 7 present numerical features were used for constructive induction.

A panel of rheumatologists selected the outcomes: death, and health status. Two health status assessment questionnaires were used: the general Medical Outcomes Study-Short Form 36 (MOS-SF36) and the RA specific Modified-Health Assessment Questionnaire (HAQ). The MOS-SF36 has eight scales: Role-Physical (RP), Physical Functioning (PF), Social Functioning (SF), Role-Emotional (RE), Bodily Pain (BP), Vitality (VT), General Health (GH), and Mental Health (MH). We dichotomized the HAQ and the MOS-SF36 scales with the median to reduce the negative effect of outliers.

4   Method

We employed clustering algorithms to find SDs. We chose these algorithms, with the labels for the transformed sets: Nearest Neighbour (*near*), Farthest Neighbour (*far*), Centroid (*centr*), Median (*media*), Average (*group*), Ward (*ward*), Minimum Spanning Tree (*desc,dist*) We looked for 10 clusters, using 5 as well for the Minimum Spanning Tree (MST).

We applied the clustering algorithms to all pairs of numerical features. This produce new features that can be easily represented and evaluated. The application of one clustering algorithm to all the pairs generates a new *set*.

We employed a postprocessing algorithm for examples whith one unknown feature to evaluate dependencies found by the MST algorithm. The label *dist* corresponds to the original dependencies and *desc* to the postprocessed ones.

We employed these ML algorithms: $C4.5$ [9], $FOIL$ [10], *InductH* [5] and T [1]. A *method* is a learning algorithm with a specified value assignation to its parameters.

Each pair $(set, method)$ represents a possible solution. We applied 10-fold cross-validation to evaluate each pair. We chose the following parameters to assess the quality of a pair: percentage of correctly classified examples (C), percentage of classified examples (P), and the overall assessment of a cross-validation iteration (V). V is the harmonic mean of C and P. We chose V to compare solutions because it combines accuracy and generality. The best solution is the one that has the highest value for the average values of V for 10 cross-validation iterations.

We selected the pair $(set, method)$ with best performance to generate the solution by applying the method to the whole set. This solution was analysed to extract the most relevant rules.

5   Results

There follows a summary of the cross validation results. From these values, we built Table 1. This table displays the best combination of transformed data set and learning algorithm for each feature.

Table 1. Cross Validation Results for Best Solutions

OUTCOME	SET	ALGORITHM	V	C	P
Death	desc.5.T	c48	93.60	88.72	99.20
HAQ	desc.10.T	c48-c80	68.68	55.79	84.33
RP	centr	t2	72.46	61.20	89.55
BP	BP	t1	69.44	55.09	94.60
RE	media	t2	69.80	58.21	89.17
PF	dist.5.T	c48	69.93	58.85	85.45
SF	media	c48	74.06	59.42	100.00
GH	desc.10.T	c48	76.58	65.54	93.42
MH	MH	t1	77.71	63.93	100.00
VT	desc.10	t2	76.67	64.70	95.02

6   Discussion and Conclusions

For 8 of the 10 outcomes studied, the models developed applying our model improved the performance of the models developed applying only a ML algorithm. They performed similarly in the other 2 outcomes, *BP* and *MH*. This shows that the constructive induction, by using stochastic dependencies, helps to achieve more accurate and reliable results.

We used several inductive learning algorithms. The algorithms that achieved the best results were $C4.5$ and T. The models developed by $Foil$ were very complex.

The bes clustering algorithm war MST, with the post-processing option and with 10 clusters. Ten clusters perform better than 5, because the higher number eliminates outliers and concentrates clusters around the real cores.

One drawback is that we used the variables that physicians selected from an initial set of 41 variables. We need to add a feature selection step to our model to overcome these potential problem. The large number of features and the small number of patients was another drawback [13]. Another factor that heightened this problem was the high percentage of unknown values for some features.

References

1. Peter Auer, Robert C. Holte, and Wolfgang Maass. Theory and applications of agnostic pac-learning with small decision trees. Technical Report NC-TR-96-034, NeuroCOLT, 1996.
2. Carla E. Brodley. Recursive automatic bias selection for classifier construction. *Machine Learning*, 20:63–94, 1995.
3. B.S Everitt. *Cluster Analysis*. Edward Arnold, London, 1993.
4. A. Famili, Wi-Min Shen, Richard Weber, and Evangelos Simoudis. Data preprocessing and intelligent data analysis. *Intelligent Data Analysis*, 1(1), January 1997.
5. Brian R. Gaines. An ounce of knowledge is worth a ton of data: Quantitative studies of the trade-off between expertise and data based on statistically well-founded empirical induction. In *Proceedings of 6th International Workshop on Machine Learning*, pages 156–159. Morgan Kaufmann, June 1989.
6. I. Kononenko, I. Bratko, and M. Kukar. Application of machine learning to medical diagnosis. In R. S. Michalski, I. Bratko, and M. Kubat, editors, *Machine Learning and Data Mining: Methods and Applications*. John Wiley & Sons Ltd, 1997.
7. T.-S. Lim, W.-Y. Loh, and Y.-S. Shih. An empirical comparison of decision trees and other classification methods. Technical Report 979, Department of Statistics, University of Wisconsin-Madison, Madison, WI, June 30 1997.
8. César Montes. *MITO: Método de Inducción Total*. PhD thesis, Facultad de Informática, UPM, 1994.
9. J.R. Quinlan. *C4.5: Programs for Machine Learning*. Morgan Kaufmann, San Mateo, CA, 1992.
10. J.R. Quinlan. Induction of logic programs: Foil and related systems. *New Generation Computing*, 13:287–312, 1995.
11. J.R. Quinlan. Improved use of continuous attributes in c4.5. *Journal of Artificial Intelligence Research*, 4:77–90, 1996.
12. J.A. Sanandrés, E. Ciruelo, J. Crespo, A. Gómez, V. Maojo, and C. Montes. Predreuma: Modelo de inducción constructiva en prognosis y clasificación en artritis reumatoide. Madrid, Abril 1997. INFORSALUD 97. II Congreso Nacional de Informática de la Salud.
13. J.H Wasson, H.C. Sox, R.K. Neff, and L. Goldman. Clinical prediction rules: Applications and methodological standards. *The New England Journal of Medicine*, 313(13):793–799, Sept 1985.

Improving Identification of Difficult Small Classes by Balancing Class Distribution

Jorma Laurikkala

Department of Computer and Information Sciences, University of Tampere,
FIN-33014 University of Tampere, Finland
Jorma.Laurikkala@cs.uta.fi

Abstract. We studied three methods to improve identification of difficult small classes by balancing imbalanced class distribution with data reduction. The new method, neighborhood cleaning rule (NCL), outperformed simple random and one-sided selection methods in experiments with ten data sets. All reduction methods improved identification of small classes (20-30%), but the differences were insignificant. However, significant differences in accuracies, true-positive rates and true-negative rates obtained with the 3-nearest neighbor method and C4.5 from the reduced data favored NCL. The results suggest that NCL is a useful method for improving the modeling of difficult small classes, and for building classifiers to identify these classes from the real-world data.

1 Introduction

Real-world data sets often have imbalanced class distribution, because many natural processes produce certain observations infrequently. For example, rare diseases in a population may result in medical data with small diagnostic groups. When some classes are heavily under-represented, statistical and machine learning methods are likely to run into problems. Cases from the rare classes are lost among the other cases during learning. The resulting classifiers misclassify new unseen rare cases, and descriptive models may give an inadequate picture of the data. The learning task is even more problematic, if a small class is difficult to identify because of its other characteristics. A small class may, for example, overlap heavily the other classes. In the following, we refer to a small and difficult class as a *class of interest*.

We balanced class distribution with data reduction before the actual analysis, because we aimed to develop a general-purpose method, whose results may be given directly to statistical and machine learning methods. The most well-known data reduction technique comes from the area of statistics, where sampling [1] is used to allow analyses which would be impractical with large populations. Data reduction has been utilized in the area of machine learning especially to accelerate the instance-based learning methods [2,3]. Recently Kubat *et al.* [4] presented one-sided selection (OSS) which uses instance-based methods to reduce the larger class when class distribution of a two-class problem is imbalanced. In this paper, we describe a new method called *neighborhood cleaning rule* that utilizes the OSS principle, but considers more carefully the quality of the data to be removed.

S. Quaglini, P. Barahona, and S. Andreassen (Eds.): AIME 2001, LNAI 2101, pp. 63–66, 2001.

2 Methods and Materials

Simple random sampling (SRS), which was used as a baseline method, is the most basic one of the sampling methods applied in statistics [1]. In SRS a sample (sub-set) S is selected randomly from the original data T so that each example in T has an equal probability to be selected into S. We applied SRS to classes that were larger than class of interest C and selected a sample with size of | C | from each of these classes. Unfortunately, the within classes SRS (SWC) may produce biased samples, because small samples may have an over-representation of outliers or noisy data.

One-sided selection (OSS) [4] reduces T by keeping all examples of C and by removing examples from the rest of data $O = T - C$. Firstly, Hart's condensed nearest neighbor rule (CNN) [3,4] is applied to select a sub-set A from T which is consistent with T in the sense that A classifies T correctly with the one-nearest neighbor rule (1-NN). CNN starts from S, which contains C and an example from each class in O, and moves examples misclassified by 1-NN from O to S, until a complete pass over O has been done without misclassifications. Secondly, examples that are noisy or lie in the decision border are removed from O. The major drawback of OSS is CNN rule which is extremely sensitive to noise [3]. Since noisy examples are likely to be misclassified, many of them will be added to the training set. Moreover, noisy training data will misclassify several of the subsequent test examples [2,3]. We also argue that data cleaning should be done before the data analysis. For example, in statistical analyses and data mining, data pre-processing is an important step before the actual analysis.

The basic idea of our *neighborhood cleaning rule* (NCL) is the same as in OSS: All examples in C are saved, while O is reduced. In contrast to OSS, NCL emphasizes more data cleaning than data reduction. Our justification for this approach is two-fold. Firstly, the quality of classification results does not necessarily depend on the size of the class. Therefore, we should consider, besides the class distribution, other characteristics of data, such as noise, that may hamper classification. Secondly, studies of data reduction with instance-based techniques [3] have shown that it is difficult to maintain the original classification accuracy while the data is being reduced. This aspect is important, since while improving the identification of small classes, the method should be able to classify the other classes with an acceptable accuracy.

Consequently, we chose to use Wilson's edited nearest neighbor rule (ENN) [3] to identify noisy data A_1 in O. ENN removes examples whose class differs from the majority class of the three nearest neighbors. ENN retains most of the data, while maintaining a good classification accuracy [3]. In addition, we clean neighborhoods of examples in C: The three nearest neighbors that misclassify examples of C and belong to O are inserted into set A_2. To avoid excessive reduction of small classes, only examples from classes larger or equal to $0.5 \cdot$ | C | are considered while forming A_2. Lastly, the union of sets A_1 and A_2 is removed from T to produce reduced data S. Fig. 1 illustrates the NCL rule. To make NCL to suit better for solving real-world problems than OSS, we utilized Heterogeneous value difference metric (HVDM) [3] and designed NCL with multi-class problems in mind.

Experiments were made with ten real-world data sets of which eight were retrieved from UCI machine learning repository [5]. Six of these data sets were medical data which is our primary application area. Female urinary incontinence [6] and vertigo [7] data sets are medical data which we have studied earlier with different methods. The characteristics of the data sets, as well as the classes of interest are reported in [8].

---

1. Split data T into the class of interest C and the rest of data O.

2. Identify noisy data A_1 in O with edited nearest neighbor rule.

3. For each class C_i in O

    if ($x \in C_i$ in 3-nearest neighbors of misclassified $y \in C$)
    and ($|C_i| \geq 0.5 \cdot |C|$) then $A_2 = \{ x \} \cup A_2$
4. Reduced data $S = T - (A_1 \cup A_2)$

Fig. 1. Neighborhood cleaning rule

We applied the three data reduction methods to the whole data as in [4] and to the training sets of 10-fold cross-validation process as in [3]. The data were classified with the three-nearest neighbor (3-NN) method (with HVDM) and C4.5 (release 8, default settings) [9]. Classification measures were accuracy, true-positive (TPR) and true-negative rates (TNR), and the true-positive rate of the class of interest (TPRC). The two-tailed Wilcoxon signed ranks test was used to test the significance of differences in the measures ($p<0.05$).

3   Results

Mean accuracies, TPRs, TNRs, and TPRCs from the original data were 76, 68, 73, 39 for 3-NN and 76, 69, 72, 40 for C4.5, respectively. Table 1 shows the changes in means of classification measures from the reduced data in comparison with the mean results from the original data. More detailed results are reported in [8]. With reduced training and test sets, the differences in accuracy, TPRs and TNRs were significant and in favor of NCL (NCL>SWC>OSS). With reduced training and original test sets, the following differences were significant in 3-NN measures: Accuracy: NCL>OSS, TPR: SWC>OSS and NCL>OSS, and TNR: NCL>SWC and NCL>OSS. In all the C4.5 measures, except TPRC, SWC>OSS and NCL>OSS were the significant differences. All statistically significant differences were in favor of NCL. There were no significant differences in TPRCs with both types of test data.

Table 1. Changes in means of accuracies (a), true-positive rates (tpr), true-negative rates (tnr) and true-positive rates for the classes of interest (c) in percents from the reduced data in comparison with mean results from the original data. Balanced (*) and original (**) test data.

Method	SWC				OSS				NCL			
	a	tpr	tnr	c	a	tpr	tnr	c	a	tpr	tnr	c
3-NN*	-7	1	-4	22	-19	-23	-17	25	11	16	13	27
C4.5*	-4	4	-1	26	-14	-13	-11	22	5	9	8	25
3-NN**	-7	1	-4	24	-8	-6	-4	25	-5	1	-1	23
C4.5**	-6	4	-3	30	-10	-8	-6	25	-6	-1	-1	20

4 Discussion

The classification results obtained from the reduced original data sets showed that the NCL method was significantly better than SWC and OSS. Only the differences in TPRCs were insignificant. All reduction methods improved clearly (22-27%) these rates in comparison with the results of original data. NCL was the only reduction method which resulted in higher accuracies, TPRs and TNRs than those of the original data sets. NCL was able to overcome the noise related drawbacks of OSS. NCL attempts to avoid the problems caused by noise by applying the ENN algorithm that is designed for noise filtering. NCL also cleans neighborhoods that misclassify examples belonging to the class of interest. The results suggest that NCL is a useful tool to build descriptive models that take better into account difficult small classes.

NCL was also the best method when the test data had the original imbalanced class distribution. All reduction methods improved clearly (20-30%) TPRCs in comparison with the results of original data. Although the other classification measures of NCL method were lower than the original ones, decrease was slight and slightly smaller in comparison with OSS. Our method may also be useful in building better classifiers for new unseen rare examples for the real-world data with imbalanced class distribution. NCL might allow us, for example, to generate classifiers that are able to identify examples of the sensory urge class [6] better than the classifiers built from the original data. This type of classifiers would be very useful in an expert system which we plan to develop to aid physicians in the differential diagnosis of female urinary incontinence [6]. In the preliminary tests with two-fold cross-validation, we have found that 3-NN classifier with NCL reduced training sets have improved on average 20% the TPRs of the difficult sensory urge class.

References

1. Cochran, W.G.: Sampling Techniques. 3rd edn. Wiley, New York (1977)
2. Aha, D.W., Kibler, D., Albert, M.K.: Instance-Based Learning Algorithms. Mach. Learn. **6** (1991) 37-66
3. Wilson, D.R., Martinez, T.R.: Reduction Techniques for Instance-Based Learning Algorithms. Mach. Learn. **38** (2000) 257-286
4. Kubat, M., Matwin, S.: Addressing the Curse of Imbalanced Training Sets: One-Sided Selection. In: Fisher, D.H. (ed.): Proceedings of the Fourteenth International Conference in Machine Learning. Morgan Kaufmann, San Francisco (1997) 179-186
5. Blake, C.L., Merz, C.J.: UCI Repository of machine learning databases [http://www.ics.uci.edu/~mlearn/MLRepository.html]. Irvine, University of California, Department of Information and Computer Science (1998)
6. Laurikkala, J., Juhola, M., Lammi, S., Penttinen, J., Aukee P.: Analysis of the Imputed Female Urinary Incontinence Data for the Evaluation of Expert System Parameters. Comput. Biol. Med. **31** (2001)
7. Kentala, E.: Characteristics of Six Otologic Diseases Involving Vertigo. Am. J. Otol. **17** (1996) 883-892
8. Laurikkala J.: Improving Identification of Difficult Small Classes by Balancing Class Distribution [ftp://ftp.cs.uta.fi/pub/reports/pdf/A-2001-2.pdf]. Dept. of Computer and Information Sciences, University of Tampere, Tech. Report A-2001-2, April 2001
9. Quinlan, J.R.: C4.5 Programs for Machine Learning. Morgan Kaufman, San Mateo (1993)

Credal Classification for Dementia Screening

Marco Zaffalon[1], Keith Wesnes[2], and Orlando Petrini[3]

[1] IDSIA, Galleria 2,
CH-6928 Manno, Switzerland
zaffalon@idsia.ch
[2] Cognitive Drug Research Ltd., CDR House, 24 Portman Road,
Reading RG30 1EA, UK
keithw@cdr.org.uk
[3] Pharmaton SA, Via ai Mulini,
CH-6934 Bioggio, Switzerland
petrini@lgn.boehringer-ingelheim.com

Abstract. Dementia is a very serious personal, medical and social problem. Early and accurate diagnoses seem to be the key to effectively cope with it. This paper presents a diagnostic tool that couples the most widely used computerized system of cognitive tests in dementia research, the Cognitive Drug Research system, with the naive credal classifier. Although the classifier is trained on an incomplete database, it provides unmatched predictive performance and reliability. The tool also proves to be very effective in discriminating between Alzheimer's disease and dementia with Lewy bodies, which is a problem on the frontier of research on dementia.

1 Introduction

Dementia is becoming recognized to be one of the leading causes for concern in the elderly, both from the perspective of their own quality of life and also the social issues concerning the hugely growing costs of caring for the rapidly growing population who require constant supervision and medical care [1,14]. The most important type of dementia is Alzheimer's Disease (AD) accounting for approximately 50% of all types of dementia. Vascular Dementia (VD) has traditionally been considered the second most common cause of dementia (up to 20% of dementias, either alone, or in combination with AD). Dementia with Lewy Bodies (DLB) is an only recently described type of dementia which is becoming recognized to be the second most common single form of dementia accounting for over 20% of all dementias [14]. It has previously often been misdiagnosed as Alzheimer's disease, as well as confused with schizophrenia. One of the major problems confronting trials with DLB is the correct diagnose of the disorder [14, 23,24,25].

There is currently no cure for any dementia although three compounds from a class of drug called anticholinesterases (galanthamine, rivastigmine and donepezil) have been registered in various countries for the mild symptomatic

S. Quaglini, P. Barahona, and S. Andreassen (Eds.): AIME 2001, LNAI 2101, pp. 67–76, 2001.
© Springer-Verlag Berlin Heidelberg 2001

relief of AD. Current research is trying to early identify AD as the hope is that these compounds may prove more effective in treating the early stages of dementia (often termed "mild cognitive impairment") and preventing rather than just reducing symptoms [27]. The first clinical trial has just been completed showing that rivastigmine can dramatically improve cognitive function in DLB [13].

Three major problems confront research in this field. On one hand, it is questionable whether or not systems are sensitive enough to detect early stages of dementia. On the other, it must still be confirmed whether or not tests are capable of differentiating different types of dementia; and measures for assessing therapeutic response to treatment must still be unequivocally determined. In this paper we focus on the first two problems. By coupling the power of emerging classification tools and the diagnostic capabilities of a well-targeted system of cognitive tests, we propose an automated diagnostic system that deals successfully with both problems.

As far as cognitive tests, we rely upon the Cognitive Drug Research (CDR) computerized assessment system. This has been designed to provide a valid, reliable and sensitive tool for assessing cognitive functions in dementia [2,16,17,20, 23,24,25,28]. The system is the *most widely* used automated system in dementia research [16] (see Sect. 2.1). We use a database describing the actual health state and the past responses to the CDR system tests for about 3,400 patients (Sect. 2.3). The data were not collected for the purpose of data mining, so they are not completely accurate, presenting a substantial amount of missing values. Missing data are recognized to be a fundamental problem in the machine learning literature [4]; treating them properly is essential to draw reliable inferences.

These challenging issues motivated us to choose the classification model called *Naive Credal Classifier* [30,31] (NCC, Sect. 2.2), a generalization of the well-known discrete *Naive Bayes Classifier* (or NBC [6]) to sets of probability distributions [26]. The NCC is currently the only classifier that takes into account the imprecision arising from prior uncertainty about the unknown distribution generating the data; and it is also robust to all the possible mechanisms of missingness. The robust Bayes classifier from Ramoni and Sebastiani presents similarities in the treatment of missing data [18], although it appears to adopt an overly conservative approach. Also, it neglects the former type of imprecision.

The characteristics of the new paradigm of credal classification enable the NCC to automatically do reliable classifications. This is the first application of credal classification to the field of dementia screening. We realize it by analyzing the predictive behavior of the NCC by an empirical study on the database, in Sect. 3. In doing this, we remarkably improve upon the diagnostic accuracy described in similar past work [12], with up to 95% correct predictions. We also show that the system is very effective in discriminating among dementias, even between the two types currently only hardly distinguishable, AD and DLB. Overall, we successfully deal with the problem of obtaining reliable inferences, which is fundamental for the application domain under consideration and it is also more critical given the incompleteness of the database.

2   Methods

2.1   The CDR System

The CDR system is a computer based system, the patient responding by using a simple response box containing just a "yes" and "no" button for each test. It takes between 25 and 40 minutes to administer the tests of the system, depending on the level of dementia shown by the patients.

Results from the CDR system have encouraged the *International Group on Dementia Drug Guidelines* to issue a position paper on assessing function in future clinical trials [10]. The working group concluded that existing testing procedures (e.g. the Alzheimer's disease assessment scale) do not properly identify all of the cognitive deficits suffered by AD patients, particularly attentional deficits, and have recommended that automated procedures should be used alongside more traditional ones to support them in this and to ultimately determine whether they should supersede traditional methods [10]. The CDR system has shown sensitivity in identifying mild cognitive impairment [17,27], has been shown capable of differentiating various types of dementia (AD, DLB, VD, Huntington's Chorea; [2,16,22,23,24,25]), of measuring therapeutic response to a variety of medications in both AD [1,9,15,19,21] and DLB [13], and has shown superior sensitivity in identifying AD and Huntington's disease to all of the most widely used non-automated procedures [16].

The CDR system is the most widely used automated system in clinical research worldwide. It is used in almost every European country, North and South America, Russia, South Africa, India, Australia and New Zealand. It is used in hospitals, universities, private and government research facilities to study the effects of new medicines, ageing, disease, trauma, dementia as well as other factors such as mobile phones, altitude and so on.

2.2   Credal Classification

Classification is a technique concerned with allocating new objects to a finite set of previously defined groups (classes) on the basis of observations on several characteristics of the objects, called *attributes* or *features* [7]. In the present application, each test of the CDR system is an attribute of the problem the values of which are the possible outcomes of the test. The class is the variable the values of which are the possible states of dementia (including the state "no dementia").

Credal classification [30] is a new way of conceiving the task of prediction that generalizes the common notion of classification: a credal classifier is defined as a function that maps an instance of a set of features to a *set of states* of a categorical class variable (a common classifier maps an instance of the features to a single class). Classifiers are usually inferred from a database. A credal classifier is a basis from which imprecision in the data can be taken into account, as generated by unobserved or rare events, small sample sizes and missing data. As a consequence, for a given state of the attributes, imprecision in the input may prevent a single output class from being obtained; then the result of a credal classifier is a set of classes, all of which are candidates to be the correct category. That is, a credal classifier recognizes that the available knowledge may not suffice to isolate a single class and thus gives rise to a set of alternatives. Reliability is thus a concept intrinsic in the definition of credal classification.

It is easy to use a credal classifier for diagnostic purposes: in the present case, the vector of responses to the CDR tests for a patient is mapped to a set of possible states of dementia by the function represented by the classifier. Credal classification is realized in this paper by the naive credal classifier [30]. The NCC is a special type of credal network [8,3] that generalizes the NBC. It maintains the good properties of the naive Bayes classifier [5], but it relaxes the assumption that the model probabilities be precise. Most importantly, it can easily and robustly be inferred from possibly small and incomplete data sets [31]. In particular, an incomplete data set is regarded as a collection of complete data sets that arises by considering all the possible replacements of the missing data with admissible values [29]. The NCC is inferred by considering the collection as a set of possible samples, so that the NCC inferences are robust to each possible mechanism of missing data. This is equivalent to considering many probability distributions be plausible given the data and to treat all of them together as a set of possible distributions, as it is common in the field of *imprecise probabilities* [26]. A set of distributions gives rise to a set of output classes in general, given an instance of the attributes, thus realizing a credal classifier.

2.3   The Database

The database is constituted by 3,385 records. Each record stores the responses to the CDR system tests for a patient. The results are expressed by either continuous or integer numbers. Each record also reports the actual health state of the patient, which is classified into 5 categories: normal, AD, to undergo Coronary Bypass Surgery (CBS), DLB and VD. Table 1 shows the percentages of patients in each class.

Table 1. Percentual distribution of the classes in the database.

	Normal	AD	CBS	DLB	VD
Percentage	67.4%	22.9%	2.4%	3.9%	3.4%

The tests are carried out in different ways according to the state of the patient. This leads to the presence of more features for the dementia patients than for the normal controls. Seven attributes are used when normal people are involved in the study (the number in parentheses is the percentage of missing values): delayed word recognition reaction time (6.4%), delayed word recognition sensitivity index (5.6%), digit vigilance false alarms (4.3%), digit vigilance reaction time (3.3%), digit vigilance accuracy (3.3%), choice reaction time (1.6%) and choice reaction time accuracy (1%). The choice reaction time is obtained as follows: either the word "no" or the word "yes" is presented on the monitor and the patient is instructed to press the corresponding button as quickly as possible. There are 20 trials for which each stimulus word is chosen randomly with equal probability and there is a varying inter-stimulus interval. We do not describe here how all other measures are obtained. The interested reader can consult the related references.

The above attributes are used in the first analysis (Sect. 3.2). The second analysis (Sect. 3.3) is based on the 1,103 units of the database restricted to the dementia group. In the second analysis we have included 18 attributes (the number in parentheses is the percentage of missing values): digit vigilance reaction time (4.6%), numeric working memory reaction time (3.9%), numeric working memory original stimuli accuracy (3.9), numeric working memory new stimuli accuracy (3.9%), numeric working memory sensitivity index (3.9), digit vigilance accuracy (3.5%), picture recognition speed (2.3%), picture recognition original stimuli accuracy (2.3%), picture recognition new stimuli accuracy (2.3%), picture recognition sensitivity index (2.3%), delayed word recognition reaction time (2.1%), delayed word recognition original stimuli accuracy (2.1%), delayed word recognition new stimuli accuracy (2.1%), delayed word recognition sensitivity index (2.1%), choice reaction time (1.5%), choice reaction time accuracy (1.5%), simple reaction time (1.1%) and age (0.2%).

3 Experiments

3.1 Experimental Methodology

The database was randomly split into a learning set and a test set. The learning set was used to infer the classifier; its size being fixed at 50% of the database size. On the remaining 50% of cases, i.e. the test set, the true classes were hidden to the classifier in order to study its predictive accuracy, i.e. the relative number of correct guesses on a set of unseen units.

As far as the NCC, it can have different degrees of caution expressed by the real parameter s [31]. The parameter plays a role analogous to the weight given to the prior in Bayesian models. This study uses $s = 1$. Further, since the NCC assumes that the attributes are categorical, the database was initially discretized by MLC++ [11], default options. The discretization was made on the basis of the learning set only.

The empirical analysis of the NCC benefits from comparing it with the NBC [31]. Several NBCs are considered, related to the Bayesian prior distribution chosen to infer them. We consider four well-known so-called noninformative priors: Haldane, Uniform, Perks and Jeffreys. We also consider other three priors obtained by modifying some of the former. In this case the original priors are required to satisfy the structural constraints implied by the special classifier under consideration. These priors are called: Uniform', Perks' and Jeffreys' (see [31] for a thorough explanation). The Bayesian classifiers were inferred by discarding, separately for each attribute, the missing values (this is possible since the NBC assumes independence of the attributes conditional on the class).

3.2 Detecting Dementia

In the first experiment the goal is to distinguish normal people from people in the dementia group. Dementias are clustered into one class so that the class variable is binary with values in: normal group (67.4%) and dementia group (32.6%). There are 7 attributes describing a patient, as reported in Sect. 2.3. The results of the experiment are shown in Tab. 2. Each row in the table refers to a different

Table 2. Results of the discrimination between normal people and people in the dementia group. A value in a cell is expressed as a percentual number ± its standard deviation.

	$C_1\%$	$N\%$	$Ns\%$	$S\%$
Haldane	94.77±0.57	92.59±0.64	72.22±3.89	9.68±0.72
Perks	94.77±0.57	92.29±0.65	69.14±4.02	9.68±0.72
Perks′	94.77±0.57	92.41±0.65	70.37±3.97	9.68±0.72
Uniform	94.77±0.57	92.41±0.65	70.37±3.97	9.68±0.72
Uniform′	94.77±0.57	92.47±0.65	70.99±3.95	9.68±0.72
Jeffreys	94.77±0.57	92.41±0.65	70.37±3.97	9.68±0.72
Jeffreys′	94.77±0.57	92.47±0.65	70.99±3.95	9.68±0.72

prior distribution for the NBC. The columns are described below. Bear in mind that the predictive accuracy is the relative number of correct guesses.

- $C_1\%$ is the accuracy of the NCC on the subset of instances where it is possible to provide a single class according to the NCC.
- $N\%$ is the accuracy of the NBC on the entire test set.
- $Ns\%$ is the accuracy of the NBC on the subset of instances for which the NCC outputs more than one class.
- $S\%$ is the percentage of instances for which the NCC outputs more than one class.

Discussion. When the credal classifier isolates a single class, it has a very high accuracy of prediction ($C_1\%$). In about 10% of cases ($S\%$), it suggests that there is not enough knowledge to isolate a single class and it outputs both, thus not giving any judgment. Note that on this subset *all* the Bayesian models have a much worse prediction ($Ns\%$) than that of the NCC. For this reason the accuracy of the NBCs on the entire test set ($N\%$) is worse than that of the NCC.

The NCC is thus able to isolate a subset of units where robust predictions are possible (despite the missing data). Note that the NBCs realize non-random predictions on the subset of instances where the NCC does not provide any judgment: the NBCs achieve about 70% accuracy that is greater than the 50% accuracy that would be obtained by randomly guessing (recall that the class is binary). This effect is due to the finiteness of the sample and does not mean that the NBCs should be applied on the subset related to $S\%$ [31]. Instead, this may suggest that the data remarkably violate the assumption of independence between attributes conditional on the class—that is made both by the NCC and the NBC—and that it might be worth trying more structured credal classifiers.

3.3 Discriminating among Dementias

In the second analysis the goal is to assign a diseased patient to the correct disease type. The class takes values in the set of 4 dementias reported in Sect. 2.3, which also reports the 18 attributes used. The results are in Tab. 3. As

Table 3. Results of the discrimination among dementias.

	$C_1\%$	$Cs\%$	$N\%$	$Ns\%$	$S\%$	Z
Haldane	94.05±1.01	98.28±1.20	91.79±1.17	83.62±3.40	21.64±1.76	2.16±0.43
Perks	94.05±1.01	98.43±1.10	89.76±1.30	75.59±3.81	23.22±1.81	2.31±0.66
Perks'	94.05±1.01	98.43±1.10	90.86±1.23	80.31±3.53	23.22±1.81	2.31±0.66
Uniform	94.05±1.01	98.43±1.10	90.86±1.23	80.31±3.53	23.22±1.81	2.31±0.66
Uniform'	94.05±1.01	98.43±1.10	91.22±1.21	81.89±3.42	23.22±1.81	2.31±0.66
Jeffreys	94.05±1.01	98.43±1.10	89.58±1.31	74.80±3.85	23.22±1.81	2.31±0.66
Jeffreys'	94.05±1.01	98.43±1.10	91.04±1.22	81.10±3.47	23.22±1.81	2.31±0.66

before, the rows of the table refer to different NBCs. (The statistics related to Haldane's prior were computed on the 98% of units only, because, since it is an improper prior, the NBC classification was undefined in the remaining 2% of cases.) There are two more columns with respect to Tab. 2:

- $Cs\%$ is the empirical probability that the actual class belongs to the set of classes proposed by the NCC. This measure is computed when the output set of the NCC is made by two classes at least;
- Z is the average number of classes proposed by the NCC. This measure is computed when the output set of the NCC is made by two classes at least.

Discussion. Again, we see that the performance of the credal classifier is very good when it isolates a single class ($C_1\%$). When it outputs more than one class, there are about 2 on average (Z); and the probability that the actual class belongs to such a set is very high ($Cs\%$). This happens about 1 time out of 4 ($S\%$). The values of $S\%$ are larger than those in Tab. 2 because now the learning set size is about 1/3 of the learning set of the first experiment and because there are more attributes; larger collections of data, or less missing values, would quickly decrease this type of indeterminacy. The considerations related to the columns $N\%$ and $Ns\%$ are similar to the case of the preceding experiment.

In order to better analyze the capability of the credal classifier to assign a patient to the actual class, we represent the *confusion matrix* in Tab. 4. We restrict attention to the 76.88% of units where the NCC suggested only one class. The cells of the confusion matrix report the empirical probabilities of the pairs of random variables representing the predicted class and the actual class, respectively, as computed from the test set: e.g. the empirical joint probability that the class predicted by the NCC is AD and the actual class is AD is 0.7571.

The confusion matrix shows that the NCC performance to assign patients to actual classes is excellent: for instance given that the NCC has predicted Alzheimer's disease, there is only a small probability that the actual disease is VD and zero probability that it is DBL or CBS. This outcome is similar for the other dementias. Most importantly, the confusion matrix shows that the NCC discriminates between AD and DLB very well. This is a very important result for research on dementias: DLB has frequently been misdiagnosed with AD. Here we show that the CDR system is capable of distinguishing them and that it is even possible to do this automatically by means of the NCC.

Table 4. Confusion matrix. The boldface values are percentages related to correct predictions.

		Predicted class			
		AD	CBS	DLB	VD
	AD	**75.71**	0.71	0.24	0.00
Actual class	CBS	0.00	**8.10**	0.00	0.00
	DLB	0.00	0.48	**5.95**	1.90
	VD	0.95	0.00	1.67	**4.29**

4   Conclusions

Cognitive tests for dementias are getting more and more important, as early diagnosis seems to be the basis for coping successfully with the diseases. This paper shows that coupling targeted cognitive tests such as the CDR computerized system with a reliable classifier such as the NCC, enables very accurate diagnoses to be automatically made. A particularly successful feature of the overall system described in this paper is the capability to discriminate between Alzheimer's disease and dementia with Lewy bodies. This is particularly important, as non-automated and non-computerized diagnoses often have problems in detecting the subtle differences in symptoms linked to the two disease types.

Diagnoses have also been shown to be robust to a non-negligible number of missing values in the database. This result is due to the powerful characteristics of credal classification, which is applied to such an important domain for the first time. The NCC enabled the difficult problem of the incomplete database to be dealt with easily and robustly.

However, the imprecision resulting from the missing data did result in less precise inferences. Future data sets with less missing values will reduce the indeterminacies in the predicted classes, and thus enable the demonstrated predictive capability of the method to be realized in all instances.

Acknowledgements. Thanks to L. M. Gambardella and C. Lepori for their kind attention and support. M. Zaffalon was partially supported by SUPSI DIE under CTI grant # 4217.1.

References

1. H. Allain, E. Neuman, M. Malbezin, V. Salzman, Guez D., K Wesnes, and J. M. Gandon. Bridging study of S12024 in 53 in-patients with Alzheimer's disease. *J. Am. Geriatr. Soc.*, 45:125–126, 1997.
2. G. A. Ayre, A. Sahgal, I. G. McKeith, C. G. Ballard, K. Lowery, C. Pincock, M. P. Walker, and K. Wesnes. Distinct profiles of neuropsychological impairment in dementia with Lewy bodies and Alzheimer's disease. *Neurology*. In press.
3. F. G. Cozman. Credal networks. *Artificial Intelligence*, 120:199–233, 2000.
4. P. Domingos. Machine learning. In W. Klosgen and J. Zytkow, editors, *Handbook of data mining and knowledge discovery*. Oxford University Press, New York. To appear.
5. P. Domingos and M. Pazzani. On the optimality of the simple Bayesian classifier under zero-one loss. *Machine Learning*, 29(2/3):103–130, 1997.
6. R. O. Duda and P. E. Hart. *Pattern classification and scene analysis*. Wiley, New York, 1973.
7. R. O. Duda, P. E. Hart, and D. G. Stork. *Pattern classification*. Wiley, 2001. 2nd edition.
8. E. Fagiuoli and M. Zaffalon. 2U: an exact interval propagation algorithm for polytrees with binary variables. *Artificial Intelligence*, 106(1):77–107, 1998.
9. T. D. Fakouhi, Jhee S. S., J. J. Sramek, C. Benes, P. Schwartz, G. Hantsburger, R. Herting, E. A. Swabb, and N. R. Cutler. Evaluation of cycloserine in the treatment of Alzheimer's disease. *J. Geriatr. Psychiatry Neurol.*, 8:226–230, 1995.
10. S. Ferris, U. Lucca, R. Mohs, B. Dubois, K. Wesnes, H. Erzigkeit, D. Geldmacher, and N. Bodick. Objective psychometric tests in clinical trials of dementia drugs. *Alzheimer Disease and Associated Disorders*, 11(3):34–38, 1997. Position paper from the International Working Group on Harmonisation of Dementia Drug Guidelines.
11. R. Kohavi, G. John, R. Long, D. Manley, and K. Pfleger. MLC++: a machine learning library in C++. In *Tools with Artificial Intelligence*, pages 740–743. IEEE Computer Society Press, 1994.
12. S. Mani, M. B. Dick, M. J. Pazzani, E. L. Teng, D. Kempler, and I. M. Taussig. Refinement of neuro-psychological tests for dementia screening in a cross cultural population using machine learning. In W. Horn, Y. Shahar, G. Lindberg, S. Andreassen, and J. Wyatt, editors, *Lecture Notes in Computer Science*, volume 1620, pages 326–335. Springer, 1999. Proc. of the Joint European Conference on Artificial Intelligence in Medicine and Medical Decision Making, AIMDM'99, Aalborg, Denmark.
13. I. McKeith, T. Del Ser, F. Spano, K. Wesnes, R. Anand, A. Cicin-Sain, R. Ferrera, and R. Spiegel. Efficacy of rivastigmine in dementia with Lewy bodies: results of a randomised placebo-controlled international study. *Lancet*, 356:2031–2036, 2000.
14. I. G. McKeith and G. A. Ayre. Consensus criteria for the clinical diagnosis of dementia with Lewy bodies. In K. Iqbal, B. Winblad, T. Nishimura, M. Takeda, and H. M. Wisnieswski, editors, *Alzheimer's Disease: Biology, Diagnosis and Therapeutics*, pages 167–178. Wiley, 1997.

15. E. Mohr, V. Knott, M. Sampson, K. Wesnes, R. Herting, and T. Mendis. Cognitive and quantified electroencephalographic correlates of cycloserine treatment in Alzheimer's disease. *Clinical Neuropsychopharmacology*, 18:23–38, 1995.

16. E. Mohr, D. Walker, C. Randolph, M. Sampson, and T. Mendis. The utility of clinical trial batteries in the measurement of Alzheimer's and Huntington's dementia. *International Psychogeriatrics*, 3:397–411, 1996.

17. C. G. Nicholl, S. Lynch, C. A. Kelly, L. White, L. Simpson, P. M. Simpson, K. Wesnes, and B. M. N. Pitt. The cognitive drug research computerised assessment system in the evaluation of early dementia—is speed of the essence? *International Journal of Geriatric Psychiatry*, 10:199–206, 1995.

18. M. Ramoni and P. Sebastiani. Robust Bayes classifiers. *Artificial Intelligence*, 125(1–2):209–226, 2001.

19. K. R. Siegfried. Pharmacodynamic and early clinical studies with velnacrine. *Acta Neurol. Scand.*, 149(10):26–28, 1993.

20. P. M. Simpson, D. J. Surmon, K. A. Wesnes, and G. R. Wilcock. The cognitive drug research computerised assessment system for demented patients: a validation study. *International Journal of Geriatric Psychiatry*, 6:95–102, 1991.

21. L. Templeton, A. Barker, K. Wesnes, and D. Wilkinson. A double-blind, placebo-controlled trial of intravenous flumazenil in Alzheimer's disease. *Human Psychopharmacology*, 14:239–245, 1999.

22. M. P. Walker, G. A. Ayre, C. H. Ashton, V. R. Marsh, K. Wesnes, E. K. Perry, J. T. O'Brien, I. G. McKeith, and C. G. Ballard. A psychophysiological investigation of fluctuating consciousness in neurodegenerative dementias. *Human Psychopharmacology*, 14:483–489, 1999.

23. M. P. Walker, G. A. Ayre, J. L. Cummings, K. Wesnes, I. G. McKeith, J. T. O'Brien, and C. G. Ballard. Quantifying fluctuation in dementia with Lewy bodies, Alzheimer's disease and vascular dementia. *Neurology*, 54:1616–1625, 2000.

24. M. P. Walker, G. A. Ayre, J. L. Cummings, K. Wesnes, I. G. McKeith, J. T. O'Brien, and C. G. Ballard. The clinician assessment of fluctuation and the one day fluctuation assessment scale. *British Journal of Psychiatry*, 177:252–256, 2000.

25. M. P. Walker, G. A. Ayre, E. K. Perry, K. Wesnes, I. G. McKeith, M. Tovee, J. A. Edwardson, and C. G. Ballard. Quantification and characterisation of fluctuating cognition in dementia with Lewy bodies and Alzheimer's disease. *Dementia and Geriatric Cognitive Disorders*, 11:327–335, 2000.

26. P. Walley. *Statistical Reasoning with Imprecise Probabilities*. Chapman and Hall, New York, 1991.

27. K. Wesnes. Predicting, assessing, differentiating and treating the dementias: experience in MCI and various dementias using the CDR computerised cognitive assessment system. In B. Vellas and L. J. Fitten, editors, *Research and practice in Alzheimer's disease*, volume 3, pages 59–65. Serdi, Paris, 2000.

28. K. Wesnes, K. Hildebrand, and E. Mohr. Computerised cognitive assessment. In G. W. Wilcock, R. S. Bucks, and K. Rocked, editors, *Diagnosis and management of dementia: a manual for memory disorders teams*, pages 124–136. Oxford Univ. Press, Oxford, 1999.

29. M. Zaffalon. Exact credal treatment of missing data. *Journal of Statistical Planning and Inference*. To appear.

30. M. Zaffalon. The naive credal classifier. *Journal of Statistical Planning and Inference*. To appear.

31. M. Zaffalon. Statistical inference of the naive credal classifier. In G. de Cooman, F. Cozman, T. Fine, and S. Moral, editors, *ISIPTA'01*, Univ. of Gent, Belgium, 2001. The Imprecise Probabilities Project. Accepted for publication.

Evaluation of Prognostic Factors and Prediction of Chronic Wound Healing Rate by Machine Learning Tools

Marko Robnik-Šikonja[1], David Cukjati[2], and Igor Kononenko[1]

[1] University of Ljubljana, Faculty of Computer and Information Science,
Tržaška 25, 1001 Ljubljana, Slovenia
`Marko.Robnik@fri.uni-lj.si,`
[2] University of Ljubljana, Faculty of Electrical Engineering,
Tržaška 25, 1001 Ljubljana, Slovenia
`David.Cukjati@fe.uni-lj.si,`

Abstract. In more than a decade of clinical use of electrical stimulation to accelerate the chronic wound healing each patient and wound were registered and a wound healing process was weekly followed. The controlled study involved a conventional conservative treatment, sham treatment, biphasic pulsed current, and direct current electrical stimulation. A quantity of available data suffices for an analysis with machine learning methods.

So far only a limited number of studies have investigated the wound and patient attributes which affect the chronic wound healing. There is none to our knowledge to include the treatment attributes. The aims of our study are to determine effects of the wound, patient and treatment attributes on the wound healing process and to propose a system for prediction of the wound healing rate.

In the first step of our analysis we determined which wound and patient attributes play a predominant role in the wound healing process. Then we investigated a possibility to predict the wound healing rate at the beginning of the treatment based on the initial wound, patient and treatment attributes. Finally we discussed the possibility to enhance the wound healing rate prediction accuracy by predicting it after a few weeks of the wound healing follow-up.

By using the attribute estimation algorithms ReliefF and RReliefF we obtained a ranking of the prognostic factors which was comprehensible to field experts. We also used regression and classification trees to build models for prediction of the wound healing rate. The obtained results are encouraging and may form a basis of an expert system for the chronic wound healing rate prediction. If the wound healing rate is known, then the provided information can help to formulate the appropriate treatment decisions and orient resources to those individuals with poor prognosis.

S. Quaglini, P. Barahona, and S. Andreassen (Eds.): AIME 2001, LNAI 2101, pp. 77–87, 2001.

1 Introduction

Skin is vital organ in a sense that loss of the substantial fraction of its mass immediately threatens life of the individual. Such a loss can result suddenly, either from a fire or mechanical accident, but can also occur in a chronic manner, as in skin ulcers.

In more than a decade of clinical use of an electrical stimulation to accelerate the chronic wound healing at the Institute of the Republic Slovenia for Rehabilitation in Ljubljana each patient and wound were registered and the wound healing process was weekly followed. At the beginning of the study in 1989, wounds were randomly assigned into four treatment groups: conservative treatment, sham treatment, biphasic current stimulation and direct current stimulation. Jerčinović et al. (1994) proved that stimulated wounds are healing significantly faster than only conservatively or sham treated wounds and Karba et al. (1997) proved that electrical stimulation with direct current is effective only if the positive electrode is placed on the wound surface, which is an invasive method, therefore only stimulation with biphasic current pulses has been in regular use ever since. However, dynamics of the wound healing process does not depend only on the type of the treatment, but depends also on the wound and patient attributes.

The aims of our study are to determine effects of the wound, patient and treatment attributes on the wound healing process and to propose a system for prediction of the wound healing rate.

So far only a limited number of studies have investigated the wound and patient attributes which affect the chronic wound healing. Skene et al. (1992) found that with the presence of the graduated compression the healing occurred more rapidly for patients with smaller initial ulcer area, shorter duration of ulceration, younger age and when no deep vein involvement was detected on photoplethysmography. The measurement of the ulcer area was found to be the strongest predictor of the ulcer healing. Birke et al. (1992) found that a time to complete the wound closure is related to the wound depth and wound diameter. Johnson (1997) found four factors influencing the vascular ulcer healing: ABpI (ankle/brachial pressure index), liposclerosis, edema, wound status and ulcer area. Lyman et al. (1970) found significant relationship between the wound healing rate and bacterial load.

None of listed studies included the treatment attributes. Presently, the quantity of available data permits the use of statistical tools and artificial intelligence methods for analysis of the healing process, as well as of the effects of different therapeutic modalities. In the first step of our analysis we determine which wound and patient attributes play a predominant role in the wound healing process. Then we investigate a possibility to predict the wound healing rate at the beginning of treatment based on the initial wound, patient and treatment attributes. Finally we discuss a possibility to enhance the wound healing rate prediction accuracy by predicting it after a few weeks of the wound healing follow-up.

The paper is organized into 5 Sections. Section 2 discusses the problem and the collected data. Section 3 describes machine learning tools and algorithms used. In Section 4 we present our findings. Final Section contains discussion.

2   The Problem and the Data Set

During more than a decade of clinical use of electrical stimulation, data concerning patients, wounds, and their treatment were collected. 266 patients with 390 wounds were recorded in computer database up to date. Unfortunately many patient and wound data are missing and not all wounds were followed regularly or until the complete wound closure which is a common problem of clinical trials. The wound case inclusion criteria was the initial wound area larger than 1cm^2 and at least four weeks (or until the complete wound closure) follow up of the wound healing process. It was were fulfilled in 300 wound cases (214 patients).

Among these 300 wound cases the observation period in 174 cases lasted until the complete wound closure and was shorter in 126 cases. In these cases the time to the complete wound closure was estimated from the wound area measurements obtained during the observation period (Cukjati et al., 2000; 2001a). No significant difference between the actual time to complete the wound closure and the estimated one (from four or more weeks of wound healing observation) was observed.

Wounds in the database are described with length, width, depth and grade. Because the time to the complete wound closure was highly dependent on the initial wound extent, a measure of the wound healing rate was defined as an average advance of the wound margin towards the wound centre and was calculated as the average wound radius (the initial wound area divided by the initial perimeter and multiplied by 2) divided by the time to the complete wound closure (Cukjati et al., 2001a):

$$\Theta = 2\frac{S_0}{p_0 T} \quad \left[\frac{\text{mm}}{\text{day}}\right] \tag{1}$$

Distribution of the wound healing rate was not normal and could not be transformed to normal distribution; non-parametric statistical analysis was therefore used. The attributes we used in our study are briefly described below, further details can be found in (Cukjati et al., 2001b).

2.1   Wound Attributes

For an evaluation of the efficacy of a particular treatment modality or for evaluation of influence of the wound and patient attributes on the wound healing it is necessary to periodically follow the wound healing process. It was demonstrated (Cukjati et al., 2001a) that following wound area is sufficient to determine wound healing process dynamics. Further it was shown that wound shape can be approximated with an ellipse and it is thus enough to periodically follow mutually perpendicular diameters (largest wound diameter and diameter perpendicular to it) of the wound. From the measured diameters the wound area, the perimeter and the width to length ratio were calculated.

The wound depth measurement is invasive, because we have to enter our measuring device into the wound. As an alternative measure of the wound, grading systems were presented. We used the four stage Shea grading system (Shea, 1975). The wound depth and grade were collected only at the beginning of the treatment. The wound depth was measured in 43% of cases and the wound grade determined in 94%. Since the wound depth was strongly correlated to the wound grade and the wound depth values were often missing, the depth was omitted from the further analysis. Also due to a strong correlation between the initial wound area and the perimeter, the perimeter was omitted from the further analysis.

Other collected wound attributes were the wound type, location (trochanter, sacrum, gluteus and other), elapsed time from spinal cord injury to wound appearance (InjuryAppear), and elapsed time from the wound appearance to the beginning of the treatment (AppearStart). The major wound aetiology was the pressure ulceration (82.7% of the cases). Other aetiologies were the arterial ulceration (1.0%), neurotrophic ulceration (6.3%), traumatic ulceration (6.0%), and vascular ulceration (3.7%).

2.2   Patient Attributes

Recorded patient attributes were age, sex, total number of wounds, diagnosis and, in the case of the spinal cord injury, the degree of spasticity. The most frequent diagnosis was the spinal cord injury (71.7%). The trauma appeared in 11.3% of cases, diabetes mellitus in 7.3%, geriatrics in 3.3%, multiple sclerosis in 3.0%, and venous diseases in 3.0% of wound cases.

2.3   Treatment Attributes

The wounds were randomly assigned into four treatment groups. 54 (18.0%) wounds received only the conservative treatment (Feedar and Kloth, 1990), while 23 (7.7%) wounds received also the sham treatment, 42 (14%) wounds received direct current and 181 (60.3%) wounds received biphasic current stimulation. In the sham treated group electrodes were applied to the intact skin on both sides of the wound for two hours daily and connected to stimulators, in which the power source was disconnected and delivered no current. The wounds treated with the direct current were stimulated with 0.6mA (Karba et al., 1997) for half an hour, an hour or two hours daily. Biphasic current stimulated wounds received biphasic, charge-balanced current pulses (Karba et al., 1991) for half an hour, an hour or two hours daily with electrodes placed on both sides of the wound.

The treatment attributes were the type of the treatment and daily duration of the electrical stimulation. The electrically stimulated wounds healed at higher rate and extent then other wounds. Over 90% of electrically stimulated wounds healed within 6 weeks. Only 70% of sham treated wounds and 72% of only conservative treated wounds healed within the same period.

2.4   Mathematical Model of Wound Healing Rate

We observed that the dynamics of changing of the wound area over time has a delayed exponential behaviour. Delayed exponential equation is therefore the structure of mathematical model of the wound healing process and by fitting this model to a particular chronic wound case, parameters of the model are calculated. We need at least four measurements (performed in at least three weeks) of the wound area before we can estimate the parameters of the mathematical model. We estimated the time to the complete wound closure from the parameters of the mathematical model (Cukjati et al., 2001a). We considered the wound healed when its estimated area was smaller than five percent of the initial value and smaller than 1cm^2. The estimated wound healing rate was calculated with Equation (1) .

The estimated wound healing rates for all wound cases were then compared to the actual ones which were calculated from the observed times to the complete wound closure. We found that the estimated wound healing rate after at least four weeks of wound follow-up did not differ significantly from the actual one (Cukjati et al., 2001b). If a wound was followed only three weeks or less the difference was significant. From the known structure of the mathematical model the wound healing rate can be predicted after at least four weeks of follow-up. In clinical trials four weeks is a short period, but in clinical practice shorter time for the treatment outcome prediction would be desirable.

3   Machine Learning Algorithms and Results

Presently, the quantity of the available data permits the use of machine learning methods. Results of the statistical analysis (Cukjati et al., 2001b) showed that the wound healing rate directly depends on the wound treatment and wound grade, while interactions of the other wound and patient attributes with the wound healing rate are not easy to determine.

We employed machine learning algorithms and built tree based models (regression and classification trees) to predict the wound healing rate based on the initial wound, patient and treatment data. We also considered the estimated wound healing rate based on the mathematical model (Cukjati et al., 2001b) and built trees for prediction of the wound healing rate after one, two, three, four, five and six weeks of follow-up. We tested several algorithms for attribute estimation which were used in a feature subset selection and for selection of splits in interior nodes of the tree based models. In the earlier stages of our data exploration we found that Relief algorithms, RReliefF (Robnik Šikonja and Kononenko, 1997) for regression and ReliefF (Kononenko et al., 1997) for classification problems, were the most effective concerning error and comprehensiveness of the learned models, so we present results only for them. The results for mean

squared error and mean absolute error as attribute estimators in regression
(Breiman et al., 1984) and Gain ratio (Quinlan, 1993) in classification are not
reported because they are inferior to the presented ones.

Relief algorithms are one of the most successful feature subset selection algorithms (Dietterich, 1997). The idea of RReliefF and ReliefF algorithms is to
evaluate partitioning power of attributes according to how well their values distinguish between similar observations. An attribute is given a high score if it
separates similar observations with different prediction values and does not separate similar observations with similar prediction values. RReliefF and ReliefF
sample the space of observations, compute the differences between predictions
and values of the attributes and form a kind of statistical measure for the proxim-
ity of the probability densities of the attribute and the predicted value. Assigned
quality estimates are in the range $[-1, 1]$, however, values below zero are assigned
to completely irrelevant (random) attributes. The quality estimate $W[A]$ of attribute A assigned by ReliefF or RReliefF can be interpreted in two ways: as the
difference of probabilities and as the proportion of explanation of the concept.

$$W[A] = P(\text{different value of A}|\text{near instance with different prediction})$$
$$- P(\text{different value of A}|\text{near instance with same prediction}) \qquad (2)$$

Equation (2) forms the basis for the difference of probabilities interpretation
of the quality estimations of the Relief algorithms: the difference of the probability that two instances have different value of the attribute if they have different
prediction value and the probability that two instances have different value of
the attribute if they have similar prediction values. These two probabilities contain additional condition that the instances are close in the problem space and
form an estimate of how well the values of the attribute distinguish between
the instances that are near to each other. As it turned out this interpretation
was quite difficult for human comprehension. Negated similarity (different values) and subtraction of the probabilities are difficult to comprehend for human
experts because they do not contain clear mental image.

Another view on attributes' estimates of ReliefF and RReliefF is possible
with the proportion of prediction values which the attribute helps to determine
(Robnik-Šikonja and Kononenko, 2001). As the number of examples n goes to
infinity the quality estimates $W[A]$ computed from m cases for each attribute
converge to the number of changes in the predicted values the attribute is responsible for (R_A):

$$\lim_{n \to \infty} W[A] = \frac{R_A}{m} \qquad (3)$$

The interpretation of Relief's weights as the proportion of explained concept is more comprehensible than the interpretation with the difference of two
probabilities as confirmed by human experts. Equation (3) has only one non
probabilistic term (a simple ratio), which can be understand taking the unlim-
ited number of examples into account. The actual quality estimates for attributes

in given problem are approximations of these ideal estimates which occur only with abundance of data.

3.1 Estimation of the Prognostic Factors

The attributes' quality estimates (see Table 1) calculated using RReliefF revealed that the initial wound area, followed by the patients' age and time from wound appearance to treatment beginning are the most prognostic attributes. Important prognostic attributes are also wound shape (width to length ratio), location and type of treatment. The attribute "Model estimation" represents the estimated wound healing rate calculated from a model of wound healing dynamics. We see (as expected) that its quality estimate increases as we add more and more observations (from 0.0 to 0.67).

Table 1. The quality of wound, patient and treatment attributes assigned by RReliefF.

Attribute	0 weeks	1 week	2 weeks	3 weeks	4 weeks	5 weeks	6 weeks
Area (mm^2)	0.135	0.168	0.171	0.161	0.127	0.123	0.122
Age (year)	0.123	0.114	0.094	0.095	0.096	0.092	0.094
AppearStart (week)	0.119	0.121	0.104	0.131	0.121	0.114	0.115
Width to length ratio	0.096	0.098	0.099	0.095	0.103	0.108	0.113
Location	0.085	0.084	0.085	0.081	0.081	0.081	0.081
Treatment	0.066	0.058	0.051	0.052	0.050	0.051	0.051
InjuryAppear (month)	0.062	0.065	0.044	0.050	0.035	0.040	0.039
Daily duration of treatment (min)	0.046	0.039	0.031	0.035	0.025	0.025	0.026
Grade	0.046	0.039	0.057	0.048	0.048	0.047	0.043
Diagnosis	0.039	0.039	0.038	0.038	0.038	0.038	0.037
Aetiology	0.027	0.025	0.026	0.024	0.024	0.0239	0.024
Model estimation	0.000	0.399	0.602	0.626	0.663	0.659	0.670

3.2 Regression Trees

We built regression trees with the improved CORE learning system (Robnik Šikonja, 1997). We used linear equations in the leaves of the tree to model the wound healing rate (we also tried k-NN, median value, mean value, and kernel regression) and stopping rule of minimal five cases in a leaf. To obtain smaller and more comprehensible trees and to get better generalization the trees were pruned. Since the sample size (n=300) was moderate, we could not afford a separate testing set but we rather used the 10-fold cross-validation as an error estimation method. An error of the regression trees was measured with the relative squared error (relative error, RE) (Breiman et al., 1984). The relative error is always nonnegative and should be less than 1 for models of reasonable quality. Trees with the relative error close to 0 produce excellent prediction of the wound healing rate and trees with the relative error around 1 or even greater than 1 produce poor prediction. Some authors are using proportion of the variance explained by the regression tree as a measure of the error. It is calculated as (1 - RE). Although the terminology is not quite appropriate (Breiman et al., 1984), we also used this measure to compare results.

Left hand side of Figure 1 summarizes predictive accuracy of the learned trees. The relative error of the prediction at the beginning of the treatment had relative squared error greater than one, i.e., the resulting regression trees were not usable. By adding the model estimate of the wound healing rate after one week of follow-up we reduced the relative squared error to 0.64, (36% of variance was explained by the tree). After two weeks 65% and after three weeks 82% of variance was explained. Accuracy was slowly approaching 94% of explained variance with six weeks of follow-up.

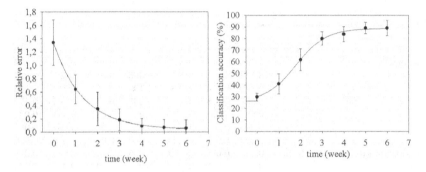

Fig. 1. The relative error of the regression trees (left) and classification accuracy of the classification trees (right) for the wound healing rate prediction as a function of observation time.

Regression trees are more useful than classification trees because the wound healing rate was estimated as continuous variable and can be directly observed in the tree. The minimal follow-up period is two weeks. After five weeks the predicted wound healing rate is equal to the healing rate estimated by the model. However, the predicted wound healing rate with shorter period of follow-up depends also on the wound, patient and treatment attributes. The regression tree built after two weeks of follow-up is presented in Figure 2. The type of the treatment is indirectly included in the regression trees as daily duration of the treatment, which was zero in case of conservative treated wounds. Important prognostic attributes seem to be the wound area, grade, shape (width to length ratio), patients age, elapsed time from the spinal cord injury to the wound appearance and elapsed time from the wound appearance to the beginning of the treatment.

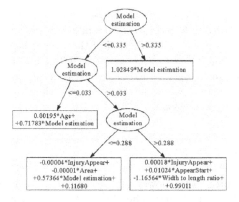

Fig. 2. The regression tree with linear equations in the leaves for prediction of the wound healing rate after two weeks of treatment.

3.3   Classification Trees

Sometimes we do not need the exact quantity of the wound healing rate so we decided to divide it into four categories (classes) according to Table 2 and then perform analysis on such classification problem.

Table 2. Dividing 300 wound cases into four classes according to their wound healing rate.

class	condition[mm/day]	no. of cases	a priori
NON HEALING WOUNDS	$\Theta \leq 0.095$	77	0.257
SLOW HEALING WOUNDS	$0.095 < \Theta \leq 0.180$	77	0.257
MEDIUM HEALING WOUNDS	$0.180 < \Theta \leq 0.300$	67	0.223
FAST HEALING WOUNDS	$\Theta > 0.300$	79	0.263

We built classification trees with ReliefF as attribute estimation measure. We used a median value of the cases as the prediction model in the leaves of the tree (we also tried k-NN and mean value) and a stopping rule of at least five wound cases in a leaf. To obtain smaller and more comprehensible trees and to get better generalization the trees were pruned. We used the 10-fold cross-validation as an error estimation method. The accuracy of the trees was measured as a proportion of the correctly classified test samples.

At the beginning of the wound treatment, only initial wound, patient and treatment data are available. The resulting classification tree accuracy at the beginning of the treatment was 30%, which is not much above a priori probability of the most probable class (26%). Adding model estimate of the wound healing rate after one week of follow-up to the data set improved the classification accuracy to 41%. With data available for two weeks the classification accuracy was 62% and with three weeks 80%. Afterwards it is slowly approaching 90% with six weeks of follow-up. Right hand side of Figure 1 summarizes the results.

In the trees built after two weeks of follow-up only the model estimate of the wound healing rate can be found in the tree nodes.

We found out that accurate prediction of the wound healing rate is possible with data available for at least three weeks of follow-up. Therefore, with classification trees we also managed to shorten the time of follow-up for one week compared to the mathematical model. Only rough estimate of the wound healing rate is possible after two weeks.

4   Discussion

We estimated the prognostic power of the wound, patient and treatment attributes with RReliefF algorithm. The obtained results revealed that the initial wound area, followed by the patients' age and time from the wound appearance to the treatment beginning are the most important prognostic attributes. Important prognostic attributes are also the wound shape (width to length ratio), location, and type of the treatment. The filed experts agree with these findings and accept this ranking because they understood the meaning of these quality estimates.

The dynamics of wound healing can be accurately predicted after at least four weeks of the wound healing process follow-up. Therefore for accurate wound healing rate estimation, wounds should be followed at least four weeks. In clinical practice the wound healing rate or the time to complete wound closure should be estimated as soon as possible to select a proper treatment and thus to improve patient care. Prediction of the wound healing rate from the initial wound, patient and treatment data collected in our database was not possible. The best prognostic factors are weekly follow-up measurements of wound area. We determined that the minimal follow-up period is two weeks. After three weeks we were able to predict the wound healing rate with 80% classification accuracy (using the classification trees), and explain 82% of the variance with the regression trees. The best results were obtained using regression trees with linear equations in the leaves. In the literature also other wound and patient attributes were reported to have prognostic value. By considering those additional attributes our prediction might be even more accurate.

The presented regression trees in combination with the mathematical model of the wound healing process dynamics possibly present a basis of an expert system for the chronic wound healing rate prediction. If the wound healing rate is known, the provided information can help to formulate the appropriate management decisions, reduce the cost, and orient resources to those individuals with poor prognosis.

References

J.A. Birke, A. Novick, C. A. Patout, and W. C. Coleman. Healing rates of plantar ulcers in leprosy and diabetes. *Leprosy Rev.*, 63:365–374, 1992.

L. Breiman, J. H. Friedman, R. A. Olshen, and C. J. Stone. *Classification and regression trees*. Wadsworth Inc., Belmont, California, 1984.

D. Cukjati, R. Karba, S. Reberšek, and D. Miklavčič. Modeling of chronic wound healing dynamics. *Med.Biol.Eng.Comput.*, 38:339–347, 2000.

D. Cukjati, S. Reberšek, and D. Miklavčič. A reliable method of determining wound healing rate. *Med.Biol.Eng.Comput.*, 2001a. (in press).

D. Cukjati, M. Robnik-Šikonja, S. Reberšek, I. Kononenko, and D. Miklavčič. Prognostic factors, prediction of chronic wound healing and electrical stimulation. *Medical & Biological Engineering & Computing*, 2001b. (submitted).

T.G. Dieterich. Machine learning research: Four current directions. *AI Magazine*, 18 (4):97–136, 1997.

J.A. Feedar and L. C. Kloth. Conservative management of chronic wounds. In L. C. Kloth and J.M. McCulloch, editors, *Wound Healing: Alternatives in Management*, pages 135–172. F. A. Davis Co., Philadelphia, 1990.

A. Jerčinović, R. Karba, L. Vodovnik, A. Stefanovska, P. Krošelj, R. Turk, I. Džidić, H. Benko, and R. Šavrin. Low frequency pulsed current and pressure ulcer healing. *IEEE Trans.Rehab.Eng.*, 2(4):225–233, 1994.

M. Johnson. Using cluster analysis to develop a healing typology in vascular ulcers. *J.Vasc.Nurs.*, 15:45–49, 1997.

R. Karba, D. Šemrov, L. Vodovnik, H. Benko, and R. Šavrin. DC electrical stimulation for chronic wound healing enhancement. Part 1. Clinical study and determination of electrical field distribution in the numerical wound model. *Bioelectrochemistry and Bioenergetics*, 43:265–270, 1997.

I. Kononenko, E. Šimec, and M. Robnik-Šikonja. Overcoming the myopia of inductive learning algorithms with RELIEFF. *Applied Intelligence*, 7:39–55, 1997.

I.R. Lyman, J. H. Tenery, and R. P. Basson. Corelation between decrease in bacterial load and rate of wound healing. *Surg.Gynecol.Obstet.*, 130(4):616–620, 1970.

J.R. Quinlan. *C4.5: Programs for Machine Learning*. Morgan Kaufmann, 1993.

M. Robnik Šikonja. CORE - a system that predicts continuous variables. In *Proceedings of Electrotehnical and Computer Science Conference*, pages B145–148, 1997.

M. Robnik Šikonja and I. Kononenko. An adaptation of Relief for attribute estimation in regression. In Douglas H. Fisher, editor, *Machine Learning: Proceedings of the Fourteenth International Conference (ICML'97)*, pages 296–304. Morgan Kaufmann, 1997.

Marko Robnik-Šikonja and Igor Kononenko. Comprehensible interpretation of Relief's estimates. 2001. (submitted).

D.J. Shea. Pressure sores classification and management. *Clin.Orthop.Rel.Res.*, 112: 89–100, 1975.

A.I. Skene, J. M. Smith, C. J. Doré, A. Charlett, and J. D. Lewis. Venous leg ulcers: a prognostic index to predict time to healing. *BMJ*, 305:1119–1121, 1992.

Making Reliable Diagnoses with Machine Learning: A Case Study*

Matjaž Kukar

University of Ljubljana, Faculty of Computer and Information Science,
Tržaška 25, SI-1001 Ljubljana, Slovenia,
`matjaz.kukar@fri.uni-lj.si`

Abstract. In the past decades Machine Learning tools have been successfully used in several medical diagnostic problems. While they often significantly outperform expert physicians (in terms of diagnostic accuracy, sensitivity, and specificity), they are mostly not used in practice. One reason for this is that it is difficult to obtain an unbiased estimation of diagnose's reliability. We propose a general framework for reliability estimation, based on transductive inference. We show that our reliability estimation is closely connected with a general notion of significance tests. We compare our approach with classical stepwise diagnostic process where reliability of diagnose is presented as its post-test probability. The presented approach is evaluated in practice in the problem of clinical diagnosis of coronary artery disease, where significant improvements over existing techniques are achieved.

Keywords: machine learning, medical diagnosis, reliability estimation, stepwise diagnostic process, coronary artery disease.

1   Introduction

In medicine we often explicitly have to deal with unreliable diagnoses. It is important to be aware of the fact that every diagnosis inherently contains some uncertainty and is therefore not completely reliable. Sometimes it is crucial to know the magnitude of diagnosis' (un)reliability in order to minimize risks for patient's health or even life. For diagnosis' reliability estimation, frequently post-test diagnostic probabilities are assessed, using the Bayesian approach. The Bayes' theorem states that the predictive value of any diagnostic test is influenced by the prevalence of the pre-test probability of the disease among the tested population, by the results of diagnostic test and by the sensitivity and specificity of the test [10]. The Bayesian approach often accompanies another common methodology, the stepwise diagnostic process.

In a stepwise diagnostic process diagnostic tests are ordered by increasing invasiveness, cost, and diagnostic accuracy. The key element is to estimate the prior (pre-test) probability of disease, and the sensitivity and specificity of different diagnostic tests. With this information, test results can be analysed by

---

* This paper represents a part of the author's doctoral dissertation.

S. Quaglini, P. Barahona, and S. Andreassen (Eds.): AIME 2001, LNAI 2101, pp. 88–98, 2001.

sequential use of the Bayes' theorem of conditional probability. The obtained post-test probability accounts for the pre-test probability, sensitivity and specificity of the test, and may later be used as a pre-test probability for the next test in sequence (Fig. 1). The process results in a series of tests where each test

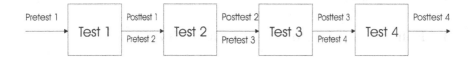

Fig. 1. Sequential tests in stepwise diagnostic process.

is performed independently. Its results may be interpreted with or without any knowledge of the other test results. However, previous test results are used to obtain the final probability of disease. Sequential diagnostic tests are performed until the post-test probability of disease's presence or absence exceeds 0.90 [1].

In our former work [6,8] we aimed to improve the stepwise diagnostic by applying Machine Learning (ML) algorithms for individual calculation of pretest probabilities and for evaluation of sequential diagnostic results. Our efforts were targeted to increasing the specificity of the entire process without decreasing the sensitivity.

In this paper we pursue a different goal. We propose a general strategy for detecting and selecting reliable diagnoses independently of the applied Machine Learning algorithms, that can be used in many practical problems.

2   Reliability of Diagnoses and Machine Learning

What exactly does the word *reliability* mean? It depends on the context, but generally it can be defined as the ability to perform certain tasks conforming to required quality standards. For our needs let us define the reliability of classification as a (sufficiently high) probability that the classification is correct.

Remark 1. In the following text we frequently (and interchangeably) use the terms *classification* and *diagnosis*. We consider diagnosis to be a special case of classification, applied in medicine.

In the usual ML setting, the concept of reliability has more than one meaning:

- It is closely connected with processing of intermediate concepts (decision tree nodes, decision rules, constructive induction, ...). Unreliable concepts are usually dumped, resulting in more compact knowledge representation and better generalization ability.
- It represents an overall estimation of method's reliability in terms of classification accuracy, sensitivity, and specificity. However, nothing can be told about reliability of single classification.

Remark 2. Most ML algorithms are able to represent their classifications as probability distribution over all possible classes. Reliability of classification can be viewed as a probability of the most probable class. However, such estimation may be heavily biased, as a consequence of the methods' inherent system error. What we are striving for is an unbiased estimation of the classification's (diagnosis') reliability.

3   Reliability as a Post-test Probability

The *post-test* probability measures the degree of certainty of the diagnosis after performing a diagnostic test. It depends on the pre-test probability (P) of disease and sensitivity (Se) and specificity (Sp) of the diagnostic test. It is calculated by the application of Bayes' theorem. The application of the theorem imposes several restrictions regarding independence of diagnostic tests [10, pp. 353-354], however it has been already successfully used in practice [1,8].

We apply the Bayes' theorem to calculate the conditional probability of the disease's presence, when the result of a diagnostic test is given [10, pp. 352]. For positive test result the probability $P(d|+) = P(disease|positive\ test\ result)$ is calculated:

$$P(d|+) \doteq \frac{P \cdot Se}{P \cdot Se + (1 - P) \cdot (1 - Sp)} \tag{1}$$

For negative test result the probability $P(\overline{d}|-) = P(no\ disease \mid negative\ test\ result)$ is calculated:

$$P(\overline{d}|-) = \frac{(1 - P) \cdot Sp}{(1 - P) \cdot Sp + P \cdot (1 - Se)} \tag{2}$$

In the stepwise diagnostic process the post-test probability after a diagnostic test serves as a pre-test probability for the subsequent test. This approach not only incorporates several test results but also the data from the patient's history. By a common agreement the diagnosis is considered reliable if its post-test probability exceeds 0.90 [1].

4   Transductive Reliability Estimation

The idea behind transductive reliability estimation leverages two approaches. The first one is based on the *iid* (identically independently distributed) assumption, usually used in statistical models and Machine Learning, and the second one is the idea of *transductive inference* [3].

In the *iid* context we assume that the training set, consisting of patients with known correct diagnoses, and the testing set, consisting of patients with unknown correct diagnoses, are independently (and randomly) drawn from the same underlying distribution function. The training set should be a random sequence with respect to the population distribution function, and so should the training set extended with a correctly classified test example [13]. If we knew how to measure the set's randomness level (or randomness deficiency), we could also measure the correctness of classification [13].

The *iid* assumption allows us to approximately calculate the extended training set's *randomness deficiency* which is a basis for Martin-Löf's generalized significance tests [9]. Thus we have a tool (though strictly speaking it is not computable and has to be approximated) that allows us to perform a significance test of classification's correctness.

A similar approach has been described in [12,13]. The main difference to our work is that their approach is based on support vector machines, while ours is completely general, and applicable to most Machine Learning classifier without modifications. The only requirement for the classifier is to represent its classifications as a probability distribution over all possible classes.

The transductive reliability estimation process [5] is described in more detail in Algorithm 1. An intuitive explanation of transductive reliability estimation is that we disturb a classifier by inserting a new example in a training set. A magnitude of this disturbance is an estimation of classifier's instability (unreliability) in a given region of its problem space.

Algorithm 1 Transductive reliability estimation

Require: Machine Learning classifier, a training set and an unlabelled test example
Ensure: Estimation of test example's classification reliability
1: Inductive step:
   - train a classifier from the provided training set
   - select an unlabelled test example
   - classify this example with an induced classifier
   - label this example with a classified class
   - temporarily add the newly labelled example to the training set
2: Transductive step:
   - train a classifier from the extended training set
   - select the same unlabelled test example as above
   - classify this example with a transduced classifier
3: Calculate a randomness deficiency approximation as a normalized *distance* between inductive and transductive classification (normalized to the [0, 1] interval).
4: Calculate the reliability of classification as $(1 - distance)$.

Remark 3. If the *iid* assumption holds, and if the classifier is close to being optimal with respect to the training data, the randomness deficiency approximation is good. This means that the classifier represents a model that accounts for all regularities in data considering the class label. If this is not the case, the approximation is not very good and has to be weighed with classifier's quality. Again, an all-inclusive assessment of classifier's quality is not computable, and we have to use feasible approximations such as classification accuracy. For the purpose of quality assessment I developed a concept of per-class post-test probabilities, a generalization of post-test probabilities for multi-class problems. In our extensive experiments on several benchmark datasets [5] it has performed very well. Per-class post-test probabilities can be estimated with an internal leave-one-out testing on the training set.

4.1   Assessing the Classifier's Quality

In the Machine Learning community the classifier's quality is usually measured in terms of its classification accuracy. In medicine the more usual measures sensitivity and specificity of the diagnostic test [10]. Unfortunately, these are limited to two-class problems. We extended the sensitivity and specificity to multi-class problems by introducing per-class sensitivities and specificities. For N-class problem they can be calculated by decomposing a problem to N two-class problems and calculating them in the usual way. We use the class sensitivities (denoted as Se) and specificities (denoted as Sp) for calculating class post-test probabilities given class's prevalence (prior probability).

Definition 1. Class post-test probability is calculated for each class C_i, given its pre-test probability $P(C_i)$, class specificity (Sp) and sensitivity (Se):

$$\text{post-test}(C_i) = \frac{P(C_i)\text{Se}(C_i)}{P(C_i)\text{Se}(C_i) + (1 - P(C_i))(1 - \text{Sp}(C_i))}$$

(3)

A big advantage of class post-test probability over classification accuracy is that it takes in account both classifier's characteristics and prevalence of each class individually. Over all classes it is also non-monotonic and therefore better describes the classifier's performance in its problem space.

4.2   Distance Metrics

There exist many different methods for measuring distance between probability distributions, such as Kullback-Leibler divergence or Hellinger distance [4]. Due to some inappropriate properties of the above distance metrics (asymmetrical, unbounded, assumption that $p_i > 0$, ...), we used a *dot product* distance (4). It achieved very good results and also accounted for classifiers' own reliability estimation in terms of assigned probability distribution.

$$d(p, \hat{p}) \;=\; 1 - p \cdot \hat{p} \;=\; 1 - \sum_{i=1}^{N} p_i \hat{p}_i \;=\; 1 - \|p\|_2 \|\hat{p}\|_2 cos\phi \qquad (4)$$

Here the $\|p\|_2$ is an Euclidean norm of the probability distribution vector p. The norms and cosine of their angle ϕ in probability distribution space are all bounded to the $[0, 1]$ interval and so is the dot product.

The motivation to use the dot product distance is that it uses not only a measure of a change between both distributions, but also takes in account classifier's trust in its classification (length probability vectors). This causes the distance between identical probability distributions to lie between 0 (for distributions of type $[0, \ldots, 0, 1, 0, \ldots, 0]$ and 0.5 (for uniform distributions $[0.5, 0.5, \ldots, 0.5]$). The dot product distance is also easy to calculate and numerically stable.

In our experiments we applied the *dot product* distance (4) multiplied by the per classification calculated class post-test probability (3). The multiplicative inclusion of class post-test probability accounts for basic domain characteristics (prevalence of classes) as well as classifier's performance.[1]

4.3   Selecting Reliable Classification

Due to non-optimal classifiers resulting from learning in noisy and incomplete datasets it is inappropriate to select *a priori* fixed boundary (say, 0.90) as a threshold for reliable classifications. We approached the problem from a different point of view. We split the whole range of reliability estimation values ($[0, 1]$) into two intervals by the boundary b. The lower interval $[0, b)$ contained unreliable classifications, while the higher interval $[b, 1]$ contained reliable classifications. As a splitting point selection criterion we used information gain maximization, aiming to maximize the intervals' purity with respect to correctness of classifications [2]. The b-split calculation was performed within leave-one-out testing on the training set, independently of the test set.

5   Case Study: A Stepwise Diagnostic Process in CAD

Coronary artery disease (CAD) is the most important cause of mortality in all developed countries. It is caused by diminished blood flow through coronary arteries due to stenosis or occlusion. CAD produces impaired function of the heart and finally the necrosis of the myocardium – myocardial infarction.

During the exercise the volume of the blood pumped to the body has to be increased, this causing the blood flow through the coronary arteries to be increased several times as well. In a (low grade) CAD the blood flow as perfusion of the myocardium is adequate at rest or during a moderate exercise, but insufficient during a severe exercise. Therefore, signs and symptoms of the disease develop only during the exercise.

There are four diagnostic levels of CAD. Firstly, signs and symptoms of the disease are evaluated clinically and ECG is performed at rest.

This is followed by sequential ECG testing during controlled exercises by gradually increasing the work load of the patient. Usually a bicycle ergometer or treadmill is used to establish the diagnosis of CAD by evaluating changes of ECG during the exercise.

---

[1] This includes class sensitivity and specificity, however it is especially useful in an automatic setting for detecting possible anomalies like default (majority) classifiers that – of course – cannot be trusted.

If this test is not conclusive, or if additional information regarding the perfusion of the myocardium is needed, myocardial scintigraphy is performed. Radioactive material is injected into the patient during exercise. Its accumulation in the heart is proportional to the heart's perfusion and can be shown in appropriate images (scintigrams). Scintigraphy is repeated at rest and by comparing both sets of images, the presence, the localization, and the distribution of the ischaemic tissue are determined.

If an invasive therapy of the disease is contemplated, i.e. the dilatation of the stenosed coronary artery or coronary artery bypass surgery, the diagnosis has to be confirmed by imaging of the coronary vessels. This is performed by injecting radio opaque (contrast) material into the coronary vessels and by imaging their anatomy with x-ray coronary angiography.

In our case study we used a dataset of 327 patients (250 males, 77 females) with performed clinical and laboratory examinations, exercise ECG, myocardial scintigraphy and coronary angiography because of suspected CAD. The features from the ECG an scintigraphy data were extracted manually by the clinicians. In 229 cases the disease was angiographically confirmed and in 98 cases it was excluded. 162 patients had suffered from recent myocardial infarction. The patients were selected from a population of approximately 4000 patients who were examined at the Nuclear Medicine Department between 1991 and 1994. We selected only the patients with complete diagnostic procedures (all four levels) [8]. In determining the pre-test probability we applied the Table 2, which we re-

Table 1. CAD data for different diagnostic levels.

Diagnostic level	Diagnostic attributes		
	Nominal	Numeric	Total
Signs, symptoms and history	23	7	30
Exercise ECG	7	9	16
Myocardial scintigraphy	22	9	31
Disease prevalence	70% positive	30% negative	

trieved from literature [11]. For each patient, the table was indexed by a subset of "signs and symptoms" attributes (age, sex, type of chest pain).

The aim of our early studies [6,7] was to improve the diagnostic performance (sensitivity and specificity) of non-invasive diagnostic methods (i.e. clinical examinations of the patients, exercise ECG testing, and myocardial scintigraphy in comparison with the coronary angiography as a definite proof of coronary artery stenosis) by evaluating all available diagnostic information with Machine Learning techniques. In this paper we aim to increase the number of reliable diagnoses after myocardial scintigraphy. This reduces the number of patients that must unnecessarily be submitted to further invasive pre-operative examinations

Table 2. Pre-test probabilities for the presence of CAD

Sex	Age	Asymptomatic patients	Nonang. chest pain	Atypical angina	Typical angina
Female	35-44	0.007	0.027	0.155	0.454
	45-54	0.021	0.069	0.317	0.677
	55-64	0.054	0.127	0.465	0.839
	65-74	0.115	0.171	0.541	0.947
Male	35-44	0.037	0.105	0.428	0.809
	45-54	0.077	0.206	0.601	0.907
	55-64	0.111	0.282	0.690	0.939
	65-74	0.113	0.282	0.700	0.943

(such as coronary angiography), that are potentially dangerous, unpleasant and very costly.

6   Experiments

In the stepwise diagnostic process we measured after each completed step the percentage (share) of reliable diagnoses (with the post-test probability over 0.90), and errors made in this process (percentage of incorrectly diagnosed patients with seemingly reliable diagnoses). We evaluated the problem in four different settings:

Case 1: Physicians. Stepwise diagnostic process is performed by physicians. Pre-test probabilities are obtained from literature. A boundary for reliable diagnoses is 0.90 (post-test probability).

Case 2: Stepwise ML. Stepwise diagnostic process is performed by Machine Learning classifiers. Pre-test probabilities are not obtained from literature, but are estimated by naive Bayesian classifier from our dataset because of special nature of our patient population. A boundary for reliable diagnoses is 0.90 (post-test probability).

Case 3: Naive Bayes. Diagnosis with all attributes available on the third diagnostic level (myocardial scintigraphy) using naive Bayes classifier. A boundary for reliable diagnoses is 0.90 (classifier's class probability).

Case 4: Reliable Bayes. Diagnosis with all attributes available on the third level using naive Bayesian classifier. Reliability of diagnosis is estimated with transductive method (Section 4). A boundary for reliable diagnoses is automatically calculated.

The comparison between physicians' and different Machine Learning performances (Table 3 and Fig. 2) gives the following results. Comparison between cases 1 and 2 (Table 3) shows improvements by 0.06 (6%) for both positive and negative patients without risk of making more errors than physicians.

Table 3. Comparison between physicians' results and different Machine Learning approaches. Remarkable improvements achieved with reliable Bayesian classifier are emphasized.

	Positive diagnoses		Negative diagnoses	
	Reliable	Errors	Reliable	Errors
Physicians	0.72	0.03	0.46	0.08
Stepwise ML	0.79	0.05	0.46	0.03
Naive Bayes	0.90	0.07	0.81	0.11
Reliable Bayes	0.89	0.05	**0.83**	**0.01**

Even larger improvements are expected when using all available attributes (case 3) for classification, since Machine Learning methods can efficiently deal with significantly larger sets of attributes than humans and are not prone to suggestibility. The predicted class probabilities were considered as post-test probabilities with the same 0.90 criterion for reliability as before. The achieved improvements were impressive (Bayes: by 0.18 (18%) for positive and even by 0.35 (35%) for negative patients), however this goes hand in hand with higher error rate (Bayes: by 0.04 (4%) for positive and by 0.03 (3%) for negative patients). In this case the physician decides whether to stay safe with relatively smaller improvements (stepwise diagnostics) or to take more risk and achieve significantly higher improvements. These results were already published in [6].

In case 4 we also used all available attributes on the third diagnostic level (myocardial scintigraphy). The tests were evaluated by naive Bayesian classifier. Classifiers diagnoses' reliability was assessed by transductive method, described in Section 4. The calculated boundary for reliable estimations was 0.9174, which is quite close to 0.90 as used in previous cases.

The overall results in case 4 were simply amazing! While the number of reliable classifications stayed on the same high level as in case 3 (naive Bayes with all attributes), the number of errors dropped significantly, even far below physicians' levels. In comparison, reliable Bayes improved the number of reliable positive diagnoses by 0.17 (17%) and the number of negative diagnoses even by 0.37 (37%)! Number of errors in positive diagnoses is slightly higher than the physicians', while number of errors in negative diagnoses dropped to under 0.01 (1%)!

Since we were mostly interesting in increasing numbers of correctly diagnosed negative patients after the third diagnostic level, we can state that our goal was achieved. Although increases in positive diagnoses are also welcome, they are not relevant for rationalization of diagnostic process, since the positive patients are always submitted for further pre-operative examinations.

7   Discussion

Experimental results of reliability estimation in CAD diagnostic process show enormous potential of our methodology. The improvements are so big that the

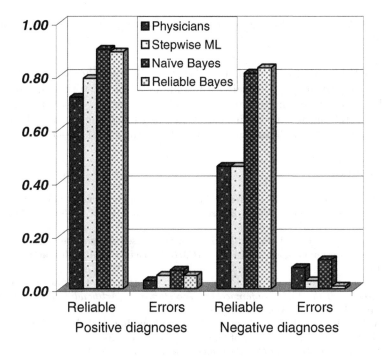

Fig. 2. Comparison between physicians' results and different Machine Learning approaches. Observe especially excellent results of reliable Bayesian classifier on negative diagnoses.

physicians are seriously considering introducing this approach in everyday diagnostic practice.

In terms of absolute numbers the 37% reduction of false positive diagnoses means that almost 12% of total population could be reliably diagnosed for CAD absence without performing coronary angiography. This means 12% less unnecessary angiographic examinations and thus shorter waiting times for truly ill patients. The 17% reduction of false negative diagnoses means that again almost 12% of total population could be reliably diagnosed for CAD presence without performing coronary angiography. However, in this case coronary angiography may still be necessary as a pre-operative examination. The total sum of almost 25% reductions is not likely to be achieved due to considerations described above. However, in practice a reduction of about 10% less patients needing to perform coronary angiography test seems reasonable.

We are aware that the results of our study are obtained on a significantly restricted population and therefore may not be generally applicable to the normal population, i.e. to all the patients coming to the Nuclear Medicine Department. Further studies are in progress to verify our findings on larger population. In particular, on-line data gathering, advocated in our previous papers, is now a part of everyday practice and may result in providing us with a more representative dataset.

Acknowledgements. I thank Dr. Ciril Grošelj, from the Nuclear Medicine Department, University Medical Centre Ljubljana, for his work while collecting the data and interpreting the results. I also thank my Ph. D. thesis supervisor prof. Igor Kononenko, for many useful comments and suggestions. This work was supported by the Slovenian Ministry of Education and Science.

References

[1] G. A. Diamond and J. S. Forester. Analysis of probability as an aid in the clinical diagnosis of coronary artery disease. *New England Journal of Medicine*, 300:1350, 1979.

[2] J. Dougherty, R. Kohavi, and M. Sahami. Supervised and unsupervised discretization of continuous features. In *Proc. ICML'95*, pages 194–202. Morgan Kaufmann, 1995.

[3] A. Gammerman, V. Vovk, and V. Vapnik. Learning by transduction. In *Proceedings of the 14th Conference on Uncertainty in Artificial Intelligence*, pages 148–155, Madison, Wisconsin, 1998.

[4] A. L. Gibbs and F. E. Su. On choosing and bounding probability metrics. Technical report, Cornell School of Operations Research, 2000.

[5] M. Kukar. *Estimating classifications' reliability*. PhD thesis, University of Ljubljana, Faculty of Computer and Information Science, Ljubljana, Slovenia, 2001. In Slovene.

[6] M. Kukar and C. Grošelj. Machine learning in stepwise diagnostic process. In *Proc. Joint European Conference on Artificial Intelligence in Medicine and Medical Decision Making*, pages 315–325, Aalborg, Denmark, 1999.

[7] M. Kukar, C. Grošelj, I. Kononenko, and J. Fettich. An application of machine learning in the diagnosis of ischaemic heart disease. In *Proc. Sixth European Conference of AI in Medicine Europe AIME'97*, pages 461–464, Grenoble, France, 1997.

[8] M. Kukar, I. Kononenko, C. Grošelj, K. Kralj, and J. Fettich. Analysing and improving the diagnosis of ischaemic heart disease with machine learning. *Artificial Intelligence in Medicine*, 16 (1):25–50, 1999.

[9] M. Li and P. Vitányi. *An introduction to Kolmogorov complexity and its applications*. Springer-Verlag, New York, 2nd edition, 1997.

[10] M. Olona-Cabases. The probability of a correct diagnosis. In J. Candell-Riera and D. Ortega-Alcalde, editors, *Nuclear Cardiology in Everyday Practice*, pages 348–357. Kluwer, 1994.

[11] B. H. Pollock. Computer-assisted interpretation of noninvasive tests for diagnosis of coronary artery disease. *Cardiovasc. Rev. Rep. 4*, pages 367–375, 1983.

[12] C. Saunders, A. Gammerman, and V. Vovk. Transduction with confidence and credibility. In *Proceedings of the International Joint Conference on Artificial Intelligence*, Stockholm, Sweden, 1999.

[13] V. Vovk, A. Gammerman, and C. Saunders. Machine learning application of algorithmic randomness. In *Proceedings of the 16th International Conference on Machine Learning (ICML'99)*, Bled, Slovenija, 1999.

A Classification-Tree Hybrid Method for Studying Prognostic Models in Intensive Care

Ameen Abu-Hanna and Nicolette de Keizer

Department of Medical Informatics, AMC-University of Amsterdam
Meibergdreef 15, 1105 AZ Amsterdam, The Netherlands
A.Abu-Hanna@amc.uva.nl

Abstract. Health care effectiveness and efficiency are under constant scrutiny especially when treatment is quite costly as in Intensive Care (IC). At the heart of quality of care programs lie prognostic models whose predictions for a particular patient population may be used as a norm to which actual outcomes of that population can be compared. This paper motivates and suggests a method based on Machine Learning and Statistical ideas to study the behavior of current IC prognostic models for predicting in-hospital mortality. An application of this method to an exemplary logistic regression model developed on the IC data from the National Intensive Care Evaluation registry reveals the model's weaknesses and suggests ways for developing improved prognostic models.

1 Introduction

Health Care is expensive and evidence for its effectiveness and efficiency is continuously sought. Many national and international quality programs have been set up to assess health care quality. For example our department is responsible for the registries on National Intensive Care Evaluation (NICE), cardiac-interventions, congenital heart diseases, and the renal registry of the European Renal Association. These registries include information about patients and outcomes of care such as mortality and comorbidity, and form vehicles for analytic tools aimed at evaluating quality of care.

Prognostic models for outcome prediction form indispensable ingredients among these evaluative tools. In Intensive Care (IC), various prognostic models to estimate in-hospital mortality[1] have been suggested such as the APACHE-II [8] and SAPS-II [10] models. Like many other prognostic models in Medicine these are statistical models that can be characterized by their use of a small set of covariates, at the heart of which is a *score* variable reflecting the patient's severity of illness, and by their reliance on the probabilistic logistic model. In Machine Learning (ML) too, various prognostic models have been suggested, many of which can be characterized by their use of an extended set of covariates and by their non-parametric and often symbolic nature [1].

---

[1] By IC mortality we mean deaths in the ICU, by in-hospital mortality we mean all deaths during the total hospital stay if an ICU admission formed part of it.

S. Quaglini, P. Barahona, and S. Andreassen (Eds.): AIME 2001, LNAI 2101, pp. 99–108, 2001.
© Springer-Verlag Berlin Heidelberg 2001

This paper builds on the merits of statistical and ML models and describes a hybrid method for studying the behavior of current prognostic models. These are exemplified by a logistic model, NSAPS, based on the SAPS-II score as its sole covariate and is developed on data from the NICE registry. The idea behind the method is to devise patient sub-populations according to a classification tree that uses the variables that *underlie* the severity of illness *score*, and scrutiny prognostic model performance on these sub-populations. The method is demonstrated in IC to reveal weaknesses of NSAPS and suggest ways to improve it.

The paper is organized as follows. Intensive Care and prognostic models are introduced in Sects. 2 and 3. Then in Sects. 4 and 5 the method of combining classification trees with local models trained on sub-populations is introduced and the IC data set is described. In Sect. 6 the results of applying this method to the IC data are provided. Section 7 concludes this paper.

2   Intensive Care and Quality Assessment

Intensive Care can be defined as *a service for patients with potentially recoverable conditions who can benefit from more detailed observation and invasive treatment than can safely be provided in general wards or high dependency areas.* The development of IC as a concept is related to the progress in the treatment of vital organ failures which started several decades ago [2]. In the Netherlands there are approximately 130,000 patients a year admitted to about 140 ICUs.

Professional ambitions, budgetary constraints and insurance regulations now have prompted physicians and managers to assess the effectiveness and efficiency of IC treatment. Since it is unethical to evaluate the effectiveness of ICU treatment in a randomized trial, information from (inter)national databases is used for appraisal of the quality of the care process by comparing outcome data such as mortality, morbidity and length of stay with *predicted* outcome values [14,7]. The predictions should take into account the characteristics of the patient population admitted to an ICU. This is called case-mix adjustment and is currently quantified by using a score of severity of illness. Prognostic models that make these case-mix adjusted predictions lie at the heart of quality assessment.

3   Prognostic Models and Their Evaluation

Various methods have been suggested for the representation of prognostic models ranging from quantitative and probabilistic approaches to symbolic and qualitative ones. Classical statistical approaches, often used in Medicine, are typically parametric and probabilistic in nature and usually tackle a regression task (the prediction of a numeric value) while ML approaches are typically non-parametric and tackle a classification task (the prediction of the class to which an instance belongs). In a quality of care assessment program one is typically interested in comparison of some outcome *summary* among patient *groups* rather than in classification of individual patients to a particular class. This emphasizes the importance of probabilistic statements about groups.

The method described in this paper uses **classification trees, logistic** and **Lowess** models which are described below along with their statistical evaluation.

3.1   Logistic Regression Models

In IC, and Medicine in general, scoring systems are used for the quantification of the severity of illness where a higher score corresponds to greater severity. Different elements contribute to this total score, for example in IC, these include physiological variables such as heart-rate, and white blood cell count; demographic variables such as age; earlier chronic history etc. Besides a means to communicate about the severity of illness of a patient, a score is usually used as a covariate in a logistic regression model to predict the *probability* of a dichotomous outcome such as mortality. A logistic regression model, $p(Y = 1|x_1, ..., x_m) = \frac{e^{g(x)}}{1+e^{g(x)}}$, computes the probability of a dichotomous variable Y having the value 1 given the values of m independent variables, x_i, $i \in \{1, .., m\}$ where $g(x) = \beta_0 + \sum_{i=1}^{m} \beta_i x_i$ is the logit function. The original SAPS-II logistic regression model which provides a mortality probability based on the SAPS-II score [10] is defined by: $g(score) = -7.7631 + 0.0737 * score + 0.9971[ln(score + 1)]$. The NSAPS model that we developed is based on this model and is reported in the results section.

Underlying these models are linearity, additivity, and distribution assumptions. The functional form of this model is fairly pre-specified and one is only required to find the appropriate β_i parameters.[2] When assumptions hold, this approach does not require much data and provides models relatively immune to overfitting: our prior knowledge allows us to search faster in a restricted space of models and compensates for idiosyncrasies in the data. If the assumptions do not completely hold, however, one introduces bias (in the statistical sense).

3.2   Non-parametric Approaches

ML and explorative statistics have suggested other methods which are not used in mainstream IC prognosis but seem to have potential to aid prognosis. In various ML approaches, for example the well known **classification trees**, very few assumptions are made about the functional form, allowing for a better fit. The downside of such non-parametric approaches, however, is that there is a lurking danger of overfitting the data (see [15]). These approaches imply requirements on the amount and quality of training data.

Another non-parametric method is Cleveland's **Lowess** [3] which has its roots in explorative statistics. In contrast to classification trees, but like the logistic model, Lowess is used in regression rather than classification. The idea behind Lowess is to smooth every scatter point based on the values of its neighbors, defined by a "window" centered around it, each with a weight inversely related to its distance from that point. In our case each patient corresponds to 0 (alive) or 1 (dead) and hence each score, which is our covariate, will correspond to a set of 0's or 1's (depending on the number of patients with the same score)

---

[2] The β_i parameters are chosen to maximize the likelihood of the data given the model.

and will be influenced by the number of 0's and 1's in its neighborhood. One could interpret the smoothed value of each point as the *probability* of mortality of patients with that score.

3.3   Model Evaluation Aspects

We are interested in a *precise* model that provides honest estimates of the *true probability* of an event rather than merely a discriminating model, the focus of the majority of work in ML, with the ability to assign the highest probability to the actual event or class.

The concepts of discrimination and precision can be put into perspective by considering the following definitions (based on [4]). For brevity we will only consider the two class case: 0 and 1. We use the following notations: $f(j|x_i)$ is the (unknown) true probability that instance x_i belongs to class j, $\widehat{f}(j|x_i)$ denotes the predicted probability that instance x_i belongs to class j, and c_i denotes the true class of instance x_i.

Accuracy is a measure of the effectiveness of the model to assign an instance to its actual class. An estimate of accuracy error is based on some summary measure of $|c_i - \widehat{f}(1|x_i)|$. Classification error rate which is used in discrimination is a special case of an accuracy error measure when one imposes a threshold on this summary measure and takes its average.

Precision is a measure of the closeness between the true and estimated probabilities. An estimate of precision error can be based on a summary measure of $|f(j|x_i) - \widehat{f}(j|x_i)|$. As $f(j|x_i)$ is unknown, some measure from the *test set* has to be obtained. This requires some grouping principle to lump instances in the test set. We distinguish between two flavors of precision: [1] **y-precision** in which one divides $\widehat{f}(1|x_i)$ in *probability groups* and compares some summary statistic within each group to its counterpart in the test set; and [2] **x-precision** in which one compares $\widehat{f}(1|x_i)$ and $f(1|x_i)$ based on instances grouped only according their similarity among their characteristics, regardless of $\widehat{f}(1|x_i)$.

Evaluation of logistic regression models such as the APACHE-II and SAPS-II models usually rely on the Hosmer-Lemeshow statistics [5] where it is referred to as calibration (see [13] for more general discussions). In our terminology these are essentially y-precision measures with *non-overlapping* probability groups. A major disadvantage of the Hosmer-Lemeshow statistics is that they have been shown to be very sensitive to the cut-off points used to form the $\widehat{f}(1|x_i)$ probability groups [6].

Performance Measures. In this work we use various measures of accuracy and precision in order to inspect the performance of prognostic models. These include the *Brier score*, also known as the mean quadratic error or $\frac{1}{n}\sum_{i=1}^{n}(c_i - \widehat{f}(1|x_i))^2$, as an accuracy measure. For precision we obtain information about $f(j|x_i)$ from the test set in two ways. The direct method uses Lowess to smooth mortality data on the *test set* and compares it, at each test point, with the $\widehat{f}(j|x_i)$ predicted by the model. The quadratic error of these "true" probabilities and

the predicted ones is used as one precision measure. In the indirect method we compare a transformation summary obtained from the predicted probabilities and from the test set. The difference between the summaries leads to a statistic that is significantly different from 0 when precision is bad. We use the logarithmic transformation [4] to obtain each summary, the difference statistic is:
$\frac{1}{n} \sum_{i=1}^{n} (c_i - \widehat{f}(1|x_i)) ln(\frac{\widehat{f}(1|x_i)}{\widehat{f}(0|x_i)})$.

These precision measures do not require division in non-overlapping probability groups in $\widehat{f}(1|x_i)$ and hence do not share the drawbacks of the Hosmer-Lemeshow statistics. Moreover these measures will be obtained on patient groups sharing various "x" characteristics (admission type and physiological variables) as described below.

4   The Classification-Tree Hybrid Method

In this section we motivate the use of a method aimed at a better understanding of the IC data and the models fitted to it. The idea is based on the following observations. A logistic model basically "distributes" the total number of events as probability estimates on the whole population. Suppose that the outcome variable is 0 or 1 if the patient lives or dies, respectively, and that there are n patients in some *training* set, then $\sum_{i=1}^{n} y_i = \sum_{i=1}^{n} \widehat{f}(Y_i = 1|x_i)$ will always hold. We believe a challenge for these models resides at patient sub-populations with very different proportions of the event. A classification tree, which minimizes entropy with respect to the event, is hence suitable for creating such groups. The idea is to use the same variables that are used in computing the severity of illness score for the tree whereas the logistic regression model will use the aggregated score (as is currently used in IC). There are at least three scenarios for experimenting with these ideas whose results are reported in Sect. 6. In each scenario the whole training set is used to grow a classification tree.

Parametric global fitting, NSAPS. In the first scenario one obtains the NSAPS model trained on the whole training set and examines its performance on each of the test subsets induced by the classification tree.

Parametric local fitting, TLR. In the second scenario one develops a logistic model, again using the SAPS-II score covariate but now on *each training subset* induced by the tree, and inspects their performances on their respective test subsets. In this scenario one could see if there is added value in training on subgroups but still using a parametric logistic model.

Non-parametric local fitting, TLW. In the third scenario, non-parametric models, using Lowess on the SAPS-II scores, are developed on the training subsets induced by the tree and their performance on the test subsets is inspected. In this scenario one can compare the performances of the parametric and non-parametric models.

Table 1. Characteristics of variables used in tree learning.

Variable name	Description	Mean±s.d.	Normal range
syst.min	minimal systolic blood pressure	92.0±32.4	100-199
urine.24	urine production in first 24 hrs	2.6±2.3	>1
heartr.min	minimum heart rate	71.2±23.0	70-119
bicarb.min	minimum bicarbonate	22.4±5.2	≥20
bicarb.max	maximum bicarbonate	25±4.5	≥20
gcs	Glasgow Coma Scale	13.8±3.2	15
wbc.max	maximum white blood cell count	12.1±11.4	1-19.9

Variable name	Description	value	Freq.	
adm.type	admission type			
	medical admission	1	45.3%	
	unscheduled surgical	2	17.7%	
	scheduled surgical	3	37.0%	

5   The Intensive Care Dataset

Data used in this analysis originates from the Dutch National Intensive Care Evaluation (NICE) registry. This includes all variables needed to calculate the SAPS-II score and includes IC and in-hospital mortality. We used NICE data from January 1998 till April 2000 and used the SAPS-II exclusion criteria. For patients with multiple ICU admissions during one hospital stay, only data from the first admission were used. The data included in this study consisted of 7803 consecutive admissions to nineteen ICUs of eight different hospitals and are characterized in Table 1. All values were obtained within the first 24 hours of IC admission. The mortality within the ICU is 15.5% and the in-hospital mortality, the dependent variable, amounts for 22.5%. The data are randomly divided into a training data set (n=5218) and a test data set (n=2585).

6   Results

This section describes the results of using our method to study the probability function within interesting IC patient sub-populations and show where weaknesses of the NSAPS model are encountered. This, we believe, will help suggest how to build an improved prognostic model for IC outcome. Our NSAPS model was developed on the training set using only the SAPS-II score as covariate (without the logarithm of the score but this has no effect on the results). The NSAPS model has the following form: $g(score) = -4.2548 + 0.0737 * score$.

6.1   Insight

We trained a binary classification tree on the training set to create the groups. The restriction to a binary tree is aimed at combating fragmentation and because all variables are either continuous or ordinal (admission type can be clinically

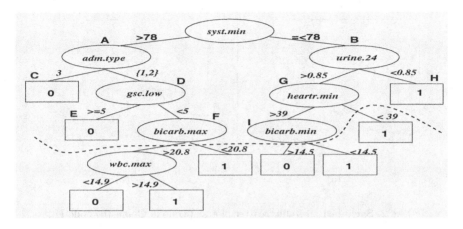

Fig. 1. The IC classification tree based on physiological variables and admission type. The leaves denote the majority class. The nodes above the dashed line will be formally inspected.

viewed this way). Information gain was used as a criterion for the variable choices in the tree. This tree is shown in Fig. 1. Note that patients with the same score could end up in different nodes in this tree as most scores can be obtained by different combinations of e.g. physiological variables.

In order to view the probability functions in the different nodes on the training set and to calculate the "true" one (on the test sets) we smooth the raw mortality data by Lowess. The Lowess smoothing makes it quite clear that there are obvious differences between the functions at different nodes. The functional form at each node turned out to be qualitatively consistent in random samples of the data set, as long as there were enough instances in each node. As an illustration consider Figs. 2(a) and 2(b) corresponding to nodes **C** and **H**. As one can see, the functions have a great deal of overlap in their SAPS-II scores but are qualitatively quite different. NSAPS would mask these differences. One way to use this insight is simply to induce the tree division within one's IC data (e.g. from a different ICU or taken at a later time) and inspect the conformance to this qualitative behavior.

6.2 Evaluation Tool

To formally inspect the model performance we obtain our performance measures for prognostic models on the tree nodes appearing above the dashed line in Fig. 1, these nodes are at depth of at most 3 and each has at least 100 patients in the test set, to avoid fragmentation.

The results are shown in Table 2 where the columns stand for the nodes considered. The rows show the performance results for the global logistic model NSAPS, and the local TLR and TLW models trained on the classification tree

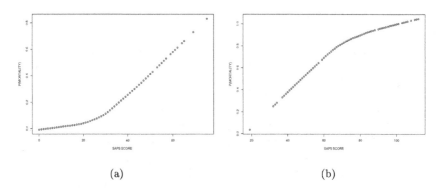

(a)　　　　　　　　　　　　　　　　　　　(b)

Fig. 2. Smoothed mortality scatter plot at (a) node **C** and (b) node **H**.

Table 2. Performance measures for the three models (all $*10^3$). Boxed values mean accuracy is better and significantly different than in the NSAPS model. Values in bold mean quadratic error precision is better and significantly different than the NSAPS model values. Underlined values mean bad precision.

Model	Msr	Node(♯instances in test set)							
		A(2072)	B(513)	C(900)	D(1172)	E(1063)	F(109)	G(402)	H(111)	I(372)
NSAPS	Brier	104.67	173.96	50.106	146.56	137.01	239.74	183.57	139.17	176.04
	Log.tr	-987.57	613.81	−3107.4	1725.1	1175.5	2528.5	1127.6	-785.28	264.57
	err	0.59	0.52	1	1.1	0.52	16.42	2.1	10.1	1.75
TLR	Brier	104.62	174.14	49.73	146.12	136.82	238.91	182.36	126.17	174.83
	Logtr	-694.4	-42.701	-537.47	-265.71	-635.82	2051	-243.46	-76.171	-784.05
	err	**0.57**	**0.34**	**0.85**	**0.35**	0.047	**15.95**	**0.4**	**0.42**	**0.35**
TLW	Brier	105.01	175.15	49.861	146.53	137.40	231.74	183.17	128.08	175.44
	Logtr	-1397.7	478.68	-1147.4	-407.25	-574.09	1633.4	398.05	-442.94	-290.18
	err	**0.42**	**0.2**	**0.88**	**0.4**	**0.3**	**11**	**0.56**	**0.91**	**0.73**

nodes. The TLR and TLW models have better Brier scores than NSAPS in nearly all cases, and at three nodes the NSAPS model has been worst and statistically significantly different than at least one of them (at the 0.05 level).

As for precision, the TLW model outperformed the NSAPS model and has been statistically significantly different than the NSAPS model at all nodes. The TLR did that in 8 cases. The difference logarithmic transformation measure has been shown to be significantly different than 0 (meaning bad precision) in two cases, both belonging to the NSAPS model.

The NSAPS model seems to have been consistently outperformed in accuracy and precision in most of the cases even when one considers multiple comparisons as we have done. Sub-populations where NSAPS shows weaknesses are:

[Node **C**] Patients with a normal to high systolic blood pressure who are admitted after scheduled surgery; these patients are relatively healthy.

[Node **F**] Patients with a normal to high systolic blood pressure who are admitted after unscheduled surgery or for a non-surgical (medical) reason and who have a very disturbed neurological status reflecting a large severity of illness.

[Node **H**] Patients with low blood pressure and low urine production reflecting possible organ failures such as heart and renal failure.

To illustrate the behavior of the models for node **C**, consider Fig. 3. The NSAPS model's predictions on the test set are shown to be consistently far from the "true" probabilities obtained from Lowess smoothing on that set. About 95% of the patients in this relatively healthy group have a score less than 35. A further examination has shown that the NSAPS model overpredicts the mortality of this group by 26 deaths compared to 8 by TLR.

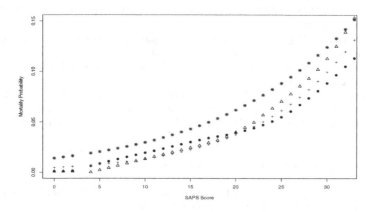

Fig. 3. Probability estimates: •: "true" probability, ∗: NSAPS predictions; △: TLW predictions; +: TLR

7   Conclusions

From this work, one can postulate that using the TLR and TLW with the NSAPS model can provide better prognostic performance instead of using the NSAPS model alone. We are experimenting with an ensemble of models to see how the performance of the models can be improved by opportunistically using the most promising model for a particular sub-population. Comparison with a logistic model enhanced with the additional variables, or dummy variables corresponding to important sub-populations, should be done. One should keep in mind, however, that any logistic model will still hide true local particularities of the data due to its underlying assumptions.

The idea of comparing (e.g. as done in [11]) or combining a classification tree with other models is in itself not new, e.g. in [9] Naive Bayes Classifiers are fit on some of the tree nodes to boost classification. The contribution of our work lies in providing a motivated synthesis of modeling and evaluation concepts tailored to the specific constraints of quality of care programs with emphasis on precision. One might conclude that the results provide proof of concept that in this era of large amounts of electronic data, there is room for a variety of modeling concepts allowing the inspection of interesting patient sub-populations as an enrichment to traditional models which were developed in different computing environments.

References

1. Abu-Hanna A, Lucas PJF. Prognostic Models in Medicine AI and Statistical Approaches, (Abu-Hanna A. and Lucas PJF, eds.). Special issue of Methods of Information in Medicine 2001, 40:1–5.
2. Bennett D, Bion J. ABC of Intensive Care. Organisation of Intensive Care. BMJ 1999; 318:1468–1470.
3. Cleveland, W. S. (1979) Robust Locally Weighted Regression and Smoothing Scatterplots. J. Amer. Statist. Assoc. 74, 829–836.
4. Hand DJ. Construction and Assessment of Classification Rules. Chichester: John Wiley and Sons, 1997.
5. Hosmer D.W., Lemeshow S. Applied Logistic Regression, Wiley, New-York, 1989.
6. Hosmer D.W., Hosmer T., Le Cessie S., Lemeshow S. A Comparison of Goodness-of-fit Tests for the Logistic Regression Model. Statistics in Medicine 1997; 16:965–980.
7. de Keizer N. An Infrastructure for Quality Assessment in Intensive Care; Prognostic Models and Terminological Systems. PhD Thesis, 2000, University of Amsterdam.
8. Knaus W, Draper E, Wagner D, Zimmerman J. APACHE II: a Severity of Disease Classification System. Crit Care Med 1985; 13:818–829.
9. Kohavi R. Scaling Up the Accuracy of Naive-Bayes Classifiers: a Decision-Tree Hybrid. Proc. of the Second Int. Conference on Knowledge Discovery and Data Mining. 1996; 202–207.
10. Le Gall J, Lemeshow S, Saulnier F. A New Simplified Acute Physiology Score (SAPS-II) Based on a European/North American Multicenter Study. JAMA 1993; 270:2957–2963.
11. Long WJ. A Comparison of Logistic Regression to Decision-Tree Induction in a Medical Domain. Compt Bio Res 1993:74–97.
12. Lucas PJF, Abu-Hanna A. Prognostic Methods in Medicine (Lucas PJF and Abu-Hanna A. eds.). Special issue of Artificial Intelligence in Medicine. 1999; 15(2):105–119.
13. Miller M.E., Hui S.L. Validation Techniques for Logistic Regression Models. Statistics in Medicine, 1991, Vol 10, pp. 1213–1226.
14. Rowan K, Kerr J, Major E, McPherson K, Short A, Vessey M. Intensive Care Society's APACHE II study in Britain and Ireland-II. BMJ 1993; 307:977–981.
15. Schwarzer G, Vach W, Schumacher M. On Misuses of Artificial Neural Networks for Prognostic and Diagnostic Classification in Oncology. Statistics in Medicine 2000; 19: 541–561.

Combining Unsupervised and Supervised Machine Learning in Analysis of the CHD Patient Database

Tomislav Šmuc[1], Dragan Gamberger[1], and Goran Krstačić[2]

[1] LIS – Rudjer Bošković Institute
Bijenička 54, 10000 Zagreb Croatia
Phone: ++385 1-4561-085, Fax: ++385-4680-114
email: smuc@rudjer.irb.hr
[2] Institute for Cardiovascular Prevention and Rehabilitation,
Draškovićeva 13, 10000 Zagreb, Croatia

Abstract. The aim of this work is twofold: to illustrate power of unsupervised data analysis approach on routinely collected diagnostic data for coronary heart disease patients and to validate findings against cardiologist's own patient classification and expert analysis. In this respect emphasis in this work is not on prediction and accuracy but rather on discovering paths to extraction of new insights and/or knowledge of the domain. The work demonstrates the use of unsupervised classification for the partitioning of the database with the aim of amplifying predictability of models describing expert classification, as well as boosting cause-and-effect relationships hidden in data.

Introduction

The main motivation behind this work is defining a novel methodology, which could facilitate discovering of 'new' or previously unknown cause-and-effect relationships, and thus support future decision making in health care management.

This is pursued through a discovery of most probable patient subgroups using both unsupervised and supervised machine learning algorithms. The role of unsupervised learning is to 'suggest' partitioning of data, prior to learning models for the original classification. In this way, different, more informative and possibly even more accurate descriptions of distinct patient subgroups are sought.

The subject of the study is a database of CHD (Coronary Heart Disease) patients. To this moment, there were numerous studies related to CHD disease, ranging from large epidemiological studies [1], to applications of novel, machine learning techniques [4], primarily for the CHD prediction. The concept of applying both unsupervised and supervised learning in extracting the knowledge out of the database correlates well with the field of *conceptual clustering* [5].

Methodology

Database of CHD (Coronary Heart Disease) patients' diagnostic data was collected in the period of 1.5 years, and contains 239 cases described by 40 parameters, from basic patient's physical characteristics to results of blood tests and heart performance measurements. This database differs from those obtained in epidemiological studies

S. Quaglini, P. Barahona, and S. Andreassen (Eds.): AIME 2001, LNAI 2101, pp. 109–112, 2001.

[1], which cover representative sample of the whole population. It represents people already suffering from CHD or having symptoms characteristic for the disease. What is important in this case is a possibility to study characteristics of patients in different stages of the disease, from early symptoms to critical stages.

The origin of the database is from everyday clinical practice and upon it cardiologist routinely performs his own classification with respect to severity of patient's overall state. This classification was already studied earlier [2,3] with respect to data quality and redundancy in applied diagnostic techniques. In these works detailed description of all individual descriptors is given. Cardiologist bases his own classification of patients mostly on results of exercise ECG and long term ECG tests, and classifies patients into five categories, from 1-healthy to 5-patients in critical stage of the disease. In this work we will refer to the results of exercise ECG and long term ECG tests as to the classification set (or test set) of descriptors and to all other descriptors as to the basic set of descriptors (these are age, weight, family history, blood tests, ECG at rest, etc.). It is important to establish significant relationships between these two sets of descriptors. These relationships are important from aspect of prevention (identifying patient risk groups), health care management (saving costs for further tests) and as insights into a genesis of the disease for different patient subgroups. This is why the final objective of this methodology are improved models of patient subgroups that use only the basic set of descriptors.

Machine learning algorithms in this work are well known implementations in freely available code package WEKA (Waikato Environment for Knowledge Analysis) developed at the University of Waikato in New Zealand [6].

We divided our analyses into three main stages as described in Figure 1. First stage is a detection of inherent major regularities in the database and is performed employing unsupervised learning algorithm (using EM - Expectation Maximization clustering algorithm). Discovered clusters in the first stage are explored and modeled in the second stage using the well-known decision tree (DT) algorithm C4.5. Based on these models, splitting descriptors and their values are decided.

Decisions about splitting of the dataset/cluster are made in stage 3, after C4.5 models for the clusters are defined. In order to simplify splitting, instead of using C4.5 model of the cluster categories as a criterion for splitting, we have used only the most important basic set descriptor from the DT model (closest to a root node) as a splitting criterion. Final evaluation of clusters and decision about splitting is based on the accuracy of models describing original classification developed separately on each cluster, as well as on cardiologist assessment of results. If the suggested split does not improve overall predictability, the splitting is not performed. Similarly, if cardiologist does not find splitting criteria interesting or sound, splitting is not performed.

After splitting of database (or cluster), a new iteration of unsupervised clustering is possible in order to further split clusters defined in the previous step. In our example we made only two iterations.

Results and Discussion

In the case of the CHD patient database, partitioning was performed in two levels. Scheme of partitioning and description of the clusters is given in Fig.1. The accuracy of the models describing original classification for the clusters is given in Table 1.

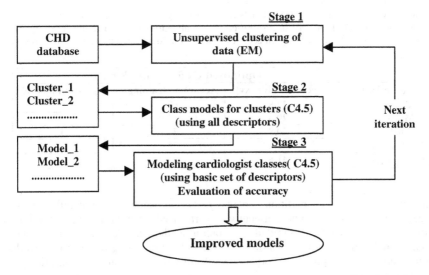

Fig. 1. Flow chart of analyses employed in the study of the CHD patient database.

First partitioning of the database was performed according to the most important basic descriptor (SEX), used in the decision tree model of clusters defined by unsupervised learning algorithm. In the second iteration partitioning was performed only for the male population, since further partitioning of the female partition did not give any improvements in predictability.

For the male partition, ST segment depression (ECG ST 1) turned out to be the most important basic set descriptor in the model describing underlying clusters.

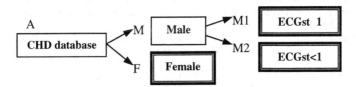

Fig. 2. Unsupervised-supervised splitting of the CHD patient dataset. Three distinct clusters (double-framed rectangles) represent optimized splitting of the dataset with respect to predictability and cardiologist evaluation.

Conclusions

This work demonstrates a combined use of unsupervised and supervised machine learning techniques in discovering important subgroups of CHD patients in different stages of the disease. Main mechanism of the methodology is partitioning of a database according to most important descriptors suggested by unsupervised clustering, followed by supervised learning of original cardiologist's patient

Table 1. Accuracy of decision tree models describing original cardiologist's classification for different database partitions. 10 fold stratified cross validation (10f sxv) results were used as criteria while pruning level was optimized. All models were developed using only the basic set of descriptors.

Model & Data	Optimized C4.5 classifier's results		
	Accuracy (10f sxv)	Accuracy (training)	Opt.pruning level
A (All)	37.8	62.1	9
M (Male)	39.6	67.0	8
F (Female)	50.8	78.1	4
M1(Male, ST 1)	42.0	75.1	5
M2(Male, ST <1	41.6	84.0	3

classification upon each partition separately. This procedure is of iterative nature (meaning that database can be consecutively partitioned several times). The level and scope of partitioning are controlled by monitoring the accuracy of generated class models, and by the expert evaluation. In this case final modeling of subgroups on the partitioned database, provided both more informative and accurate descriptions of patient subgroups.

References

1.   Dawber TR. The Framingham Study. The epidemiology of atherosclerotic disease. Cambridge, Harvard Univ. Press, 1980.
2.   Gamberger, D., Krstačić, G., Šmuc, T. (2000). Medical Expert Evaluation of Machine Learning Results for a Coronary Heart Disease Database. In *Proc. Medical Data Analysis (ISMDA'2000)*, pp.159-168.
3.   Gamberger, D., Krstačić, G., Šmuc, T. (2000). Inconsistency Tests for Patient Records in a Coronary Heart Disease Database. In *Proc. Medical Data Analysis (ISMDA'2000)*, pp.183-189.
4.   Kukar, M., Grošelj, C. (1999). Machine Learning in Stepwise Diagnostic Process. In *Proc. Joint European Conference in Medicine and Medical Decision Making (AIMDM'99)*, pp.315-325.
5.   Michalski, R.S., Kaufman, K.A., (1997). Data Mining and Knowledge Discovery: A Review of Issues and a Multistrategy Approach, Chapter 2 of: *Machine Learning and Data Mining: Methods and Applications* (Michalski, R.S., Bratko, I. and Kubat, M. eds), John Wiley and Sons
6.   Witten, I.H., Eibe, F. (1999). Data Mining - Practical Machine Learning Tools and Techniques with Java Implementations. Morgan Kaufmann Publishers, San Francisco.

Coronary Heart Disease Patient Models Based on Inductive Machine Learning

Goran Krstačić[1], Dragan Gamberger[2], and Tomislav Šmuc[2]

[1] Institute for Cardiovascular Prevention and Rehabilitation,
Draškovićeva 13, 10000 Zagreb, Croatia
[2] Rudjer Bošković Institute, Bijenička 54,10000 Zagreb, Croatia
E-mail: dragan.gamberger@irb.hr

Abstract. The work presents a model construction process which is a combination of the inductive learning based detection of interesting subgroups, comparative statistical analyses of risk factors for these groups, and expert knowledge interpretation of the results. The induced models describe population subgroups with unproportionately high rate of the disease what might be helpful in the prevention process.

1 Introduction

Atherosclerotic coronary heart disease (CHD) is one of the world's most frequent causes of mortality and an important problem of medical practice. Many extensive epidemiological studies have been performed with intention to detect and evaluate factors that increase the risk of this cardiovascular disease. It was also detected that coexistence of risk factors increases the disease rate [2]. Today prevention of the CHD relies practically on two significantly different concepts. The first is general education of the whole population about known risk factors while the other is prevention based on risk factor screening in the general practice.

In this work a few CHD patient models are presented which should help general practitioners to recognize CHD or even to detect it before the first symptoms based on data available in typical primary practice. The intention is not to substitute existing decision methods but to enable easy detection of important risk groups in the population. In Section 2 is the overview of the methodology used for patient modeling and in Section 3 is the presentation of the induced models for the CHD.

2 Model Induction Process

The development of the CHD patient models in this work has been done by a novel approach which is a combination of the inductive learning based detection of interesting subgroups and statistical analyses of the detected subgroups. Expert knowledge is included into the approach so that both the process of the subgroup detection and the statistical analysis are directed by the domain expert. Final result analysis is also based on the expert knowledge.

S. Quaglini, P. Barahona, and S. Andreassen (Eds.): AIME 2001, LNAI 2101, pp. 113–116, 2001.
© Springer-Verlag Berlin Heidelberg 2001

The first step in the inductive modeling is subgroup detection based on the confirmation rule concept [1] implemented in the ILLM (Inductive Learning by Logic Minimization) system. The properties of the concept are: for the dataset few independent rules are induced, each rule has the form of a conjunction of conditions, and conditions can be only significant properties of the subgroup. In the second step statistical analysis of all risk factors for induced subgroups is performed. The used statistical techniques are standard ones and they include mean values, medians, deviations, and typical ranges. Statistical values are computed for two populations: the reference are the healthy subjects and the target are properties of the CHD patients included into the subgroup. Interesting are those risk factors which have significantly different statistical values for the two populations. Among them are always conditions used in the rule for subgroup definition (*called principle risk factors*), but often there are some additional, which are called *supporting risk factors*. The final step in inductive modeling is expert description of the obtained results. Its most important part is expert knowledge based interpretation of potential connections among detected supporting characteristics. Sometimes even nonexistence of a supporting risk factor may be interesting if it is contradictory with the existing medical expectations.

The importance of the presented approach to inductive modeling is that it is applicable also to other medical, and perhaps not only medical problems. Its significant difference to other modeling experiments is that the domain expert and its knowledge has the central role in the process which is a combination of the machine learning and the statistical data analysis.

In this work the described model induction process has been applied on a database representing typical medical practice in CHD diagnosis. The descriptor set includes anamnestic data (level A with 10 items), laboratory test results (level B with 6 items) and the resting ECG data (level C with 5 items). The available database is in no case a good epidemiological description of the CHD in a typical population. But it is very representative for different types of the disease with about 50% cases representing CHD patients. The included negative cases are also not randomly selected persons but people with some subjective problems or people detected by general practitioners as potential CHD patients.

3   Induced Patient Models

A few important models for CHD patients could be constructed using the described methodology and the available patient data. As it was described in the second section, there are three typical levels A-C in the risk factor screening process. The intention was to construct at least one model for every level. Figures 1 and 2 present patient distributions in respect to the age.

Model A1 for men ⇒ *positive family history* **AND** *age over 46 years*
Main supporting characteristic is psychosocial stress, but important are also cigarette smoking, hypertension, and overweight.

Model A2 for women ⇒ *body mass index over 25 kgm^{-2} (typically 29)* **AND** *age over 63 years*

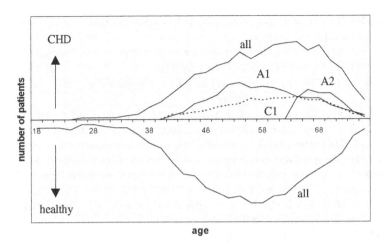

Fig. 1. Distribution of CHD patients and healthy subjects with respect to age in years. Curves A1, A2, and C1 present corresponding model properties. Model A1 is for men, model A2 is for women, and model C1 presents patients with left ventricular hypertrophy. About 60% of CHD patients detected by model C1 are also described by models A1 and A2.

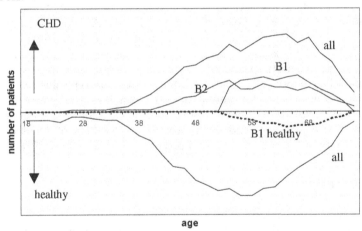

Fig. 2. Same as Figure 1 but for models B1 and B2. Model B1 are elderly people with increased total cholesterol values while model B2 are patients with increased fibrinogen and total cholesterol values. Dashed line presents healthy people included into model B1. Models B1 and B2 have about 70% of patients in common.

This simple model is very good for female population with sensitivity about 50%. Supporting characteristics are positive family history and hypertension. Women in this model will typically have slightly increased LDL cholesterol values and normal but decreased HDL cholesterol values.

Model B1 $\Rightarrow$ *total cholesterol over 6.1 mmolL^{-1} (typically 7.2, normal 3.6 to 5.0)* [3] **AND** *age over 53 years*
This model is characteristic for the older part of the population, especially for women. Typical age of the people in this model is 65 years for women and 61 years for men. The only supporting risk factor is increased triglycerides value which is more often detected for men.

Model B2 $\Rightarrow$ *total cholesterol over 5.6 mmolL^{-1} (typically 6.6, normal 3.6 to 5.0)* **AND** *fibrinogen over 3.7 mmolL^{-1} (typically 4.4, normal 2.0 to 3.7)*
This is a CHD patient model with similar properties for men and women. Typical patients do not have problems with overweight, hypertension and cigarette smoking but do have positive family history very often. Very high body mass index is contraindication for this CHD patient model. Although the main model properties are similar for both sexes, representative woman in this model is about 66 years old while a man has 10 years less.

Model C1 $\Rightarrow$ *left ventricular hypertrophy*
This model is important both for men and women above the age of 55 years. Left ventricular hypertrophy is a well known risk factor which includes many other known CHD risk factors like hypertension and obesity. The main supporting risk factor detected for this model is positive family history. Often the patients of this CHD model have problems with hypertension and diabetes mellitus.

The described models have estimated specificity between 73% and 94% and they can not be used as final diagnostic decision rules. Their primary function is early detection of CHD from anamnestic data and routine laboratory tests as well as definition of the risk population groups which should undertake non-invasive cardiovascular diagnostic procedures before first disease symptoms. Sensitivity of the models is between 23% and 50%. Such values are typically unacceptable for prediction models but for prevention purposes and for the type of data used at levels A-C these are impressive values. Additionally, for a concrete person it is enough that a CHD problems are suspected by at least one of the used models and sensitivity of the combination of 5 presented models is above 70%.

References

1. Gamberger, D. and Lavrač, N. (2000) Confirmation rule sets. In *Proc. of 4th European Conference on Principles of Data Mining and Knowledge Discovery (PKDD2000)*, pp.34–43.
2. Goldman, L., Garber, A.M., Grover, S.A., Hlatky, M.A. (1996) Cost-effectiveness of assessments and management of risk factors. *Journal of American College Cardiology* **27**:1020-1030.
3. Maron, D., Ridker, P.M, Pearson A.T. (1998) Risk factors and the prevention of coronary heart disease. In *Wayne A.R., Schlant R.C., Fuster V. : HURST'S: The Heart*, 1175-1195. McGrawc Hill, NY.

Prediction of Protein Secondary Structures of All Types Using New Hypersphere Machine Learning Method

Markku Siermala

Department of Computer Science, 33014 University of Tampere, Finland
Markku.Siermala@uta.fi

Abstract. In this paper, we present a new hypersphere machine learning method and use it to predict all protein secondary structures. It finds sequences with sufficiently high homology. Prediction accuracy of the new method with protein secondary structures was good (average 89.3%). However, the method could not classify all test cases.

1   Introduction

Biological sequence data can be very problematic to the machine learning methods, because variables in the multidimensional space are categorical. Moreover, a direction is a difficult concept in such a space and lengths of sequences may vary strongly.

Almost all prediction methods for secondary structure form a function between a set of sequences (1-dimensional information) of a certain length and a set of structures (3-dimensional information). The methods are called local prediction. The newest and most efficient methods are based on neural network approaches [1 - 3], but, of course, there are also other viewpoints to look at this task. Also the postprocessing of the prediction helps to increase prediction accuracies [4]. Unfortunately, the local prediction approach has a strong boundary that limits prediction accuracy [5, 6]. In the literature there are no earlier prediction results for the infrequent secondary structure types and we believe that the reason for that is the inability of statistical methods to handle biased distributions between the frequencies of several secondary structure types. Usually, the whole sequence data is separated to three groups: α and β structures and coil group. The best prediction results with these groups are over 70 %, but stay clearly below 80 % [6].

In this study, we present a hypersphere machine learning method that belongs to the family of the instance based methods and have relations to the nearest neighbor method. We aim to predict accurately all types of secondary structures (known in DSSP [7]), that may be a hard task for the conventional machine learning methods.

2   Hypersphere Method

The basic condition for the hypersphere method is that the method should produce a hypothesis that is consistent with training data [8]. Therefore, the learning algorithm

S. Quaglini, P. Barahona, and S. Andreassen (Eds.): AIME 2001, LNAI 2101, pp. 117--120, 2001.

must form a sphere for each learning instance, where inside the sphere it is more probable to classify the case correctly than outside the sphere. We assume that the best radius is such that the hypersphere stays away from learning cases which come from another class, but can include all query cases which with high probability belong to the same class. For this reason, we set the radius of the hypersphere to stretch halfway from the cases which come from the other class. In this paper, we will denote these examples as enemies (see Algorithm 1).

```
for each class i
    for each case j in class i (case_ij)
        c = the closest enemy
        e = distance(case_ij, c)
        r_ij = e/2
```

Algorithm 1. Hypersphere learning algorithm.

In the learning process to the class i, the algorithm detects the nearest enemy to the case j and obtains the distance e. Then, the radius r is calculated to form a sphere over the case j. If the learning material contains cases which are situated in the same location, but come from different classes, the algorithm sets radiuses to be zero for these cases. Finally, a complex volume has been built over the cases that came from class i and every query case that belongs to this volume is classified into this class.

For example, when a neural network with winner takes all method meets two cases in the same location, it has to make a compromise and both cases are classified into the same class. The hypersphere method avoids decision making in this area by restricting its generalization.

Prediction is a simple operation where, for each query case, the method tries to find a hypersphere that can include the case (see Algorithm 2). The query case is classified into the class of a hypersphere that includes the case. Hypersphere volumes that belong to the different classes, cannot intersect each other.

```
for each query case q
    for each class i
        for each case j in the class i
            if(distance(case_q, case_ij) < r_ij)
                classify case_q into the class i,
                start new query from case_{q+1}
```

Algorithm 2. Hypersphere prediction algorithm.

3   Prediction of Protein Secondary Structures with Hypersphere Method

The data of this study was taken from Protein Data Bank [9]. The pruning work has been described in [10]. We present results for eight different secondary structures. Six of them are named like those in the DSSP files [8] and one special structure is polyproline type II-structure (PPII) [11] that we have studied earlier [10]. The last class is the coil class, which includes the sequences that do not belong to any other class.

We used the hypersphere method to predict a secondary structure that lies in the middle of a 13-length sequence as in the conventional secondary structure predictions (see [3,4,7,10]). Distance function in 13 length sequence data is number of amino acids that differ in the same position and a multidimensional hypersphere (S,d) with an amino acid sequence is defined as a set of sequences S' that can be changed to the sequence S by replacing at most d amino acids.

Prediction accuracy $pa = tp/(tp+fp)$, (tp = number of true positive, fp = number of false positive cases). Recognition accuracy $ra = tp/n_c$, (n_c = number of cases which belong to the same class and get a classification). Misclassification rate $mr = fn/n_p$ (n_p = number of cases in the class p).

There were about 324000 13-length sequences in the database. More precisely, there were 61464 coil cases, 3823 PPII cases, 99221 H (α-helix) secondary structure cases, 39520 T cases, 71696 E (β-sheet) cases, 31577 S cases, 4327 B cases and 12421 G cases. Table 1 shows average accuracies for hypersphere method (10 x crossvalidation) and Table 2 shows average accuracies of the 1-nearest neighbor algorithm (10 x crossvalidation).

Table 1. Accuracies in percents for the hypersphere method: prediction accuracy, true positive rate, recognition accuracy, and misclassification rate for all secondary structures.

	coil	PPII	H	T	E	S	B	G	average
pa [%]	92.3	78.9	97.7	88.7	96.7	87.0	85.7	87.0	**89.3**
ra [%]	92.1	70.5	97.9	89.7	97.0	85.2	85.6	87.9	**88.2**
mr [%]	2.5	8.9	0.7	3.3	1.0	4.8	4.7	3.8	**3.7**

Table 2. Accuracies in percents for the 1-nearest neighbor method: prediction accuracy, true positive rate, and misclassification rate for all secondary structures.

	coil	PPII	H	T	E	S	B	G	average
pa [%]	56.4	40.7	66.1	54.2	63.1	50.1	46.8	49.5	**53.4**
ra [%]	53.2	30.7	75.1	49.7	64.4	43.6	37.2	38.2	**49.0**
mr [%]	46.8	69.3	24.9	50.1	35.6	56.4	62.8	61.8	**51.0**

4   Discussion

The prediction accuracies for hypersphere method were high for all secondary structures. The results showed that, if the method restricts uncertain generalization, prediction results are good. Unfortunately, the method could classify approximately only 30% of all the query cases. However, in the secondary structure prediction highly accurate prediction is seen to be more important than identification of all cases. It must be noted that, with more separate classes or with less noisy in the data, we can expect much less unclassified cases. For example, average results for female urinary incontinence data were $pa = 94.6\%$ and $ra = 59.7\%$ [12].

Since H is a well-known α-helix, we can compare this to the bound of 78 %, which was presented to be the upper bound for neural network predictions [5]. Clearly, using the hypersphere method prediction accuracy was better.

Although, the nearest neighbor method gave classification to whole test material, the accuracies strongly decreased. Moreover, *tpr* of the rare PPII and B secondary structure types were almost as small as with hypersphere method.

To summarize, the hypersphere method with protein secondary structures concentrated on finding sequences that had enough homology to make classifications. This means that many a case remained without classification, but prediction accuracy was high for the data applied. Moreover, it means that we can make accurate predictions for all secondary structures and this is entirely new.

Acknowledgements. The author wishes to thank the University of Tampere, Tampere Graduate School in Information and Engineering (TISE), and Academy of Finland for financial support.

References

1. Baldi P., Brunak S., Frasconi P., Soda G., Pollastri G.: Exploiting the Past and the Future in Protein Secondary Structure Prediction. Bioinformatics **15** (1999) 937-946
2. Rost B.: A Neural Network for Prediction of Protein Secondary Structure. In Fiesler, E. and Beale, R. (eds.), Handbook of Neural Computation. IOP Publishing and Oxford University Press (1997), pp. G4.1:1-9.
3. Ruggiero C., Sacile R., Rauch G.: Peptides Secondary Structure Prediction with Neural Networks: A Criterion for Building Appropriate Learning Sets. Trans. Biomed. Eng. **40** (1993) 1114-1121.
4. Guermeur Y., Geourjon C., Gallinari P., Deleage G.: Improved Performance in Protein Structure Prediction by Inhomogeneous Score Combination. Bioinformatics **15** (1999) 413 – 421
5. Hayward S., Collins J.: Limits on α-Helix Prediction With Neural Network Models. Proteins **14** (1992) 372-381
6. Baldi P., Brunak S. (eds.): Bioinformatics: The Machine Learning Approach. The MIT Press, London (2000)
7. Kabsch W., Sander C.: Dictionary of Protein Secondary Structure: Pattern Recognition of Hydrogen-Bonded and Geometrical Features. Biopolymers **22** (1983) 2577-2637
8. Mitchell T.: Machine Learning. McGraw-Hill, Singapore (1997)
9. Berman H, Westbrook J., Feng Z., Gilliland G., Bhat T., Weissig H., Shindyalov I., Bourne P.: The Protein Data Bank. Nucleic Acids Research **28** (2000) 235-242.
10. Siermala M., Juhola M., Vihinen M.: Neural Network Prediction of Polyproline Type II Secondary Structure. In Hasman et al. eds. Medical Infobahn for Europe, Proceedings of MIE2000 and GMDS2000, IOS Press **77** (2000) 475-479
11. Adzhubei A., Sternberg M.: Left-handed Polyproline II Helices Commonly Occur in Globular Proteins, J. Mol. Biol. **229** (1993) 472-493
12. Laurikkala, J., Juhola, M., Lammi, S., Penttinen, J., Aukee, P.: Analysis of the Imputed Female Urinary Incontinence D67ata for the Evaluation of Expert System Parameters. Comput. Biol. Med., (2001) 31(4).

Integrating Different Methodologies for Insulin Therapy Support in Type 1 Diabetic Patients

Stefania Montani[1], Paolo Magni[1], Abdul V. Roudsari[2], Ewart R. Carson[2], and
Riccardo Bellazzi[1]

[1] Dipartimento di Informatica e Sistemistica Università di Pavia, Pavia, Italy
stefania@aim.unipv.it
[2] MIM Center, City University, London, UK

Abstract. We propose a Multi Modal Reasoning (MMR) methodology designed to provide physicians with knowledge management and decision support functionality in the context of type 1 diabetes mellitus care. The MMR system performs a tight integration of Case Based Reasoning (CBR), Rule Based Reasoning (RBR) and Model Based Reasoning (MBR), with the aim of suggesting a therapy properly tailored to the patient's needs, overcoming the single approaches' limitations. This methodology allows the exploitation of the implicit knowledge embedded in patients' visits (past cases) and in monitoring data through Case Based retrieval. Moreover the explicit domain knowledge is formalized in a set of production rules and in a mathematical model. The system has been preliminary tested both on simulated and on real patients' data.

1 Introduction

The interest in reasoning approaches that integrate different methodologies is recently increasing through various application areas [1], including medical decision support. These Multi Modal Reasoning (MMR) paradigms offer the opportunity of taking advantage of all the available information, thus providing help in decision making in the light of both well-established, explicit knowledge, and of the know-how collected in the single organization where the application will be deployed. This is a particularly important issue in the medical domain, where the introduction of Hospital Information Systems (HIS) into clinical practice has led to the memorization of a huge quantity of data, extracted from day by day activity, thus making available pieces of operative information, which embed the unarticulated experience of individual workers.

From a methodological viewpoint, Case Based Reasoning (CBR) [2] comes out to be a suitable means for implementing the Knowledge Management (KM) task [3] when dealing with operative knowledge. CBR is a problem solving paradigm that utilizes the specific knowledge of previously experienced situations, called cases. It basically consists in retrieving past cases that are similar to the current one and in reusing (by, if necessary, adapting) past successful solutions; the current case can be retained and put into a case library. The case

S. Quaglini, P. Barahona, and S. Andreassen (Eds.): AIME 2001, LNAI 2101, pp. 121–130, 2001.

library enables one to keep track of the organization expertise, and can be continuously and easily upgraded through the addition of new cases and (possibly) the deletion of old ones that proved to be out of date. Rule Based Reasoning (RBR) and Model Based Reasoning (MBR) are instead helpful strategies for representing and managing explicit knowledge. A MMR methodology that integrates CBR with RBR or MBR (or with both) offers the possibility of managing all the available information within the organization, and of relying on it for automatic reasoning support. In the literature, the combination of CBR with RBR has received particular attention, since rules are truly the most successful explicit knowledge representation formalism for intelligent systems. Different levels of integration between the two paradigms are described. Usually RBR and CBR are applied in mutually exclusive ways, where RBR deals with knowledge on standard or typical problems, while CBR faces exceptions. In this view, CBR is exploited to retrieve similar cases from a library of peculiar and non-standard situations only when RBR has failed to produce a solution [4,5]. Other approaches rely on CBR for instantiating and providing suitable contexts to rules, while rules are used to assist CBR by permitting the extraction of more general concepts from concrete examples [6]. It is possible to select which methodology to apply first in a dynamic way, depending on the situation at hand [6,7]. In particular, the rule base and the case memory can be searched in parallel for applicable entities. Then the best entity (i.e. rule or case) to reuse (and therefore the reasoning paradigm to apply) can be selected on the basis of its suitability for solving the current problem [7]. Finally, RBR can support CBR in adapting the past retrieved solutions to the current problem: if the memory does not contain suitable examples of adaptations to situations similar to the current one, the system will employ some general adaptation rules [8]. A few examples of a MMR strategy that integrate all the three methodologies under examination can be found as well. In Sary's work, for instance, RBR is applied to routine problems, MBR to more complex ones, and CBR on the few remaining cases, to improve system performances [9].

The common basis of all the above approaches (except perhaps the work in [6]) is that the methodological elements are used in a quite exclusive way. On the contrary, only a very tight integration, taking place within the general problem solving cycle, is able to overcome the intrinsic limitations the three reasoning paradigms may show, that can be summarized as follows: (i) on the one hand, classical RBR systems don't have the capability of specializing the explicit knowledge embedded in the rules, by resorting to contextual knowledge (e.g. the single patient's features). The risk one may incur is the definition of a very large rule base, meant to deal with as many peculiar situations as possible (the so-called *qualification problem* [10]); (ii) on the other hand, CBR just relies on the implicit knowledge stored in the case library. A misleading indication on how to solve the current problem may emerge when the number of cases is too small, or when the retrieved information is polarized on too specific examples. The capability of filling such a *competence gap* is crucial especially in medical applications, since final decisions should always be based on established knowledge; (iii) finally, defining a suitable model to work with may be very critical, especially when the available data are few or of poor quality, in a word inadequate to be relied upon in the model identification phase.

In previous years, we have defined a methodology that integrates CBR and RBR, designed to provide support for managing knowledge and making decisions in the field of type 1 diabetes mellitus management. In our MMR system, Case Based retrieval results are used to specialize the behaviour of a set of production rules, thus tailoring the therapeutic suggestion to the situation at hand. An added value of a MMR system is also the possibility of exploiting it in a modular way: in our application, in particular, the physician is allowed to rely on the CBR tool alone, to navigate the case library, and rebuild the patients' clinical histories over time. CBR can therefore be seen as an independent operative KM methodology. Additional details of this work can be found in section 2.3, and are fully described elsewhere (see for example [11]). In this paper, we present an evolution of the MMR strategy, that incorporates also a model of the patient's metabolic behaviour, as a mean for computing the optimal therapeutic suggestion. The method is currently in a preliminary testing phase within the decision support tools under study in the EU funded telemedicine project M^2DM (Multi Access Services for the Management of Diabetes Mellitus). The results that will be presented in the following sections are some of the ones that we have got during this testing phase.

2   MMR for Type 1 Diabetes Management

2.1   The Application Domain

Diabetes mellitus is one of the major chronic diseases in the industrialized countries, involving up to 3% of the population. Seven to 20% of the total number of diabetic patients are affected by type 1 diabetes, and need to undergo Intensive Insulin Therapy (IIT), consisting in 3 to 4 injections of exogenous insulin every day, in order to regulate blood glucose, and to reduce the risk of later life complications. A correct implementation of IIT requires patients to perform a strict self-monitoring: they have to test Blood Glucose Level (BGL) before every injection, and to record the measurements on hand-written diaries, together with the insulin doses really injected, and with additional information about their diet and lifestyle. Every 2-4 months they undergo periodical control visits, during which the physician evaluates also the diary data, and defines a suitable insulin administration protocol to be implemented, in order to optimize the patient's metabolic behaviour. The major long-term intervention trial on type 1 diabetic patients, the DCCT [12], has clearly shown that the definition and realization of an appropriate individual therapeutic goal, customized on the single patient's needs, is the key to effective diabetes care. Defining a proper therapy is therefore a relevant decision problem to be addressed, that starts from the interpretation of a huge amount of information.

2.2   A New Probabilistic Model of the Glucose/Insulin System

In this paper, we have exploited a stochastic extension of the model proposed in the UTOPIA system [13]. This model assumes that a patient reaches a daily cyclo-stationary behaviour in response to a certain insulin protocol. The change in the daily steady state values of BGL caused by a change in the therapeutic protocol is described by a linear differential equation, whose solution assumes the following form:

$$BGL(t_i, R2) = -S \int_{t_i-24}^{t_i} [(1-r(t))Iarel(t)exp(-k(t_i-t))]dt + BGL(t_i, R1) \quad (1)$$

where $BGL(t_i, R_j, j = 1, 2)$ is the steady state value of BGL at day time i, in response to insulin therapy regimen R1 or R2, $Iarel$ is the change of the daily insulin activity profile moving from R1 to R2, $r(t)$ is a function with values in [0 1] that expresses the different insulin resistance that may occur during the day, and k and S are the patient specific model parameters. One basic problem in the application of this model is the need to extract a set of point estimates that describe the daily behaviour of a diabetic patient, i.e. a *single* daily profile as a summary of the patient's response to a certain therapy (i.e. the modal day). As a matter of fact, a point-based representation of patients' behaviour does not take into account the intra-patient variability, that is caused by a variety of factors, ranging from physiological reasons to a day-by-day change in the patient's life-style.

To overcome such limitation, we have extended the model (1) in a probabilistic framework. The daily cyclo-stationary profile of the patients (BGL modal day) has been represented through a collection of H probability distributions, each one describing the measurements' variability at a certain time of the day, or time slice. By assuming that the measurements are taken approximately at the same time for the monitoring period, and by discretizing the BGL in L values, we can estimate with a Bayesian approach the probability of the l-th BGL discrete level, with $l = 1, \ldots, L$ in the h-th probability distribution, with $h = 1, \ldots, H$ as

$$P_h^l = \frac{n_h^l + m_h^l}{N_h + M_h} \quad (2)$$

where N_h is the number of data available in the h time slice, while n_h^l is the number of data in the h time slice belonging to the l-th discretization interval; m_h^l and M_h are values defining the a-priori probability distribution.

Having obtained a probabilistic description of the patient's cyclo-stationary behaviour in response to a given therapy regimen R1, that we will denote as $\Pi(R1) = \{\pi(R1, h), h = 1, \ldots, H\}$, it is possible to obtain a forecast $\Pi(R2)$ on the effect of a new therapeutic regimen R2 by resorting to the model (1). If we run the model at each time slice by taking as initial value the central value of each discretization interval, we obtain a collection of H probability transition matrices M_h, that are able to compute $\Pi(R2)$ by multiplying M_h and $\pi(R1, h)$

for all h. It is important to note that the matrices M_h do not depend only on the change in the therapy regimen, but also on the values assumed by the model parameters S and k, that should be inferred from the data. In our case, we fixed the value of k on the basis of available knowledge, and we resorted to a probabilistic description of the parameter S. In particular, we have discretized S in a fine grid of S_d values. By applying Bayesian statistics on a Dirichlet-multinomial model, it is possible to use $\Pi(R)$ of two consecutive periods to derive the posterior distribution of S. Since each M_h is a function of S, also M_h turns out to be stochastic, so that for each discrete value of S, s_d, there is a correspondent deterministic (i.e. only 0 and 1 values) transition matrix $M_h(s_d)$ whose probability is $P(S = s_d)$. Given the change in the therapeutic regimen, it is therefore possible to obtain the posterior estimate of M_h as the mean value of $P(M_h)$. The model presented here is able to obtain a probabilistic forecast of the effect of a therapy change on the BGL stationary behaviour. Once a certain $\Pi(R)$ is obtained, it is possible to apply standard utility theory to derive the optimal regimen, by minimizing the expected cost (EC):

$$EC(R) = \sum_{h=1}^{H} \sum_{l=1}^{L} P_h^l C_l \qquad (3)$$

where C_l is a suitable cost associated with each BGL discretization level.

In this paper, we have studied the problem with 3 time slices ($H = 3$), i.e. Before Breakfast (BR), Before Lunch (LU) and Before Dinner (D), 5 discretization values ($L = 5$) for BGL, 20 discretization levels for S, $k = 0.125$ $hours^{-1}$ and the cost function defined in DIAS [14]. It is finally crucial to remark that such new model may present two basic problems in its application: (i) the identification procedure may lead to a very flat probability distribution for S. This may be due to an insufficient change in insulin regimen related to the data exploited for identification, or to the inadequacy of the model in describing the data themselves; (ii) the dose optimization procedure may be extremely time-demanding. Therefore, the use of the model should always be coupled with the use of suitable heuristics to reduce the search space. In the following, we will see how these difficulties have been overcome within our MMR system.

2.3   The System Architecture

In the field of type 1 diabetes care, the therapy revision process is typically articulated in four consecutive tasks; in our implementation, the completion of the process is scheduled by a RBR system, within which each task is mapped to a specific set of rules, fired through a forward chaining mechanism. In detail, the reasoning paradigm proceeds as follows:

1. **Data analysis**: to interpret the effects of a therapy, we resorted to the probabilistic description of the *typical day* of the patient described in the previous section. In more detail, we extract the typical day by calculating the BGL modal day, through a generalization of the equation (2) able to handle missing data

(see [15]), after a discretization and aggregation of BGL values performed on the basis of Temporal Abstraction concepts [11];

2. Problem identification: the results of the modal day extraction trigger the identification of hyperglycaemia or hypoglycaemia problems in the different periods of the day. The RBR system can complete this task independently, or its behaviour can be specialized resorting to the integration with Case Based retrieval. The concept of *case* is mapped to the one of periodical control visit. We structured the case library resorting to a taxonomy of prototypical classes, representing the most common diseases associated with diabetes, or clinical course conditions which paediatric patients may incur. Each case belongs to one and only one class. It was thus possible to implement Case Based retrieval as a two-step procedure: (i) classification of the input case as belonging to a precise class in the taxonomy, and (ii) retrieval of past similar cases, on the reduced search space found by classification. In particular, in the problem identification task, only classification results are exploited (see figure 1), to tune specific rule parameters, thus tailoring the identification of metabolic alterations to the single patient's needs (see [11] for details);

3. Suggestion generation and selection: for each detected problem, a set of suggestions on how to modify the current insulin therapy are proposed; the most effective ones are selected resorting to the concept of insulin *competence*. The most competent insulin, that has the stronger effect on the moment of the day in which the problem has been found, is identified. Competence is evaluated relying on the pharmacokinetics of the different insulin types [16];

4. Therapy revision: the RBR system proposes an adjustment to the current insulin therapy, in accordance with the selected suggestions. It is meant to be general enough to be safely applicable in a variety of different situations: therefore, it typically proposes small variations to the current protocol insulin doses, quantitatively speaking. Even though the RBR behaviour was judged correct and quite satisfactory in a formal evaluation study [17], it came out to be sometimes not sharp enough to promptly face the patient's alterations. A way of overcoming this weakness is by integrating the RBR results with MBR or with CBR. In particular, we propose to use the model described in section 2.2 to calculate the optimal insulin doses increase or decrease, in the direction identified by the generated suggestions. Unfortunately, as mentioned before, not always does the model turn out to give reliable predictions, in particular when a clear causal effect of insulin doses on the BGL cannot be identified in the data (for example because of the presence of "brittle control" or "Somogyi effect"). To detect this problem, a two-level strategy is applied: (i) first, during the model parameter identification phase, we evaluate if the posterior distribution of S is quite uniform: in this case, since it is not possible to identify a value for S that is more reliable then the others, we conclude that the model is not able to correctly represent the specific patient situation, and it is not exploited in the MMR process; (ii) second, if the application of the therapy adjustments suggested by the model does not succeed in ameliorating the patient's metabolic behaviour, as it can be verified observing that the expected cost assumes a higher value then the one obtained from the initial data, the system rolls back, and again does not make use of the model suggestions. When this situation holds, the integration process goes on by performing the CBR retrieval step, restricted to the most probable class(es) identified during the problem identification phase. Some simple statistics are calculated on the retrieved cases, to set the insulin adjustments width that will then be applied to the current protocol. Therefore, MBR and Case Based retrieval are used in a mutual exclusive way to specialize the rules behaviour (see figure 1). In any case, if the system is not able to retrieve a sufficiently large number of past similar cases, integration with CBR will not take place, and the reasoning process will be completed relying only on RBR.

As stated in the introduction, CBR can also be seen as an independent implicit KM tool. From an implementation viewpoint, each case in the library is linked to the previous and to the following ones, in terms of time, by two chains of pointers; in this way, it is easy for the user to navigate the whole patient's history, and to visualize the transitions from one class to another, together with the therapeutic choices that made possible the transitions themselves. Moreover, the classification procedure provides an added value: the identification of the most probable class(es) for the input case allows to detect a suitable context for interpreting the case itself; the metabolic alterations experienced can be evaluated in the light of the patient's features, and the therapeutic suggestion can be adapted to them. Finally, classification focuses the attention only on the relevant parts of the case library, thus speeding up retrieval of past cases and making it more efficient.

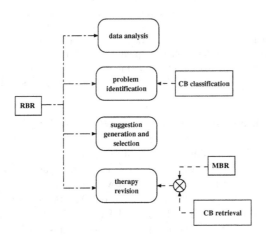

Fig. 1. Implementation of the integration between RBR, CBR and MBR in the automatic reasoning process for therapy revision

3   Preliminary Results

We evaluated the MMR system performance both prospectively on simulated data, obtained through a realistic diabetic patient simulator [18], which underlying model is not related to the UTOPIA one, and retrospectively on real patients data.

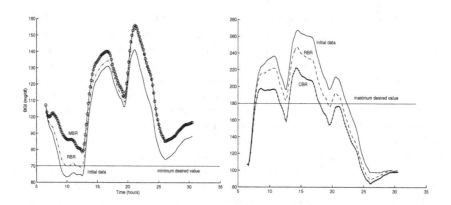

Fig. 2. Daily simulated BGL profiles (24 hours) in response to different therapeutic regimens. (a): Comparison between RBR and MBR-RBR in stabilizing a simulated patient in the clinical remission phase. Both methods suggest therapy changes that ameliorate the initial metabolic behaviour, but the use of the model allows a total recovery from hypoglycaemia (b): Comparison between RBR and CBR-RBR in stabilizing a simulated patient suffering from typical puberal problems. Rules specialization through CBR results leads to larger adjustments in the competent insulin doses in comparison to the application of RBR alone, and thus to a more significant metabolic improvement.

Prospective evaluation. To perform prospective evaluation, for each test 21 days of BGL measurements were generated; then the therapeutic suggestions proposed by the RBR system, and the ones obtained by specializing rules resorting to MBR or to CBR, were collected. Finally, an additional period of 21 days, following the application of each therapy, was simulated: in this way, it was possible to compare the performance of different MMR solutions. In particular, figure 2(a) shows the comparison between RBR and MBR-RBR integration, on a simulated patient entering the clinical remission phase, affected by hypoglycaemia problems in the morning and over night. Both the methodologies suggest therapy changes that ameliorate the initial metabolic behaviour, but the model proves to be much more sharp, since it totally recovers from hypoglycaemia. A second test was performed by simulating a patient suffering from typical puberal problems, leading to frequent hyperglycaemia. This time, the application of the model suggestions led to an unidentifiability situation, in which also the expected cost function was higher than the actual one; therefore, as described in section 2.3, the MMR system identified a condition of non-applicability of the model, and rolled back, exploiting the CBR-RBR integration. Figure 2(b) shows the comparison between the therapy suggested by applying RBR, and the one obtained by specializing the rules through past cases retrieval. CBR clearly improves the efficacy of the rules, allowing for larger adjustments in the competent insulin doses.

Retrospective evaluation. The MMR system was retrospectively evaluated on 10 real patient cases, in order to verify the model applicability. On 4 cases, the model was not able to describe the patient's situation (see section 2.3), while Case Based retrieval results could be applied to specialize the rules. On the remaining 6, we evaluated the potential effectiveness of the different strategies through the prediction of the BGL values that can be obtained exploiting our model. In these cases a slight amelioration of the initial metabolic behaviour can be obtained through RBR, the CBR-RBR integration proposes a wider improvement, and the MBR-RBR integration obviously leads to the optimal solution. Therefore, in more then 50% of the examples, the model was applicable. When the model could not be effectively used, the possibility of exploiting past cases similar to the current one was very helpful for the definition of a proper therapy: CBR-RBR integration represents a way for obtaining a sub-optimal therapeutic advice.

4   Conclusions

In this paper, we have presented an upgrade to the MMR strategy for supporting insulin therapy revision we developed in the previous years. While the existing methodology was based on CBR-RBR integration, the new system incorporates also a model of the patient's metabolic behaviour, as a mean for specializing the rules. A first evaluation procedure was carried out resorting both to simulated data, and to real patients' ones, provided by the Paediatric Department at Policlinico S. Matteo hospital in Pavia. Even though the results have to be interpreted as very preliminary, it is clear that, when applicable, the model leads to the identification of the optimal therapeutic strategy for the situation at hand. Non-applicability can be highlighted during the model identification phase, or can be verified *a posteriori*, when the application of the MBR suggestions does not succeed in reducing the cost function in comparison with the initial data. The MMR strategy is able to automatically detect these situations, and then to specialize rules relying on Case Based retrieval results. When a sufficiently large number of past similar cases can be retrieved, CBR-RBR integration represents a way for obtaining sub-optimal therapeutic advice. When the case library content is poor, the retrieval results may lead to an unfit rule specialization. In this condition, the MMR system will exploit RBR alone, thus providing a reliable (even if "conservative") solution. Moreover, the CBR methodology enables easy storing and upgrading of knowledge. Therefore we believe that the overall system will automatically improve its competence if introduced into routine clinical practice: in this way new cases will be stored in the HIS without imposing an additional work load on the physicians, and will contribute to reduce the competence gaps in the case library. The system will thus learn how to cope with more and more complex situations, and to effectively specialize rules also when the model cannot be relied upon.

References

1. Aha, D., and Daniels, J. (eds.): Proc. AAAI Workshop on CBR Integrations, AAAI Press (1998)
2. Kolodner, J.L.: Case-Based Reasoning. Morgan Kaufmann (1993)
3. Steels, L.: Corporate knowledge management. Proc. of ISMICK '93, Compiegne (1993) 9–30
4. Surma, J., Vanhoff, K.: Integrating rules and cases for the classification task. In: LNAI 1010, Proc. ICCBR, Springer Verlag (1995) 325–334
5. Xu, L.D.: An integrated rule- and case-based approach to AIDS initial assessment. International Journal of Biomedical Computing 40 (1996) 197–207
6. Branting, L.K., Porter, B.W.: Rules and precedents as complementary warrants. Proc. AAAI 91, Anaheim (1991)
7. Bichindaritz, I., Kansu, E., Sullivan, K.M.: Case-based reasoning in CARE-PARTNER: gathering evidence for evidence-based medical practice. In: LNAI 1488, Proc. 4th EWCBR, Springer Verlag (1998) 334–345
8. Leake, D.B.: Combining rules and cases to learn case adaptation. Proc. 17th International Conference of Cognitive Science Society, Pittsburgh (1995)
9. Sary, C., et al.: Trend analysis for spacecraft systems using multimodal reasoning. Proc. AAAI Spring Symp. on Multi-modal Reasoning, AAAI Press (1998) 157–162
10. Russel, S., Norvig, P.: Artificial Intelligence, a modern approach. Prentice Hall (1995)
11. Montani, S., Bellazzi, R., Portinale, L., Stefanelli, M.: A Multi-Modal Reasoning Methodology for Managing IDDM Patients. International Journal of Medical Informatics 58-59 (2000) 243–256
12. The Diabetes Control and Complication Trial Research Group: The effect of intensive treatment of diabetes on the development and progression of long-term complications in insulin-dependent diabetes mellitus. The New England Journal of Medicine 329 (1993) 977–986
13. Deutsch, T., Roudsari, A.V., Leicester, H.J., Theodorou, T., Carson, E.R., and Sonksen, P.H.: UTOPIA: a consultation system for visit by visit diabetes management. Medical Informatics 21 (1996) 345–358
14. Andreassen, S., Benn, J., Hovorka, R., Olesen, K.G., Carson, E.R.: A probabilistic approach to glucose prediction and insulin dose adjustment: description of metabolic model and pilot evaluation study. Computer Methods and Programs in Biomedicine 41 (1994) 153–165
15. Ramoni, M., Sebastiani, P.: The use of exogenous knowledge to learn Bayesian Networks for incomplete databases. In: Liu, X., Cohen, P., and Berthold, M. (eds.): Advances In Intelligent Data Analysis, Springer Verlag, Berlin (1997) 537–548
16. Hovorka, R., Svacina, S., Carson, E.R., Williams, C.D., Sönksen, P.H.: A consultation system for insulin therapy. Computer Methods and Programs in Biomedicine 32 (1996) 303–310
17. Nucci, G., et al.: Verification phase final report, T-IDDM deliverable 5.2. http://aim.unipv.it/projects/tiddm/ftp.html
18. Cobelli, C., Nucci, G., Del Prato, S.: A physiological simulation model in type I Diabetes. Diabetes nutrition and Metabolism 11 (1998) 78

Diagnosing Patient State in Intensive Care Patients Using the Intelligent Ventilator (INVENT) System

Stephen E. Rees[1], Charlotte Allerød[2], Søren Kjærgaard[2], Egon Toft[3], Per Thorgaard[2], and Steen Andreassen[1]

[1] Department of Medical Informatics and Image Analysis, Aalborg University, Denmark
[2] Department of Anaesthesia, Aalborg Hospital, Denmark
[3] Department of Cardiology, Aalborg Hospital, Denmark.

Abstract. A method is presented to estimate parameters describing ICU patients' ventilatory, circulatory, and metabolic state from simultaneous solution of models of O_2 and CO_2 transport. This method is shown to provide a consistent and reasonable picture of data from 5 ICU patients even without a pulmonary arterial catheter.

1 Introduction

Several systems have been developed to advise on appropriate ventilation for patients residing in the intensive care unit using either protocols or rules, rules combined with physiological models, or physiological models combined with utility functions in a decision theoretic approach [1]. The intelligent ventilator (INVENT) system [2] uses the latter of these approaches, finding the ventilator settings which result in predicted physiological variables incurring the lowest total penalty.

As a first stage in this process INVENT is used to assess the patients' pathophysiological state. This is far from trivial and involves obtaining values of parameters describing the ventilatory, circulatory, and metabolic systems. For severely ill patients invasive measurement techniques can be justified and many of these parameters can be directly measured. In patients with less severity of illness many parameters cannot be measured and obtaining a physiological parameter based description of the patient from a reduced and inaccurate data set, is much more difficult. This paper presents an approach to estimating parameters describing patients' pathophysiological state from measurements typical to an ICU. The paper investigates whether simultaneous solution of models of O_2 and carbon dioxide (CO_2) transport can give parameter estimates that give a consistent and reasonable picture of the patient even without invasive measurements from a pulmonary arterial (PA) catheter.

2 Methods

Figure 1 illustrates the INVENT data collection and parameter estimation screen. Data is collected for all tables on the left hand side of figure 1. i.e. *Patient/ processing details*: a) the type of catheter, i.e. PA or central venous; b) the pulmonary gas exchange model, i.e. models including pulmonary shunt and either ventilation/perfusion mismatch (V/Q), or alveolar oxygen diffusion resistance (Rdiff) [3]; and c) the ventilator mode. *Arterial (a)*

S. Quaglini, P. Barahona, and S. Andreassen (Eds.): AIME 2001, LNAI 2101, pp. 131–135, 2001.
© Springer-Verlag Berlin Heidelberg 2001

and mixed venous (mv) or central venous (cv) blood: Blood samples are taken and used to measure: pH, CO_2 pressure (PCO_2), O_2 pressure (PO_2), haemoglobin (Hb) concentration (tHb), O_2 saturation (SO_2), fraction carboxyhaemoglobin (FCOHb), and fraction methaemoglobin (FMetHb). *ALPE data:* An automated procedure taking 10-15 minutes is performed where inspired O_2 fraction (FIO_2) is varied in 4-6 steps to give SaO_2 from 90 to100%. At each FIO_2 ventilation and SaO_2 are measured from blood (SaO_2) or pulse oximetry (SpO_2). Measurements of ventilation are: end tidal O_2 fraction (FEO_2), (FIO_2), end tidal CO_2 fraction ($FECO_2$), tidal volume (VT) and respiratory frequency (f). The positive inspiratory pressure (PIP), positive end expiratory pressure (PEEP), and the ratio of the duration of inspiration to expiration (I:E), are also recorded. Figure 1 illustrates data from patient 1 (table 1). This patient had a central venous catheter and was pressure control ventilated.

These measurements are used with mathematical models of O_2 and CO_2 transport [3,4], to estimate shunt, fA2, dead space (VD), Q, and the dynamic compliance (Comp) and resistance (Res) of the lung; and to predict values (p) of mixed venous blood gasses (pHmvp, PCO_2mvp, SO_2mvp), end tidal CO_2 fraction ($FECO_2p$), VO_2 (VO_2p), CO_2 production (VCO_2p) and the respiratory quotient (RQp). Values of Comp and Res are estimated from a one compartment model of lung mechanics. Other parameters are estimated using the following 8 step algorithm:

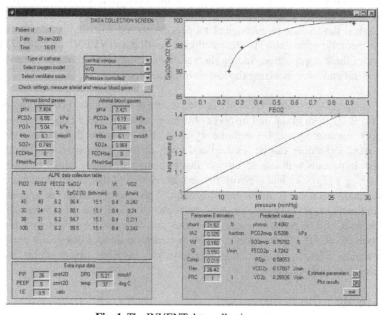

Fig. 1. The INVENT data collection screen.

Step 1: Values of VD and Q are selected and used with the current ventilator settings to calculate VO_2p, i.e. $VO_2p = f (VT - VD) (FIO_2 - FEO_2)$. *Step 2*: The ALPE data and the current values of VD and Q are used to calculate pulmonary gas exchange parameters [3], resulting in estimates of shunt and either fA2 or Rdiff which give a fit to the ALPE data illustrated in the FEO_2 v SaO_2/SpO_2 plot, figure 1. *Step 3*: Measurements of arterial blood are used with a model of acid-base chemistry [4] to calculate state variables describing the arterial blood. These are: total CO_2 concentration (taCO$_2$), base excess (BEa), total O_2 concentration (taO$_2$), and Hb concentration (tHba). *Step 4*: Calculated values of shunt, fA2 and taCO$_2$, plus the values of VD and Q are then inserted into the equations illustrated in figure 2. These equations are uniquely solved to predict values of VCO_2p, $FECO_2p$ and the total CO_2 in mixed venous blood (tmvCO$_2p$). *Step 5*: Other state variables for mixed venous blood (i.e. BEmvp, tHbmvp, and tmvO$_2p$) are then calculated i.e. assuming no net addition of strong acid or Hb from the arterial to the venous blood then BEmvp= BEa and tHbmvp = tHba. Total oxygen in the mixed venous blood (tmvO$_2p$) is calculated by solving the Fick equation i.e. $VO_2p = Q$ (taO$_2$ – tmvO$_2p$). *Step 6*: The four predicted state variables needed to fully describe the acid-base chemistry of mixed venous blood (tmvCO$_2p$, BEmvp, tmvO$_2p$, tHbmvp) are then inserted into the model of acid base chemistry [4] and used to calculate pHmvp, PCO$_2$mvp, PO$_2$mvp and SO$_2$mvp. *Step 7*: Calculated values of pHmvp, PCO$_2$mvp, SO$_2$mvp and $FECO_2p$ are then inserted used to calculated the error for the current values of VD and Q using:

$$\text{Error} = ((pHmvp - pHv) / SD_{phv})^2 + ((PCO_2mvp - PCO_2v) / SD_{PCO_2v})^2 +$$
$$((SO_2mvp - SO_2v) / SD_{SO_2v})^2 + ((FECO_2 - FECO_2p) / SD_{FECO_2})^2 \qquad (1)$$

The standard deviation of measured central venous blood values and end tidal CO_2 are assumed to be SD_{phv} =0.01, SD_{PCO_2v} = 0.1 kPa, SD_{SO_2v} = 0.5%, SD_{FECO_2} = 0.001. *Step 8*: A gradient descent optimization algorithm chooses new values of VD and Q, so as to lower the calculated error, and steps 1-8 are repeated, terminating when a minimum for the error function is found.

Five patients, four male, were studied using this method. All patients were, according to clinical opinion, haemodynamically stable and presented with a history of respiratory insufficiency described by bile acid inspiration (Pt. 1), or signs of atelectasis on X-ray (Pts. 2-5). Patients receiving vaso-active drugs other than dopamine were excluded. All patients had a central venous catheter. Ethical approval was obtained from the ethics committee of North Jutland and Viborg. Informed written and oral consent was obtained from the patients' relatives in all cases.

3 Results

Table 1 includes parameter estimates and measured and predicted blood gas values for all 5 patients. Predicted mixed venous pHmvp, PCO$_2$mvp, SO$_2$mvp levels were almost identical to central venous measurements. Predicted values of FECO2p were also very close to those measured, except in patient 1, where fitting the model including Rdiff produced a good fit to the data. Values of shunt (range 22-50%, normal 5%) and fA2 (range 0.3-0.58, normal 0.9) were consistent with abnormal gas exchange. Shunt values were also consistent with atelectasis seen on X-rays in patients 2-5. Estimates of Q and VD were reasonable giving VD/VT ratios close to healthy anaesthetised patients (normal range VD/VT = 0.3-0.35) in all but patient 5. Predicted values of VO_2 and VCO_2p were reasonable in patients 1-4. The respiratory quotient was within the physiological range (0.7- 1.0) in patients 2,4 and 5, and only slightly outside this range in patients 1 and 3.

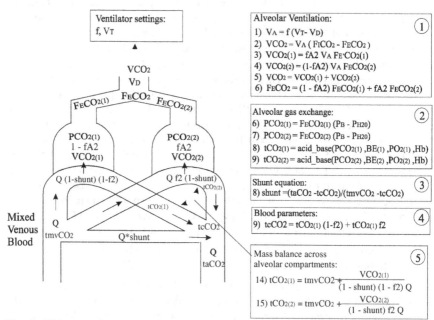

Fig. 2. CO2 transport across the lungs. All variables are described in the text except for f2, which is a fraction of non-shunted blood flow and is fixed at f2=0.9. The function acid_base seen in equations 8 and 9 is a solution of the acid base model of blood described previously [4].

Table 1. Parameters estimates and predicted (p) and measured (m) blood values in patients 1-5.

	Pt. 1		Pt. 2		Pt.3		Pt. 4		Pt. 5	
Shunt (%)	21.5		26.0		42.0		24.0		49.9	
fA2	0.33		0.40		0.58		0.48		0.30	
V_D (l)	0.16		0.18		0.28		0.3		0.5	
V_D / V_T	0.40		0.28		0.36		0.36		0.69	
Q(l/min)	9.6		6.5		11.0		9.0		7.0	
Comp (l/cmH20)	0.019		0.032		0.033		0.055		0.052	
Res (cmH20/l/s)	26.4		25.3		6.5		5.7		5.3	
Rq	0.59		0.83		1.1		0.80		0.81	
VCO_2 (l/min)	0.171		0.244		0.279		0.313		0.121	
VO_2 (l/min)	0.289		0.294		0.251		0.393		0.150	
pHa (m)	7.421		7.459		7.411		7.39		7.289	
PCO_2a (kPa) (m)	6.19		4.83		5.37		4.18		7.61	
SO_2a (%) (m)	96.4		96.2		96.1		95.8		92.7	
PHcv (m/p)	7.404	7.408	7.419	7.425	7.369	7.381	7.347	7.363	7.273	7.273
PCO_2cv (kPa) (m/p)	6.55	6.53	5.56	5.53	6.16	5.97	5.03	4.80	8.03	8.09
SO_2cv (%) (m/p)	74.8	75.8	69.6	68.3	78.2	78.5	74.2	70.7	78.3	78.1
$FECO_2$ (%) (m/p)	6.2	4.7	3.7	3.3	4.4	4.4	3.1	3.2	4.7	4.9

4 Discussion

This paper presents the approach included in INVENT for estimating parameters describing patients' ventilatory (shunt, fA2, VD, Comp, Res), circulatory (Q), and metabolic (VO_2, VCO_2) state from measurements typical in an ICU. The method assumes that there are single values of these parameters describing the transport of both O_2 and CO_2, so that a simultaneous fit of models of both these systems should provide a consistent picture of the patients' pathophysiological state. The method has been shown to provide reasonable parameter estimates and fit for the data of five ICU patients.

The method presented here might be used to monitor changes in physiological parameters due to therapy, or to justify placing a PA catheter. In the haemodynamically stable patients presented here central venous blood might approximate mixed venous [5]. In cases of cardiac or septic shock perfusion of the inferior and superior caval veins may be altered and this may no longer be true [5]. A PA catheter is then required to estimate Q. The method presented here may be used to justify the placement of this catheter, i.e. it is only required if no reasonable parameter values can be found which explain all the data. This is illustrated in patient 5 where extremely low values of VO_2 and VCO_2 are consistent with either abnormal tissue metabolism, or central venous blood gasses not reflecting mixed venous. Both interpretations suggest that the patient is severely ill and that a PA catheter may be justified. Ideally, to test this method studies should be conducted comparing parameters obtained using invasive and non-invasive measurements. This is difficult, as placement of a PA catheter in stable patients is somewhat unethical. Newer methods of estimating Q based upon partial CO_2 rebreathing or thermodilution with femoral arterial sampling may provide alternative measurements of Q by which to compare the method presented here.

Acknowledgements. This work was supported by the Danish Technical Research Council.

References

1.   Rudowski R, East TD, Gardener RM. Current status of mechanical ventilation decision support systems: a review. Int. J. Clin. Monit. Comput. 1996; 13:157-166.
2.   Rees S.E., Andreassen S, Freundlich M, et al. Selecting ventilator settings using INVENT, a system including physiological models and penalty functions. AIMDM'99 - Joint conference of European societies of Artificial Intelligance in Medicine and Medical Decision Making. Workshop, Computers in Anaesthesia and Intensive Care, 20-24th June 1999.
3.   Kjærgaard S, Rees SE, Nielsen JA, et al. Modelling of hypoxaemia after gynaecological laparotomy. Acta Anaesthesiol. Scand. 2001; 45(3):349-3564 .
4.   Rees S E, Andreassen S, Hovorka R et al. A dynamic model of carbon dioxide transport in the blood. In: D. Linkens and E.R.Carson (Eds). Proceedings of the 3rd International Federation of Automatic Control (IFAC) symposium on Modelling and Control in Biomedical Systems, Elsevier (1997), 63-68.
5.   Vincent JL. Does central venous oxygen saturation accurately reflect mixed venous oxygen saturation? Nothing is simple, unfortunately. Int. Care Med. 1992; 18:386-387.

A User Interface for Executing Asbru Plans

Robert Kosara and Silvia Miksch

Institute of Software Technology
Vienna University of Technology, Austria
{rkosara, silvia}@ifs.tuwien.ac.at
http://www.ifs.tuwien.ac.at/~{rkosara, silvia}/

Abstract. Asbru is a language for specifying treatment plans. These plans are then used by an execution unit to give advice to the medical staff what actions to take (open-loop system). In order to do this, the execution unit has to monitor patient data and needs to be informed about the duration and success of actions.

This communication requires a flexible and adaptive user interface that 1) makes it possible to understand which information is currently needed most urgently, and 2) allows the user to tell it the outcome of treatment steps he or she has performed. It must also be possible to simulate patient parameters for testing treatment plans prior to actual clinical trials.

We present a user interface, called AsbrUI, that meets these criteria.

1   Introduction

Asbru [5,6] is a plan-specification language for defining clinical protocols. A clinical protocol is usually translated into many Asbru plans that contain small units of the treatment and information about how they work together. This knowledge acquisition and translation is supported by a visual tool named AsbruView [3].

The execution of these plans is monitored and controlled by an execution unit that gives advice to medical staff based on the procedures laid down in Asbru plans. This is called an *open-loop system*, as opposed to a *closed-loop system* where no human is involved who can check proposed settings or steps before they are performed.

The execution unit needs information about the patient, only a part of which can be acquired automatically. It also needs information about actions the medical staff has performed, and their outcome. The user interface for the execution unit is called AsbrUI, and is described in this paper. Because we are still in the design phase of AsbrUI, all images presented in this paper are mock-ups.

2   Related Work

There is a user interface for PROforma [1], which allows the definition and execution of plans. But it does not show when a data item that it requests is needed, nor does it provide a way of aborting or suspending user actions.

S. Quaglini, P. Barahona, and S. Andreassen (Eds.): AIME 2001, LNAI 2101, pp. 136–139, 2001.
© Springer-Verlag Berlin Heidelberg 2001

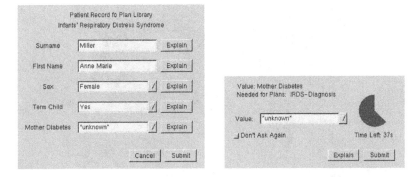

Fig. 1. Patient record input windows. Left: The complete patient record as shown when the first plan ist started. Right: The execution unit asks for a specific value.

There is also a strict distinction between diagnosis and treatment phases in PROforma, which is the reason for parameter input during plan execution not being supported in this interface. To the best of our knowledge, there is no runtime support appropriate for the medical staff for either GLIF [4] or the Arden Syntax [2].

3 Data Acquisition

Two different types of data are acquired by AsbrUI: Entries in the patient record and parameters.

Patient Record. In Asbru, the patient record not only contains information like the name, date of birth, etc. of the patient, but can also contain additional information like if the patient has a genetic predisposition to a certain disease. A form (Figure 1, left) is shown at the start of the first plan, where the information for the current patient can be entered. Information that is not entered here but is later on needed is requested with the form shown in Figure 1, right.

Manual Parameters. Parameters are all data that comes from the patient, rather than being generated in the execution unit (program variables). Manual parameters are parameters that cannot be acquired automatically. The execution unit asks the user interface for values, and gives it the latest point in time, when the value must be available. This "latest point in time" is determined depending on the context the parameter is used in. For example, if a parameter has a certain sampling period, the end of the current sampling interval is the deadline for this value. AsbrUI then provides an input mask (Figure 2a, right) which tells the user about the time constraint and allows input of the value and the time when the value was actually acquired (this is important for tests that take longer, like blood samples). The users are warned if the deadline for a value is less than a certain pre-specified amount of time away. This is done by displaying a circle

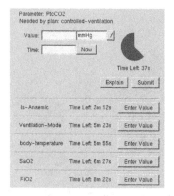
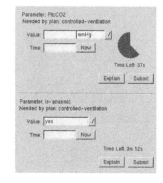

a) The list of currently needed parameters (left) and input fields for single values (right)

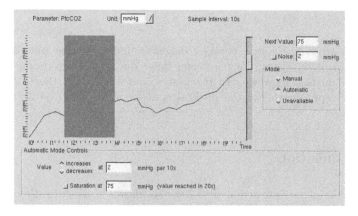

b) The environment simulator in automatic mode.

Fig. 2. Parts of AsbrUI: manual parameters and the environment simulator.

for each minute in that time span, with the last one being "cut" to reflect the amount of seconds still left in that minute.

Usually, of course, there will be more than just one parameter that the execution unit is waiting for. AsbrUI sorts the list of asked parameters by their urgency (Figure 2, left) and also lists the plans that need that parameter, so that the user knows what the value is needed for.

Automatic Parameters and the Environment Simulator. Automatic parameters are usually acquired by devices rather than entered manually. For testing of plans, it is useful to be able to also control the values of these parameters, so that different paths through the plan can be tried out. Each automatic parameter is displayed in the environment simulator (Figure 2b) as a function over time. The value that will be fed into the abstraction unit at the next sampling point can be set manually, automatically, or be set to "unavailable".

4   Plan Execution Control

Manual plans need approval by a user before they can be started. AsbrUI displays simple dialog boxes for this case, where the user can allow or deny a plan from running. This is more complicated when such plans are part of a parallel plan. In this case, a dialog is shown that allows the user to select which subplans of that parallel plan to start (not shown due to space restrictions).

The execution unit monitors patient data while a user-performed plan is active, but does not necessarily know when it is complete or when it has to be aborted, because not all conditions might be filled with enough information or the user might decide to abort or complete a plan regardless of fulfilled conditions. For this purpose, AsbrUI uses a dialog that allows the user to suspend, abort and complete user-performed plans (not shown due to space restrictions).

5   Conclusions and Future Work

We have presented a part of a user interface design for the execution of Asbru plans. It is able to provide the user with information he or she needs to make needed data available on time, and to control the control flow for manual plans.

The obvious next step is to implement AsbrUI and test it together with the execution unit that is in development in real-world scenarios.

Acknowledgments. This work is part of the Asgaard Project, supported by "Fonds zur Förderung der wissenschaftlichen Forschung" (Austrian Science Fund), grant P12797-INF.

References

1. John Fox and Subrata Das. *Safe and Sound: Artificial Intelligence in Hazardous Applications.* MIT Press, 2000.
2. George Hripcsak, Peter Ludemann, T. Allan Pryor, Ove B. Wigertz, and Paul D. Clayton. Rationale for the Arden syntax. *Computers and Biomedical Research,* 27:291–324, 1994.
3. Robert Kosara and Silvia Miksch. Metaphors of movement: A visualization and user interface for time-oriented, skeletal plans. *Artificial Intelligence in Medicine, Special Issue on Information Visualization in Medicine,* 22(2):111–131, 2001.
4. Lucila Ohno-Machado, John H. Gennari, Shawn Murphy, Nilesh L. Jain, Samson W. Tu, Diane E. Oliver, Edward Pattison-Gordon, Robert A. Greenes, Edward H. Shortliffe, and G. Octo Barnett. The guideline interchange format: A model for representing guidelines. *JAMIA,* 5(4):357–372, 1998.
5. Andreas Seyfang, Robert Kosara, and Silvia Miksch. Asbru's reference manual, Asbru version 7.2. Technical Report Asgaard-TR-2000-3, Vienna University of Technology, Institute of Software Technology, 2000.
6. Yuval Shahar, Silvia Miksch, and Peter Johnson. The Asgaard project: A task-specific framework for the application and critiquing of time-oriented clinical guidelines. *Artificial Intelligence in Medicine,* 14:29–51, 1998.

Improving HISYS1 with a Decision Support System

David Riaño[1] and Susana Prado[2]

[1] Universitat Rovira i Virgili, Carretera de Salou s/n, 43006 Tarragona, Spain,
drianyo@etse.urv.es,
[2] Informática El Corte Inglés, Bolivia 234, 08020 Barcelona, Spain
susana_prado@ieci.es

Abstract. HISYS1 is an information system that physicians, hospital managers and health-care administrations can use to analyze the data about the evolution of the admitted patients in a hospital. The system is enriched with a learning procedure that is able both to extract knowledge about the hospital departments, and also to organize that knowledge in a module-based Decision Support System (DSS) that is used to predict the evolution of the new patients. We have tested the system with six primary diagnoses at the Hospital Joan XXIII in Tarragona (Spain).

1 Introduction

Hospitals are complex systems in which patients, physicians, hospital managers, and public health-care administrations interact.

Whereas patients and physicians are concerned about the best medical care, managers and public administrations go after the cost reduction, mainly. These two points of view give rise to faced up decisions as whether an expensive drug must be prescribed or whether a medical test must be done or not. Therefore, many hospital decisions are a trade off between excellence and cost.

As far as the application of computers in hospitals is concerned, these two points of view divide computer software applications in medicine into those which are based on the database technologies [1], and those which are based on artificial intelligence [2][3].

The evolution of the patients uses to be represented by a sequence of records that show a *dynamic* appearance of the data. Moreover, medical *cost evaluation*, *quality measurement* and *path analysis* can be not only calculated but also predicted if some artificial intelligence methodologies as *intelligent data analysis* are used to work with the dynamic data.

The organization of this paper is as follows. Section 2 broadly describes the system HISYS1 [5] which is used to host some intelligent data analysis abilities that are introduced in section 3. This section is also introduces the automatic construction of a decision-support system that is evaluated with the data of the patients of the Hospital Joan XXIII in Tarragona (Spain). The results are given in section 4. Finally, section 5 shows the conclusions.

S. Quaglini, P. Barahona, and S. Andreassen (Eds.): AIME 2001, LNAI 2101, pp. 140–143, 2001.
© Springer-Verlag Berlin Heidelberg 2001

2   The HISYS1 System

Hospitals store data about the admitted patients. *Static data* is the information that do not depend on a particular admission: *personal data* as age, sex, address, phone number, bank account, etc. or *clinical data* as the case history and the antecedents. *Dynamic data* is related to a particular admission; for example, the *admission number*, the *primary diagnosis*, and the *primary procedure* that patients receive when they are admitted.

HISYS1 [5] is a tool that combines the static and the dynamic data of the patients. HISYS1 represents the patient transitions as a path in a flowchart where nodes are admissions, hospital services and discharge reasons, and arrows are patient transitions within the hospital. Each node stores information about the number of patients visiting the node, the number of days and cost of all the stays, and the sets of secondary diagnoses, procedures and physicians involved. Each arrow stores the detailed static and dynamic data of the patients that pass through it. Moreover, HISYS1 has operations to handle the flowcharts, see [5].

Physicians and managers use HISYS1 to find out the patient circuits, detect bottlenecks and anomalies, see the patient final destination, analyze marginal costs, to highlight re-admissions and effective treatments, calculate the effective average stay in a hospital service, and predict the new patient transitions, etc. Many of these uses could not be achieved with a database approach, therefore HISYS1 extends and eases the analysis of the hospital costs and quality [6].

3   Improving HISYS1 with a DSS

In spite of the benefits that HISYS1 gives to the hospital staff, there are some additional improvements that can increase the abilities of HISYS1. These improvements come from the application of machine learning and knowledge organization to the patient information stored in the arrows of the flowcharts.

3.1   The Learning Process

A HISYS1 flowchart represents the evolution of all the patients which are admitted with a particular primary diagnosis, in a selected period of time.

For each non terminal node of a flowchart, a data matrix is generated that contains the static and dynamic data of all the patients leaving the node. Outgoing arrows are used to distinguish patient types, so a supervised data matrix is obtained. Then, the CN2 [4] inductive learning algorithm is applied and a set of unordered rules is extracted. These rules represent the next transition of the patients that have passed through a flowchart node. Rules predict the future transitions of the new patients arriving.

3.2   The Knowledge Organization

Actually, the hospital Joan XXIII has 57 services and a catalogue of 14,091 feasible diagnoses attended in the hospital. Although not all of them have enough cases as to deserve a data analysis with HISYS1, the number of feasible uses of the learning process explained in 3.1 is high.

Rule sets are organized in a knowledge-base system. The process is divided into four automatic stages. *Relation*, the user chooses the diagnoses $d_1, ..., d_k$ that he wants to study. *Graphic*, a flowchart is generated for each diagnosis. For all the initial nodes of all the flowcharts, the learning process is applied and k rule sets $C_1, ..., C_k$, describing initial admissions, are obtained. For all the intermediate nodes of the flowcharts, the learning process is also applied. *Learning*, a rule set is filled with the distribution rules IF primary_diagnosis = d_i THEN class = C_i, $(i = 1, ..., k)$. Finally, the last stage makes a hierarchy with all the rule sets. On the top, the distribution rules decide the initial C_i that HISYS1 must apply. In the second level, the initial C_i indicates which is the hospital service that will attend the patient (intermediate rule sets). Then, the rules indicate the transfer between hospital services until the patient is discharged.

3.3   The Decision-Support System

HISYS1 has been modified to integrate the above hierarchy of rule sets in order to use it as a decision-support system (DSS). Figure 1 shows the new DSS window of HISYS1 which was obtained with the rule sets of all the patients of the hospital that were admitted in 1999 with the diagnoses that table 1 codifies.

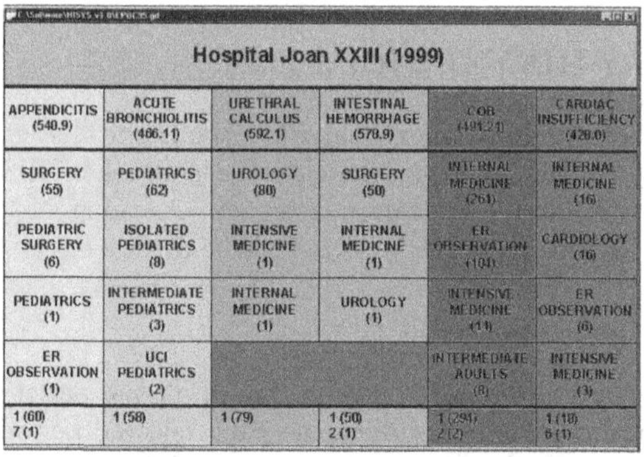

Fig. 1. DSS for the Hospital Joan XXIII in 1999.

All the blocks are sensitive and they are input points to the DSS. Whenever a block is pressed, a template is displayed to collect the data of a new patient. Then, a prediction is made for this patient with the rule set related to the block pressed. Predictions can be chained in a temporal sequence.

Physicians and hospital managers use the DSS to detect patient patterns, abstract common features of patient subgroups, obtain explanations about the patient and hospital transitions, study the hospital casuistry (*case mix*), and compare the activities of two hospitals.

4   Tests and Results

Two DSS were generated with the patients of the Hospital Joan XXIII (Spain) for the diagnoses of appendicitis (540.9), acute bronchiolitis (466.11), urethral calculus (592.1), intestinal hemorrhage (578.9), COB (491.21), and cardiac insufficiency (428.0). The first DSS was trained with the patients in 1998 and tested with the patients in 1999, and the second DSS the opposite. The DSS accuracies were studied separately for the hospital services and globally for the whole treatment. Table 1 shows the global accuracies.

Table 1. Global accuracy in 1998 and 1999.

year	540.9	466.11	592.1	578.9	491.21	428.0
1998	98.30%	87.25%	98.75%	96.01%	73.50%	70.15%
1999	96.30%	100.0%	97.50%	93.50%	71.10%	63.67%

Structural changes between the 1998 and the 1999 protocols of the *internal medicine* and *ER* services affected the cardiac insufficiency and COB results which showed low accuracies. The rest of predictions show high accuracies.

5   Conclusions

AI can be used to analyze the internal activity of the hospitals. Whereas static data is suitable to discover domain and diagnostic knowledge, dynamic data is useful to obtain predictive and hospital functioning knowledge.

Here, we describe a new functionality of HISYS1 that applies CN2 [4] to make rules that predict transfers within a hospital. The rules are organized in a hierarchical module-based DSS that is tested with real data.

This work was supported by the CICyT project SMASH (TIC96-1038-04), IECISA and the *Hospital Joan XXIII*. The authors want to express gratitude to Dr. X. Allué, head of the Pediatric Service, to Dr. Olona, head of the Epidemiology Unit, and to D. Pi.

References

1. Dick, R. S., Steen, E. B.: The computer-based record. Institute of Medicine. National Academic Press. Washington (1991)
2. Lavrač, N.: Selected techniques for DM in medicine. AI Med. **16** (1999) 3–23
3. Miksch, S.: Plan management in the medical domain. AI Com. **12** (1999) 209–235
4. Clark, P., Niblett, T.: The CN2 induction algorithm. ML **3**(4) (1989) 261–283
5. Riaño, D., Prado, S.: A DM alternative to model hospital operations: filtering, adaptation, and behaviour prediction. LNCS **1933** (2000) 293–299
6. Riaño, D., Prado, S.: The analysis of healt care data with HISYS1. Submited to the International Conference on Medical Information, MedInfo, London (2001)

Diagnosis of Iron-Deficiency Anemia in Hemodialyzed Patients through Support Vector Machines Technique

Paola Baiardi[1], Valter Piazza[2], and Maria C. Mazzoleni[1]

[1] Salvatore Maugeri Foundation, IRCCS , Medical Informatics Unit, Via Ferrata 8, 27100
Pavia, Italy
{pbaiardi, cmazzoleni }@fsm.it
[2] Salvatore Maugeri Foundation, IRCCS , Nephrology Unit, Via Ferrata 8,
27100 Pavia, Italy
vpiazza@fsm.it

Abstract. Support Vector Machines (SVMs) technique is a recent method for
empirical data modelling applied to pattern recognition problems. The aim of
the present study is to test SVMs performance when applied to a specific medical classification problem – diagnosis of iron-deficiency anemia in uremic patients - and to compare the results with those obtained by traditional techniques
such as logistic regression and discriminant analysis. Models have been compared both in learning and validation phases. All methods performed well (accuracy > 80%). Sensibility of SVMs is always higher than the ones of the other
models; specificity and accuracy are lower in one repetition over three. Within
the limits of the present study, we can say that the SVMs can constitute an innovative method to approach clinical classification problem on which to further
invest.

1 Introduction

Patients with chronic renal failure treated by maintenance hemodialysis frequently
suffer from iron-deficiency anemia. In order to evaluate iron status in uremic patients,
serum ferritin (SF) is reported to be the best indicator of body iron stores even if some
patients, when given iron therapy, do not improve anemia in spite of low SF levels.
Other iron status values such as corpuscular indexes, serum iron, transferrin saturation
are advocated by some authors as more reliable parameters to iron deficiency [1]. The
correct classification of iron status may then be treated as a pattern classification
problem, in which iron-deficiency anemia should be revealed starting from a series of
independent variables. Potential usefulness of analytic methods can be considered and
tested in an attempt to better predict response to iron therapy in uremic patients.

The aim of the present study is to test SVMs performance, a recent technique for
empirical data modelling developed by Vapnik [2], when applied to a specific medical
classification problem, and to compare the results with those obtained by traditional
techniques such as logistic regression and discriminant analysis.

S. Quaglini, P. Barahona, and S. Andreassen (Eds.): AIME 2001, LNAI 2101, pp. 144–147, 2001.
© Springer-Verlag Berlin Heidelberg 2001

2   Methods

Ninety-two uremic patients on chronic hemodialysis at our Centre were enrolled. Eligibility criteria were: hemoglobin (Hb) concentrations in the 8-10 g/dl range and SF levels below 100 µg/L. Exclusion criteria were: assumption of erythropoietin or androgen therapy, presence of inflammatory and hepatic diseases and transfusion in the previous months. Subjects received 1 mg/kg of i.v. iron at the end of 20 dialytic sessions; for each patient the study period lasted 4 months, inclusive of 7 weeks of iron therapy and of the follow-up period. Patients were classified as suffering or not from iron-deficiency anemia according to their response to iron therapy, being the response evaluated as difference from baseline of peak Hb value in the follow-up period.

A dichotomic response was identified:

-No Response (NR, no iron-deficiency) if Hb values were reduced, stable or improved of less than 1 g/dl (31 subjects)

-Response (R, iron-deficiency) if Hb levels were steadily improved of at least 2 g/dl (61 subjects).

Ten variables were identified by the medical staff according to literature [1]: log transformed serum ferritin (SF), hemoglobin (Hb), red cells (GR), mean corpuscolar volume (MCV), serum iron (SI), total iron binding capacity (TIBC), hematocrit (HT), mean corpuscolar Hb (MCH), mean corpuscolar Hb concentration (MCHC), transferrin saturation (TSAT).

The problem of classification was faced using the theory of the SVMs with linear approach. Peculiarity of Vapnik technique [2] is its promising generalization performance obtained by minimizing an upper bound on the expected risk (structural risk minimization principle (SRM)) instead of minimizing the error on the training data (empirical risk minimization principle (ERM)). For linear classifier [3], the SRM principle is implemented by determining a hyperplane, named *Optimal Separating Hyperplane* (OSH) which maximize the minimum distance between the two classes (called *margin*) minimizing the classification error. Among all the points of the training set, only a subset is critic in determining the OSH. These points are called the *Support Vectors* (SV). In removing the training patterns that are not SV the solution is unchanged. From a numerical point of view, the SRM principle reduces to solve a constrained optimization problem in which a cost function associated to misclassification is introduced. The OSH can vary according to the variations of a parameter C (regularization parameter of the cost function): OSH maximizes the margin when $C \to 0$ and minimizes the number of misclassified points when $C \to \infty$. A compromise solution occurs for in-between values. It can be demonstrated [4] that it is possible to partition the positive real axis $\Re^+$ in a finite number of disjoined intervals, each characterized by a fixed set of SV and in which the OSH is completely determined.

The first step of our application was to investigate the dependence of OSH on the changes of C. For this purpose, the whole date set was used [4]. Once identified a C value for which the OSH is fixed, such value was used to validate the model.

Since no independent data-set for the testing phase was available, the sample was randomly divided into three subsets subsequently combined two by two to obtain three subsamples for the training phase (about 60 cases) and three independent subsamples for the testing phase (about 30 cases). The SVM model was compared with the linear discriminant and the logistic regression models. Method performances were evaluated in terms of sensibility, specificity and accuracy, both in learning and in validation phase. The software used for the implementation of the SVM model is based on MATLAB routines by Steve Gunn [5] (http://svm.first.gmd.de). Discriminant analysis and logistic regression were performed by SAS software (Proc DISCRIM and Proc LOGISTIC)

3   Results

Univariate (unpaired t test) and multivariate comparisons between R and NR groups showed statistically significant differences between the groups for all the variables (p<0.001) except hemoglobin and hematocrit.

As in literature, when C   the number of classification errors decreased to a minimum (accuracy 91%) and the number of SV is maximum (60 points), while when C 0 the opposite situation occured (48 SV and accuracy 82%). For C>50, SV and accuracy didn't improve any longer, hence C=100 was used for the validation phase.

Sensibility, specificity and accuracy were estimated for both learning and validation phases in three repetitions for each model. Table 1 reports the results.

Table 1. Ranges of sensibility (SE) specificity (SP), classification error (1-accuracy) (CE), False Negative (FN) and False Positive (FP) rates in the three repetitions for the three methods in the training and testing phases.

	Learning			Validation		
	SVM	Discrim	Logistic	SVM	Discrim	Logistic
SE	82.9 - 95.4	80.0 - 93.0	82.8 – 95.4	80.8 – 94.1	69.2 – 83.3	73.1 – 88.2
SP	72.2 - 96.1	72.2 - 88.9	66.7 - 88.5	69.2 - 80.0	69.2 - 84.6	46.1 - 84.6
FN	4.6 - 17.1	7.0 - 20.0	4.6 - 17.2	5.9 - 19.2	16.7 - 30.8	11.8 - 26.9
FP	3.9 - 27.8	11.1 – 30.8	11.5 – 33.3	20.0 – 30.8	15.4 - 30.8	20.0- 53.9
CE	11.3-11.5	11.3 - 16.4	12.9 - 14.7	16.6 - 19.3	16.1 - 29.0	16.1 – 30.0

In general all the methods showed good performances in identifying iron-deficient subjects. SE values were almost always greater than 80%. It must be noted that SVM technique reached the highest values for SE in the validation phase. With the exception of the second test, in which all the methods showed the same performances, SE for SVM methods was 10% higher in both first and third testing.

In terms of SP, lower performances occurred for all the methods. In validation phase the SVMs showed comparable performance with those of the other models, even if inferior in the second testing.

4   Discussion and Conclusion

Statistical methods could turn out to be useful in order to support medical diagnostic process, once an exhaustively validated model is available. The models here tested confirmed that contemporary evaluation of all the indexes of iron status supplies useful contribute to the problem of the correct diagnosis of iron-deficiency anemia in hemodialyzed population. Our results seem to confirm the best performances of the SVMs in comparison with those of the other tested models, when linear relationship is superimposed among the input variables.

Some considerations should however be done. First, the hemodialyzed population is, for nature, limited: our hemodialysis unit takes care of 150 patients whose turnover is quite low. These patients, during their dialytic life, can be affected by problems of anemia more than once. Building the dataset for this study, only the first occurrence of anemia for each patient was considered in order to preserve the independence of the observations, leading to the limited number of recruited cases and the lack of independent data-sets for the evaluation phase. Second, the application of a re-sampling method would constitute, in absence of independent large data-sets, a better approach to evaluate generalization performance of the investigated models.

Next steps could be the planning of a multi-center study to enlarge the samples and to evaluate the opportunity of modifying the SVM model, in order to consider an ordinal response to iron therapy instead of the dicothomic one.

Within the limits of the present study, we can say that the SVMs can constitute an innovative method to approach clinical classification problem on which to invest. The greatest limitations to the use of such techniques may derive from 1) the complexity of calculation involved when the sample size increases (millions of SV), and 2) the implementation of non-linear relationships [6].

References

1. Allegra V., Mengozzi G., Vasile A. *Iron deficiency in maintenance hemodialysis patients: assessment of diagnosis criteria and of three different iron treatments.* Nephron 57: 175-182, 1991.
2. Vapnik V. *The Nature of Statistical Learning Theory.* Springer-Verlag, 1995.
3. Cortes C. e Vapnik V. *Support Vector Networks.* Machine Learning 20:273-297, 1995.
4. Pontil M., Verri A. *Properties of Support Vector Machines.* Neural Computation 10: 955-974, 1998.
5. Gunn S.R. *Support Vector Machines for Classification and Regression. Technical Report.* Image Speech and Intelligent Systems Research Group, University of Southampton, 1997.
6. Scholkopf B., Simard P., Smola A., Vapnik V. *Prior knowledge in support vector kernels.* In: M. Jordan, M. Kearns and S. Solla eds, Advances in Neural Information Processing Systems 10, Cambridge, MA, MIT Press, 1998.

A Visual Tool for a User-Friendly Artificial Neural Network Based Decision Support System in Medicine

Mauro Giacomini, Raffaella Michelini, Francesca Deantoni,
and Carmelina Ruggiero

Dept. of Communication Computer and System Science - University of Genova
Via Opera Pia 13 16145 Genova Italy
giacomin@dist.unige.it

Abstract. A system has been set up in which data obtained from previously treated patients and stored into a data base are used to enable medical doctors to set up decision support systems based on artificial neural networks.The system contains a graphical interface in Visual Basic, a graphical interface in Matlab and a Visual Basic Tool for an easy to understand visualization of neural network outputs. The system has been tested using data from patients treated in the Esophageal Surgical Unit of School of Medicine of University of Genova in the period 1996 - 2000.

1 Introduction

One of the major issues in IT-strategy is the Electronic Patient Record (EPR) implementation in hospitals, as EPR is expected to become the driving force in a process leading to improved efficiency and better quality of health care. However, improved efficiency and quality of health care is not an automatic consequence of introducing IT-applications like EPR. Several prerequisites related to organisational development and individual competencies are necessary in order to make most EPR systems efficient [1]. One way to innovate health care is to consider information as a fourth resource ranking equally with the traditional three key resources: people, money and physical resources [2]. Medical decision is a difficult and complex task, largely empirically based and poorly understood. During the last three decades a great amount of research has been devoted to the development of methodologies able to cope with complex problems such as medical decision making [3]. One of the recent developments in this area is the integration of clinical decision support systems and EPR [4]. The basic idea behind computer-assisted medical problem solving is to use data obtained from the clinical study of previously treated patients to predict the most likely diagnosis and treatment alternatives in new patients [5] [6]. We have many tools for EPR collection and for applied decision support systems, but their use in a clinical environment is quite limited, above all for research purposes. The aim of the paper is the description of a set of tools for a user friendly management of clinical decision making based both on data base management systems, for data collection, and on artificial neural networks for data classification.

S. Quaglini, P. Barahona, and S. Andreassen (Eds.): AIME 2001, LNAI 2101, pp. 148–151, 2001.
© Springer-Verlag Berlin Heidelberg 2001

2   Materials and Methods

The system can be divided into four main parts:

- A graphical interface in Visual Basic to help insert and control data in a Microsoft Access database
- A graphical interface in Visual Basic for extracting data in order to organize a file for artificial neural network learn/test.
- A graphical interface in Matlab to make artificial neural network running easier.
- A Visual Basic tool for an easy to understand visualization of artificial neural network's output.

2.1   The Artificial Neural Network

The combination of clinical and algorithm diagnosis can contribute in the decrease of doubtful and incorrectly classified patients and add weight to the work of the physician in the vast majority of cases. There are three important rules to observe in choosing medical data to form a good learning set: they should be **Homogeneous**, **Significant** and **Representative**. The system has been designed in order to use both supervised and unsupervised type of networks. The interaction between physician and the neural network begins with a Matlab graphical interface made of two main buttons for each type of network: LEARN and TEST. Before starting the learning process it is necessary to set up network properties: some fields are read only and others are connected to properties which can be tuned up such as the number of learning epochs, visualization frequency, number of neurons(in each row for Kohonen network and hidden neurons for supervised), error goal, starting eta and transfer function. To prevent improper values of these parameters a control mechanism has been implemented which, through a series of error messages, does not allow the user to start the network if everything is not set properly. Moreover, a set of default values has been given. When the test is completed the weights and all other network parameters are saved in a standard Matlab data file. This file will allow the user to apply the learnt network for further use. During the test period Matlab asks the user to choose two files: the first containing weights that have been stored during the learning phase and the second containing data to classify. When the test is completed the outputs of the network are stored in a results file. This file maintains Matlab format which can be considered as cryptic by most of physicians, so we decided to set up another part of our system in order to make the network results easily readable for everybody.

2.2   The Automatic Interpreter

As data interpretation needs to rely on information stored into database the implementation has been directly performed in Visual Basic. Supervised network produces an output table. Its interpretation consists in building up a new table with additional information. Specifically, an identification column and two result columns: the first containing the chosen class, the second its reliability based on the differences between the first and second neuron highest output value. Kohonen network's output is a three column table:

- The first row contains the index of the considered pattern in the input list, in order to assign to this pattern the correct key which identifies it within the database
- The second row contains the number of neurons to which the pattern has been assigned
- The third row contains the reliability of the assignment of the pattern to the considered neuron.

The output table formalism is then translated into a more understandable map (in Microsoft Excel) in which the 2D structure is maintained. The user can chose which type of information the system should store in these maps, typically it can be patient Id or some features that can be classified by the network (for example the species in a taxonomy application). Homogeneous areas of the map are then colored in order to increase the intelligibility of the output.

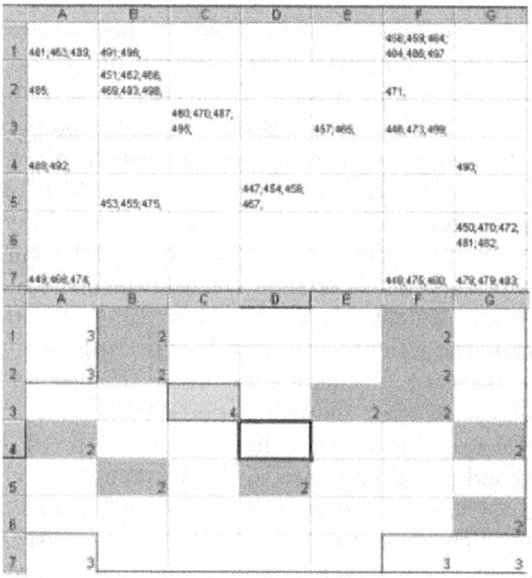

Fig. 1. The first half contains the map with patients identification numbers while the second half represents the security level of the considered pirosis symptoms.

3   Results

The system is still in its implementation phase. Nevertheless, a prototype framework has already been tested in a pre-release version at the Esophageal Surgical Unit of School of Medicine of the University of Genova to find possible qualitative correlations between Gastro Esophageal Related Disease (GERD) symptoms and functional results from esophageal manometry and 24 -hour esophageal-gastric pH - monitoring. Patients, aged between 20 and 85 years were requested to answer an anamnestic questionnaire and were submitted to esophageal manometric and pH - metric testing. A relational database records both instrumental results, collected with specific direct connections, and symptoms represented within the database with a semi quantitative scale filled by the clinician who perform the direct examination. Also, in order to test the decision support part of the system we selected 53 patients from a group of 500 with the following features:

- date of treatment: between the 1st of January, 2000 and the 31st of December, 2000
- presence of G.E.R.D. symptoms
- absence of esophageal and gastric surgical operations

The result maps are shown in fig. 1

4   Conclusions

The present paper joins together database, clinical record and artificial neural network based approaches into a comprehensive decision support system. The system has been designed in order to overcome problems often faced by medical doctors who lack understanding of the methods used by the system when using computer aided diagnosis. In this respect the learning from example features of artificial neural networks are used to obtain high user friendly feature for the system.

References

1. Kokol, P., Zupan, B.,Stare, J., Premik, M., and Engelbrecht, R., editors. Clinicians Must Invest Resources when Implementing Electronic Patient Records. 1999; 824 p. Studies in Health Technology and Informatics.
2. Best DP. Best DP, editors. The fourth resource.Information and his management. Aslib/Gower; 1996; 1,Business Process and Information Management.
3. Y. Reisman "Computer-Based Clinical Decision Aids. A Review of Methods and Assessment of Systems". Medical Informatics, 1996, vol. 21, n. 3, pp. 179-197
4. J.C. Wyatt "Clinical Data System, Part 1: Data and Medical Records". Lancet, 1994, vol. 344, pp. 1543 - 1546
5. W.W. Daniel "An introduction to computer-assisted diagnosis". Journal of Medical Association Georgia, 1979, vol 68, n. 4, pp. 285-289
6. C.A. Kulikowski "Computer systems that learn: classification and prediction methods from statistic, neural net, machine learning and expert system" Morsa Kaufmann 1980 (San Matteo - CA - USA).

Modeling of Ventricular Repolarisation Time Series by Multi-layer Perceptrons

Rajai El Dajani[1,2], Maryvonne Miquel[1,2], Marie-Claire Forlini[2], and Paul Rubel[1,2]

[1] INSA de Lyon,LISI, Bat 501, 20 avenue Albert Einstein, 69621 Villeurbanne, France
rmourid@lisi.insa-lyon.fr
miquel@if.insa-lyon.fr
rubel@insa.insa-lyon.fr
http://lisi.insa-lyon.fr
[2] INSERM ERM107, 28 avenue Doyen Lépine, 69500 Bron, France
forlini@insa.insa-lyon.fr
http://www.inserm.fr

Abstract. The QT interval measured on the body-surface Electrocardiogram (ECG), corresponds to the time elapsed between the depolarization of the first myocardial ventricular cell (beginning of the Q wave) and the end of the repolarisation of the last ventricular cell (end of the T wave). Predictive models of the QT dynamical behavior are believed to be a useful tool to detect abnormalities in QT adaptation for heart rate changes. In this paper, patient specific predictive models based on a Multi Layer Perceptrons are presented and their predictive performances are tested on real and artificial data.

1   Introduction

One of the main reasons for the cardiologists increasing interest in measuring the QT interval on the ECG is that its prolongation might trigger cardiac arrhythmias like ventricular fibrillation and *torsades de pointes,* the main causes of sudden death [1].

The QT duration is influenced principally by the inverse of the heart rate, measured by the RR duration between two successive heart beats. None of the formulas previously proposed for the adjustment of QT for changes in heart rate provide satisfactory correction [2].

The conception of non-invasive predictive models of the QT dynamics in function of the changes of RR should allow to detect life-threatening variations of the QT duration by comparing the predicted value (the expected one) to the real measured one. But up to now the only way for studying the ventricles response to sudden heart rate changes are invasive electrophysiology techniques.

In this paper we propose to model the QT dynamic behaviour in function of the history of RR intervals by means of Multi Layer Perceptrons (MLP), chosen for their capacity to approximate any non-linear function with excellent accuracy. The networks will be trained to learn the following non-linear patient specific relationship:

$$QT_i = f(RR_i, RR_{i-1}, ..., RR_{i-M+1}, RR_{i-M})   \tag{1}$$

where M is a time delay.

S. Quaglini, P. Barahona, and S. Andreassen (Eds.): AIME 2001, LNAI 2101, pp. 152–155, 2001.

2   Methods

2.1   Multi-layer Perceptron

To determine the value of the delay M and the number of neurons in the hidden layer, two 20 minute duration ECG sequences belonging to patient "Clav" were selected. These sequences, recorded at 4:25 am and at 6:05 am, were used respectively as training and test sets. The measure used for the evaluation of the performance of the training was the mean square error (MSE).

Several MLPs have been trained by varying the delay M from one minute up to eight minutes and the number of hidden neurons from 1 to 22. The best results in learning the training set and in predicting the test set were obtained for an MLP with 120 entry neurons (M=4 minutes) and 10 hidden neurons.

2.2   Real and Artificial Data Description

Several 20 minute duration ECG sequences were chosen within a set of six 24 hour Holter recordings from six patients without heart disease. The RR and QT time series of the corresponding ECG sequences were calculated using the "Lyon System" and the "Caviar" methods [3], low-pass filtered at 0.05Hz to eliminate the high frequency (HF) and low frequencies (LF) components corresponding to the parasympathic (HF) and the sympathic (LF) activities [4], and resampled at 0.5 Hz.

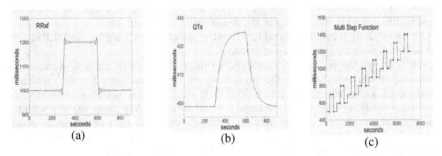

Fig. 1. Artificial data: (a) RRsf: step impulse filtered at 0.05Hz; (b) QTs: simulated first order one minute time constant response; (c) eight step functions centered on several RR values.

The neural networks were trained on two night sequences of patients Clav and Gard and tested on the other night sequences of these patients and on the night sequences of the other 4 patients. The prediction capacities of the two neural models have also been tested on artificial data simulating several additional RR and QT time series, build to cover all possible RR and QT ranges of variation usually found in invasive electrophysiology settings. Examples of simulated data are displayed in figure 1.

3   Results

Learning was performed on an original signal sequence of patients "Clav" and "Gard", respectively recorded at 4:25 and 05:54 am, giving rise to two predictive models, respectively called CC and GD.

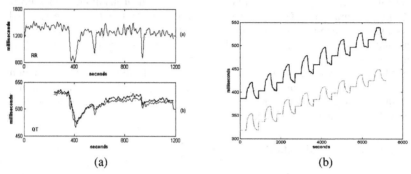

Fig. 2. Prediction results for the CC model: (a) real RR and QT in full line and predicted QT in dotted line; (b) predicted QT in full line and simulated multi step QT response in dotted line.

Figure 2(a) shows the result of the CC network prediction for the Clav RR sequence recorded at 7:35 am. The dynamic behavior of the predicted QT (QTp) follows closely the real QT variations, with a standard deviation of the prediction error of 3.5 msec. The vertical shift between the two signals is due to a different time recording and to differences in the activity of the neurovegetative system [4].

From figure 2(b), it can be noticed that the step response predicted by the MLP is very close to a first order system step response.

Table 1 shows the prediction results for a subset of the tested night sequences. All standard deviations (StD) of the prediction error are less than 5 msec, which is considered as an acceptable result. This 5 msec limit was set experimentally, by carefully verifying each predicted sequence and by comparing them visually with the original recordings. The best prediction results are obtained when applying the neural network models on sequences belonging to the same patient for which the training was preformed, CC on Clav sequences and GD on Gard sequences.

Table 1. Standard deviations (StD) of the prediction error for night sequences belonging to non-pathological patients. Data in bold italic correspond to the learning sets, the other to the test sets. All values are in msec.

Patient	Sex	Age	Time of Recording	CC model StD	GD model StD
Clav	F	22	03:45	3.40	3.52
			04:25	*2.25*	3.32
			06:05	2.86	3.80
			07:35	3.51	4.50
Gard	F	27	00:45	2.79	2.28
			01:37	3.34	2.29
			02:25	1,93	1.47
			05:54	4.03	*1.90*

4   Discussion

The main finding of the study is that, thanks to the MLPs, we could obtain the same type of step impulse information from ambulatory ECG recordings as the one that are usually obtained during invasive tests [1]. The 4 minutes time delay is coherent with the fact that the step response of a one-minute time constant first order system will reach 98% of the expected amplitude after 4 minutes. The main limitation however is in the difficulty of selecting the most appropriate training sets. The selected ECG sequences should display a large amount of RR and QT variations, and using the totality of the 24H recording for the training won't solve this problem. Automatic methods need to be developed to select RR and QT sequences covering a wide range of variation.

Another feature is the vertical shift between the predicted and the measured QT. This shift depends on the time of the day and on the activity of the central nervous system, and is in itself a valuable measurement that is expected to have a diagnostic importance. The same yields for several additional clinically useful measurements that could be computed for the predicted QT intervals, such as the amplitude of the step impulse response, the time constant of the response and the symmetry of the rising and the falling edges.

5   Conclusions

Although preliminary, our results indicate that Multi Layer Perceptrons are able to approach the non-linear aspects of the patient specific QT-RR relationship, and can model both the dynamic behaviour (response to a step impulse) and the steady state dynamic behaviour QT=f(RR) (response to different, fixed RR intervals).

The difference between the measured QT interval and the predicted one could be used to trigger an alarm each time a given threshold is passed. Further studies however are needed to determine such thresholds and to assess their predictive value as well as the value of the features that can be derived from the step impulse responses.

References

1. Lee, JA., Attwell, D.: The effect of heart rate on the QT interval and its relationship to arrhythmias causing sudden death. In: Butrous, GS., Schwartz, PJ., (eds.): Clinical aspects of ventricular repolarisation. Farrand Press London (1989) 323-329
2. Rubel, P., Fayn, J., Mohsen, N., Girard, P.: J Electrocardiol. New methods of quantitative assessment of the extent and significance of serial ECG changes of the repolarisation phase. (1988) 177-182
3. Arnaud, P., Rubel, P., Morlet, D., Fayn, J., Forlini, M.C.: Method Inform Med. Methodology of ECG interpretation in the Lyon program (1990) 393-402
4. Presciuttini, B., Duprez, D., De Buyzere, M., Clement, DL.: Acta Cardiol. How to study sympatho-vagal balance in arterial hypertension and the effect of antihypertensive drugs? (1998) 143-152

Expert Knowledge and Its Role in Learning Bayesian Networks in Medicine: An Appraisal

Peter Lucas

Dept. of Computing Science, University of Aberdeen, Aberdeen AB24 3UE, UK
`plucas@csd.abdn.ac.uk,lucas@cs.uu.nl`

Abstract. A major part of the medical knowledge concerns diseases that are uncommon or even rare. The uncommon nature of these disorders renders it impossible to collect data of a sufficiently large number of patients to develop machine-learning models that faithfully reflect the subtleties of the domain. An alternative is to develop a Bayesian network with the help of clinical experts. Lack of data is then compensated for by eliciting the structure with its associated local probability distributions from the experts. The resulting network can be subsequently evaluated using the available dataset. One may also consider adopting very strong independence assumptions, such as in naive Bayesian models. Normally not all subtleties of the interactions among the variables in the domain are reflected in such models. Yet, a relatively small dataset suffices to obtain an acceptably accurate model. This paper explores the trade-offs between modelling using expert knowledge, and machine learning using a small clinical dataset in the context of Bayesian networks.

1 Introduction

There exists considerable experience in medicine in analysing data of diseases with high prevalence, such as lung cancer and myocardial infarction. Most of the evidence underlying current medical practice is based on such analyses. The frequent occurrence of these disorders renders it practically feasible to collect data of large numbers of patients. Typically, datasets collected in the context of clinical studies of these disorders may include many thousands of patient records. Such datasets are quite attractive for evaluating machine-learning techniques, and, in fact, have been used for that purpose by many researchers.

However, for more than 90% of medical disorders, the picture is quite different: these disorders do only occur occasionally or rarely, and, as a consequence, even clinical research datasets may only include data of a hundred to a few hundred patients. Developing decision-support systems that assist clinicians in handling patients with these disorders is thus scientifically challenging, because there may not be sufficient data available. Systems covering such disorders would be practically useful, as many doctors will lack knowledge and experience to deal with patients affected by uncommon disorders effectively.

Machine-learning literature in medicine not only tends to consider only problems for which much data are available, but in addition it focuses on models

S. Quaglini, P. Barahona, and S. Andreassen (Eds.): AIME 2001, LNAI 2101, pp. 156–166, 2001.

capable of performing single tasks, such as classifying patients in particular disease or prognostic categories to assist clinicians with the tasks of diagnosis or treatment selection. However, medical management cannot be captured in terms of single, simple tasks. As a consequence there appears to be a mismatch between common task-specific computer-based models and the complexity of the field of medicine. Bayesian networks have the virtue of being declarative models that can be reused for different tasks [6]. They can also be employed to look at particular problems from different angles, just by varying the supplied evidence and the questions posed to the model. However, developing such models is challenging, both in terms of the amount of probabilistic information required and modelling effort. When it comes to handling uncommon or rare disorders, where only small volumes of data will be available, it is unclear whether such effort is worthwhile. Developing simple linear discriminators like naive Bayesian classifiers and logistic regression models seems a more obvious choice, as it is straightforward and requires datasets with relatively few cases [1,3,4].

This paper attempts to provide answers to a number of questions related to the issues mentioned above, based on our experience in developing declarative prognostic models of non-Hodgkin lymphoma of the stomach, gastric NHL for short. Gastric NHL is a typical example of an uncommon, although not extremely rare disease. The following questions are addressed:

– Does additional structure enhance the learning of knowledge?
– Can the structure of a Bayesian network be learnt, either completely or partially, from the data of a small dataset?

The remainder of this paper is organised as follows. In the next two sections, a number of different Bayesian-network models of gastric NHL are introduced. Section 4 pays attention to their evaluation, whereas in Section 5 some results of checking the structure of a Bayesian network are presented. The paper is rounded off by a discussion of what has been achieved.

2   Preliminaries

A *Bayesian network* $\mathcal{B}$ is defined as a pair $\mathcal{B} = (G, \Pr)$, where G is a directed, acyclic graph $G = (V(G), A(G))$, with a set of vertices $V(G) = \{V_1, \ldots, V_n\}$, representing a set of stochastic variables $\mathcal{V}$, and a set of arcs $A(G) \subseteq V(G) \times V(G)$, representing conditional and unconditional stochastic independences among the variables, modelled by absence of arcs among vertices [5]. The basic property of a Bayesian network is that any variable corresponding to a vertex in the graph G is conditionally independent of its non-descendants given its parents; this is called the *local Markov property*. On the variables $\mathcal{V}$ is defined a joint probability distribution $\Pr(V_1, \ldots, V_n)$, for which, as a consequence of the local Markov property, the following decomposition holds: $\Pr(V_1, \ldots, V_n) = \prod_{i=1}^{n} \Pr(V_i \mid \pi(V_i))$, where $\pi(V_i)$ denotes the conjunction of variables corresponding to the parents of V_i, for $i = 1, \ldots, n$. In the following, variables will be denoted by upper-case letters,

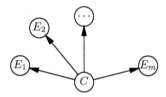

Fig. 1. Independent-form Bayesian network.

e.g. V, whereas a variable V which takes on a value v, i.e. $V = v$, will be abbreviated to v. When it is not necessary to refer to specific values of variables, we will usually just refer to a variable, which thus stands for any value of the variable.

Bayesian-network models conforming to the topology shown in Fig. 1 correspond to the situation where a distinction is made between *evidence variables* E_i and a *class variable* C, with the evidence variables assumed to be conditionally independent given the class variable. In the following such a network will be called an *independent-form Bayesian network*, by way of analogy with the special form of Bayes' rule, called its independent form, for which the same assumptions hold. The independent form is used to compute the a posteriori probability of a class value c_k given the evidence $\mathcal{E} \subseteq \{e_1, \ldots, e_m\}$ [5]:

$$\Pr(c_k \mid \mathcal{E}) = \frac{\Pr(\mathcal{E} \mid c_k)\Pr(c_k)}{\Pr(\mathcal{E})} = \frac{\prod_{e \in \mathcal{E}} \Pr(e \mid c_k)\Pr(c_k)}{\sum_{j=1}^{q} \prod_{e \in \mathcal{E}} \Pr(e \mid c_j)\Pr(c_j)}$$

where class variable C has q mutually exclusive values, and $\Pr(\mathcal{E}) > 0$. The model is normally used for classification of cases, i.e. as a classifier. Note that $\Pr(\mathcal{E}|c_k) = \prod_{e \in \mathcal{E}} \Pr(e \mid c_k)$ holds, because of the assumption that the evidence variables E_i are conditionally independent given the class variable C. Furthermore, $\Pr(\mathcal{E}) = \sum_{j=1}^{q} \Pr(\mathcal{E} \mid c_j)\Pr(c_j)$ follows from marginalisation and conditioning.

An independent-form Bayesian network may lack important probabilistic dependence information, hence its nickname: *naive Bayesian model*. However, the model has the advantage that assessment of the required probabilities $\Pr(E_j \mid C)$ and $\Pr(C)$ is straightforward, and can be carried out with a relatively small dataset. Determination of the a posteriori probabilities $\Pr(C \mid \mathcal{E})$ is computationally speaking a trivial task under the mentioned assumptions. One would expect that adopting such strong simplifying assumptions may be at the expense of reduced performance. However, Domingos and Pazzani have convincingly shown that the independent form yields a surprisingly powerful classifier, much more robust than previously thought [3]. These features of the independent form of Bayes' rule explain why it is becoming increasingly popular, after having fallen into disgrace two decades ago.

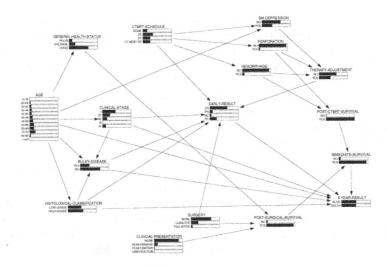

Fig. 2. Bayesian-network model as designed with the help of medical experts.

3   Bayesian Models of Gastric Non-Hodgkin Lymphoma

In the following, a number of declarative and independent-form Bayesian models
for gastric NHL are analysed to shed some light on the issues mentioned above.

3.1   The Models

A Bayesian-network model incorporating most factors relevant for the management of gastric NHL was developed in collaboration with clinical experts from
the Netherlands Cancer Institute (NKI). The resulting model, shown in Fig. 2,
includes variables like age of the patient and clinical stage of the tumour. Some of
the included variables concern patient information obtained from diagnostic procedures, which will be available prior to treatment selection. We shall refer to this

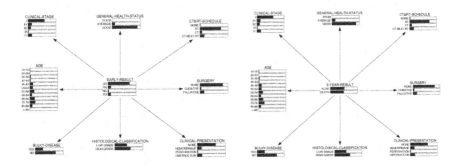

Fig. 3. Independent-form models for EARLY-RESULT (left) and 5-YEAR-RESULT (right).

information as *pretreatment* information. Another part of the model variables will only become available following treatment; examples are EARLY-RESULT and 5-YEAR-RESULT. It is called the *posttreatment* part of the model. Finally, the model includes the *treatment* variables SURGERY and CT&RT-SCHEDULE. Note that this declarative model of gastric NHL can indeed be used in the context of different tasks, such as prediction of prognosis, treatment selection – possibly using utility information – and generation of patient profiles [6].

Two independent-form Bayesian networks, depicted in Fig. 3, were derived from the network shown in Fig. 2. In one of those, the variable EARLY-RESULT was taken as a class variable; the other includes 5-YEAR-RESULT as class variable. Their probability distributions were also derived from that of the complete Bayesian network. In both models, all pretreatment and treatment variables, and a single posttreatment variable were included. As the other posttreatment variables would typically be unknown, it would not make sense to include them as well. This illustrates one difference between a declarative Bayesian model, as shown in Fig. 2, and task-specific models, as shown in Fig. 3.

3.2   Patients

Taking the topologies of the three networks as fixed, the probability distributions of the three models mentioned above were also learnt. Learning and evaluation took place using a dataset with patient data from the Netherlands Cancer Institute, comprising 137 cases, with some missing data. Since in 4 patients the early result of treatment was unknown, we used only 133 cases when studying the performance of the models concerning the class variable EARLY-RESULT. See Table 1 for a description. A brief description of the individual models is given in Table 2. Models with the letter S in their name are declarative or structured models; models with the letter I in their name are independent-form Bayesian networks. The superscript *er* indicates that EARLY-RESULT was the class variable; the superscript *5y* is used to denote models with 5-YEAR-RESULT as a class variable. The subscript E indicates that a model is based on subjective probability assessment by an expert.

Missing data were either ignored or distributed uniformly among the values of the variable for which a value was missing, indicated by the subscript u.

Table 1. Characteristics of the datasets.

Class	Patients (n)	Class	Patients (n)
5-YEAR-RESULT		EARLY-RESULT	
alive	70	CR	102
death	67	PR	14
		NC	4
		PD	13
Total	137	Total	133

Table 2. Bayesian models.

Model	Description	Topology	Missing Data
S_E	expert-assessed model	declarative	—
S	learnt model	declarative	ignored
S_u	learnt model	declarative	uniform distribution
I_E^{er}	derived from S_E	independent form	—
Ier	learnt model	independent form	ignored
I_u^{er}	learnt model	independent form	uniform distribution
I_E^{5y}	derived from S_E	independent form	—
I^{5y}	learnt model	independent form	ignored
I_u^{5y}	learnt model	independent form	uniform distribution

4 Evaluation

4.1 Methods

The a posteriori probability distributions $\Pr(\text{EARLY-RESULT} \mid \mathcal{E})$ and $\Pr(\text{5-YEAR-RESULT} \mid \mathcal{E})$ were computed, where $\mathcal{E}$ was the available evidence for each of the 133 and 137, respectively, patients with gastric NHL, restricted to values of all pretreatment and treatment variables. The value v^* of the class variable V with largest probability was taken as the resulting classification:

$$v^* = \mathrm{argmax}_v\{\Pr(V = v \mid \mathcal{E})\}$$

However, a disadvantage of this straightforward method of comparing the quality of the Bayesian models is that the actual a posteriori probabilities are ignored. A more precise impression of the behaviour of the Bayesian models is obtained when the resulting probabilities are taken into account as well. For example, if a patient Q is known to have survived more than 5 years following radiotherapy, and a Bayesian model has predicted this event with probability 0.8, this conclusion would seem intuitively better than the conclusion of another model which predicted this event with a probability of 0.6. One of the simplest scoring rules that measures this effect is the *logarithmic scoring rule* defined below [2].

Let D be a dataset, $|D| = p$, $p \geq 0$. With each prediction generated by a Bayesian model for case $r_k \in D$, with actual class value c_k, we associated a score (the entropy) [1]: $S_k = -\ln\Pr(c_k \mid \mathcal{E})$, which has the informal meaning of a penalty: when the probability $\Pr(c_k \mid \mathcal{E}) = 1$, then $S_k = 0$ (actually observing c_k generates no information); otherwise, $S_k > 0$. The total score for database D is now defined as the sum of the individual scores: $S = \sum_{k=1}^p S_k$. Since S is a stochastic quantity, it can be characterised further by means of central moments, such as the average E_k: $E_k = -\sum_{i=1}^q \Pr(c_i \mid \mathcal{E})\ln\Pr(c_i \mid \mathcal{E})$, with total average $E = \sum_{k=1}^p E_k$, and the variance V_k: $V_k = -\sum_{i=1}^q \Pr(c_i \mid \mathcal{E})(\ln\Pr(c_i \mid \mathcal{E}))^2 - E_k^2$, with total variance $V = \sum_{k=1}^p V_k$.

Three additive components make up the error in classifying: (1) the intrinsic error due to noise in the data, (2) the statistical bias in the model, and (3) the variance (model's sensitivity to the characteristics of the dataset) [1,3].

Table 3. Results for different Bayesian models for EARLY-RESULT and 5-YEAR-RESULT. Percentages were computed by dividing the number of correct conclusions by the number of classified cases.

Model	Total	Classified (n)			Missing Data
		Incorrect	Correct	(%)	
		EARLY RESULT			
S_E	133	31	102	(76.7)	—
S	133	20	113	(85.0)	ignored
S_u	133	18	115	(86.5)	distributed among values
I_E^{er}	133	35	98	(73.7)	—
Ier	133	22	111	(83.5)	ignored
I_u^{er}	133	24	109	(82.0)	distributed among values
		5 YEAR RESULT			
S_E	137	43	94	(68.6)	—
S	137	22	115	(83.9)	ignored
S_u	137	20	117	(85.4)	distributed among values
I_E^{5y}	137	40	97	(70.8)	—
I^{5y}	137	40	97	(70.8)	ignored
I_u^{5y}	137	39	98	(71.5)	distributed among values

One would expect a large statistical bias for the naive Bayesian classifier, as its independence assumptions are almost always not satisfied. On the other hand, experimental evidence shows that the naive Bayesian classifier has a low variance [3]. Methods with a greater representational power have a greater ability to respond to the dataset, i.e. they have a large *information-storage capacity*, and tend to have a lower bias and higher variance [1]. These properties one would expect to hold for the structured Bayesian network [4].

4.2   Upper-Bound Evaluation Results

As an initial experiment, the performance of the various models was investigated by determining predictions for the patient data, either for the expert-based models (S_E, I_E^{er}, and I_E^{5y}) without learning, or after learning the joint probability distribution from the data. The results obtained for the nine models (three S models and six I models, three concerning EARLY-RESULT and another three concerning 5-YEAR-RESULT) are shown in Table 3. Note that for the non-expert assessed models, learning and performance evaluation was accomplished using the same dataset.

Prediction of 5-year survival is medically speaking more difficult than predicting the early result of treatment. Note that according Table 1, the two classes for 5-YEAR-RESULT are approximately uniformly distributed, i.e. the prior probability of correct classification is about 50%, with lower bound of about 0%. The distribution of EARLY-RESULT, however, is skewed towards CR (complete remission) with an upper bound of 76.7% and a lower bound of 53.4% when using a random classification scheme that respects the frequency of occurrence

Table 4. Logarithmic scores: (a) and (b) describe upper-bound evaluation results; (a) Model S_E has no scores for the variable EARLY-RESULT, as for some cases the probability of the class value was equal to 0; (c) Results obtained by cross validation.

Model	S	E	V
	EARLY RESULT		
S_E	–	–	–
S	65.72	75.04	58.63
S_u	49.32	73.13	67.72
I_E^{er}	92.66	114.29	85.75
Ier	53.98	43.15	45.32
I_u^{er}	57.41	54.33	56.63

(a)

Model	S	E	V
	5 YEAR RESULT		
S_E	81.28	71.47	30.65
S	57.05	65.93	25.65
S_u	48.92	58.88	25.91
I_E^{5y}	75.43	73.91	29.91
I^{5y}	67.50	51.31	28.20
I_u^{5y}	69.50	54.07	31.99

(b)

Model	S	E	V
	EARLY RESULT		
S	116.14	127.36	68.21
S_u	116.95	129.37	74.48
Ier	118.00	54.72	63.18
I_u^{er}	115.64	53.30	62.06
	5 YEAR RESULT		
S	92.23	87.57	11.42
S_u	90.51	87.07	12.49
I^{5y}	86.81	55.11	31.85
I_u^{5y}	88.87	57.53	33.01

(c)

of classes in the dataset. This is reflected in the results obtained by the models, in the sense that the percentage of correctly classified cases is higher for the class variable EARLY-RESULT than for the variable 5-YEAR-RESULT. The performance of the declarative model S_E, with its associated derived independent Bayesian models I_E^{er} and I_E^{5y}, which incorporate expert-assessed probabilities, were lowest. The Bayesian networks S and S_u, having the same topology as S_E, but with joint probability distributions learnt from data, yielded the best results. As might be expected, the expert-based models were inferior to the other models due to the subjective nature of their underlying probability distributions.

The various independent-form Bayesian networks yielded results that were always below those of the two trained declarative models S and S_u. The Bayesian models in which missing values were uniformly distributed among values yielded sometimes slightly better results than the other models, with one exception, due to the artificial increase in sample size. The logarithmic scores shown in Table 4(a)-(b), however, indicate that this results in a slightly decreased accuracy of the a posteriori probability for the independent-form Bayesian model; in contrast, the accuracy of the a posteriori probabilities of the declarative model was improved. The last effect is likely due to their greater information-storage capacity.

Finally note that the performance of the structured models for 5-YEAR-RESULT was only slightly less than for EARLY-RESULT. This may be taken as evidence for overfitting of the structured models.

4.3   Cross Validation

For six of the models, excluding the three expert-based models, cross validation was carried out, using the leave-one-out method [1]. The results are given in tables 5 and 4(c).

The most significant result was a drop in performance of the structured Bayesian networks, in comparison to the upper-bound results discussed in the

Table 5. Results for different Bayesian models for EARLY-RESULT and 5-YEAR-RESULT using the leave-one-out method. Only correctness percentages are given.

Model	Total	Classified (n)			Missing Data
		Incorrect	Correct	(%)	
		EARLY RESULT			
S	133	40	93	(69.9)	ignored
S_u	133	40	93	(69.9)	distributed among values
Ier	133	36	97	(72.9)	ignored
I_u^{er}	133	37	96	(72.2)	distributed among values
		5 YEAR RESULT			
S	137	56	81	(59.1)	ignored
S_u	137	53	84	(61.3)	distributed among values
I^{5y}	137	47	90	(65.7)	ignored
I_u^{5y}	137	48	89	(64.7)	distributed among values

previous section, between 13-17%, whereas the drop in performance of the independent form models was only between 5-10%. While in the first study the performance of the structured models was better than that of the independent form models, here the order was revered. This is a clear indication that the original high performance of the structured models was due to their large information-storage capacity. Furthermore, note that the logarithmic scores give quite similar results, but that the mean and variance of the score S indicate that the independent-form Bayesian models are less sensitive to variation in the data. Dealing with the missing data had again little effect on the performance results. Finally, note that the performance of the expert-based models S_E, I_E^{er} and I_E^{5y} was superior to all other models.

5   Checking the Topology

Experiments with a network topology selection algorithm were carried out in order to obtain more insight into how far one gets with such algorithms, given a small uncommon disease dataset. Use was made of the Bayesian Knowledge Discoverer system (BKD), which implements a heuristic search method for finding the Bayesian-network structure S that best fits the data D according to the ratio $\Pr(D, S)/\Pr(D, S')$, where S' is an alternative structure [8]. The system incorporates an interval midpoint algorithm for dealing with missing values [7].

The resulting Bayesian network is shown in Fig. 4. Only 6 of the 30 arcs as suggested by the experts were identified correctly; the arcs between the vertex GENERAL-HEALTH-STATUS and BULKY-DISEASE is clinically incorrect. The arc between HISTOLOGICAL-CLASSIFICATION and BULKY-DISEASE was reversed. Finally, the arc between the vertex CLINICAL-STAGE and CT&RT-SCHEDULE is correct, but omitted by the expert, because therapy is always selected.

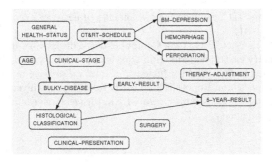

Fig. 4. Bayesian-network structure as learnt using BKD.

6   Discussion

In this paper, we have investigated the relative merits of machine-learning approaches versus knowledge acquisition and modelling in the clinical context of relatively uncommon or rare disorders. In addition, the pros and cons of structured versus unstructured Bayesian networks were studied, in order to gather experimental evidence that the development of structured Bayesian networks is worthwhile. The study was carried out against the background of a rising popularity of the naive Bayesian classifier and its variants [3,4].

The results achieved in this paper suggest that acquiring both structure and joint probability distributions from domain experts may result in robust classifiers, even though Bayesian networks are normally developed as declarative, reusable models, and not purely for the purpose of classification.

This research also extends results previously reported in the machine-learning literature, in which the naive Bayesian classifier was shown to outperform non-Bayesian classifiers in many circumstances. A similar effect was shown to exist for structured Bayesian networks. The naive Bayesian classifier and its variants offer the best choice when learning from a small dataset; the additional structure in the declarative models seem to be of little help in this respect.

Finally, although learning the structure of a Bayesian network from a small dataset is not feasible, checking its structure might offer some insight.

References

1. M. Berthold and D.J. Hand (Eds.). *Intelligent Data Analysis: an Introduction.* Springer, Berlin, 1999.
2. R.G. Cowell, A.P. Dawid, D. Spiegelhalter. Sequential model criticism in probabilistic expert systems. *PAMI* 15(3) (1993) 209–219.
3. P. Domingos and M. Pazzani. On the optimality of the simple Bayesian classifier under zero-one loss. *Machine Learning* 29 (1997) 103–130.
4. N.I.R. Friedman, D. Geiger and M. Goldszmidt. Bayesian network classifiers. *Machine Learning* 29 (1997) 131-163.

5. P.J.F. Lucas and L.C. van der Gaag. *Principles of Expert Systems*. Addison-Wesley, Wokingham, 1991.
6. P.J.F. Lucas, H. Boot, B.G. Taal. Computer-based decision-support in the management of primary gastric non-Hodgkin lymphoma. *Meth Inf Med* 37 (1998) 206–219.
7. M. Ramoni and P. Sebastiani. *Efficient Parameter Learning in Bayesian Networks from Incomplete Data*. Report KMi-TR-41, KMI, Open University, 1997.
8. M. Ramoni and P. Sebastiani. *Bayesian Knowledge Discoverer: reference manual*. KMI, Open University, 1997.

Improving the Diagnostic Performance of MUNIN by Remodelling of the Diseases

Steen Andreassen[1], Marko Suojanen[1], Björn Falck[2], and Kristian G. Olesen[1]

[1]Department of Medical Informatics and Image Analysis, Institute of Electronic Systems,
Aalborg University, Fredrik Bajersvej 7 D, DK-9220 Aalborg, Denmark
{sa, ms}@miba.auc.dk, kgo@cs.auc.dk
[2]Department of Clinical Neurophysiology, Turku University Hospital, Finland
bjorn.falck@tyks.fi

Abstract. The paper describes a revision of the structure of MUNIN, a causal probabilistic network that specifies a stochastic model of the relations between a range of neuromuscular diseases and the findings associated with these diseases. The stochastic model was revised 1) to achieve a more flexible specification of the anatomical distribution of findings associated with the diseases, 2) to allow diagnosis of diseases or groups of diseases (e.g. polyneuropathies and motor neuron diseases) previously lumped under the common concept of diffuse neuropathy and 3) to model the correlation between carpal tunnel syndrome on the left and right side. Minor adjustments were also made to some of the conditional probabilities used to specify the pathophysiology of the diseases.

The diagnostic capability of the revised model was evaluated by letting MUNIN diagnose 30 cases. The evaluation showed that the revised model performed better with a sensitivity of 94% and a specificity also of 94%.

1 Introduction

MUNIN (Muscle and Nerve Inference Network) is a prototype decision support system for diagnosing peripheral muscle and nerve diseases [1], [3], [6]. MUNIN is implemented as a Causal Probabilistic Network (CPN), also known as a Bayesian Network [8], [2], [5]. MUNIN calculates the probability that the patient has a given disease, and in addition it provides a more detailed description of the disease. It provides a description of the severity of the disease, and for most diseases several other attributes are given. For example, in local nerve lesions it will describe the severity of the lesion, the pathophysiology (axonal or demyelinating) and the time course, that is whether it is acute, subacute or chronic. The diagnostic performance of MUNIN has previous been evaluated using a set of 30 cases collected by leading European neurophysiologists [4]. Although the group that evaluated MUNIN concluded that "...MUNIN performed at the level of an experienced neurophysiologist.." the evaluation also made it clear that MUNIN had a number of problems that had to be dealt with before the system could be considered ready for clinical use. Three major problems identified at that time were: 1) The computer

S. Quaglini, P. Barahona, and S. Andreassen (Eds.): AIME 2001, LNAI 2101, pp. 167–176, 2001.

memory size required to run the entire MUNIN CPN was many orders of magnitude greater than can be conveniently handled by available computers. 2) It was not conceptually clear which disease prevalences should be used to specify a priori probabilities for the diseases:should it be the prevalences found in the general population or prevalences found in the group of patients referred for electrodiagnostic consultations 3) The anatomy of the current MUNIN prototype, the so-called microhuman, is too small. The anatomy of the prototype only covers a sensory nerve, a motor nerve, two mixed nerves and three muscles on each side of the body.

The first two of these problems have now been solved. The first problem was solved by considering subsets of diseases instead of all diseases simultaneously. This method provides results that are essentially identical to those that would have resulted from considering all diseases simultaneously, but it reduced the memory requirements to a level that can easily be handled by a PC and reduced computation times per case to a level that is compatible with clinical practice [7], [9]. Two different versions of the method were developed. The results given below refer to the version where "soft conditioning" [11] was used.

The second problem with the choice of disease prevalences was solved by introducing the concept of the FIDL-factor [10]. FIDL is an acronym for Found In Doctors Lab, and it can be seen as a summary of all the reasons that have led to the referral of the patient to the EMG examination. The introduction of the FIDL-factor made it possible to use the much smaller prevalences from the general population (e.g. 1.5% of the prevalences in the population seen in the EMG lab), and this in turn solved a problem with what we call the false positive probability mass: Although the diagnostic capability of the original MUNIN prototype was satisfactory in the sense that it in 29 out of the 30 cases had a "silver standard" diagnosis as the most probable diagnosis [4], it had the problem that a number of other diseases had probabilities significantly larger than zero. The sum of these probabilities for other diseases was called the false positive probability mass, and it averaged 81% over the 30 cases considered [10]. The introduction of the FIDL factor reduced the average false positive probability mass to 19% [11]. The false negative probability mass was defined as the difference between the probability of a disease and 100% for the disease (or diseases) listed as the "silver standard" diagnosis (or diagnoses) for that case. The average false negative probability mass over the 30 cases increases a little, from 17% to 23%, but due to the large reduction in the false positive probability mass, the introduction of the FIDL-factor must be considered a major improvement.

The solution of the problems with memory size and computation time has paved the way for the next step, the expansion of the microhuman anatomy to a size that will be clinically interesting. However, we decided that before this expansion, we would inspect the modelling of both the generalized diseases and the local nerve lesions to see if there were areas where the models could be improved. We used the 30 cases previously used to test MUNIN to help us identify areas where the models might need revisions. This paper reports on the revisions performed and on the resulting improvements in diagnostic performance.

2   Remodelling the Diseases of MUNIN

Fig. 1 shows the diagnostic results, as obtained by Suojanen et al. [11] after introduction of the FIDL-factor. The diseases have been arranged in 8 different groups, and it can be seen that there are cases with large false positive or false negative probabilities in most of the groups, with the exception of the myotonic dystrophies, polyneuropathies and the patients with no diseases, where the false positive probability masses reflect the expectation that 75% of the patients referred for an EMG examination have a neuromuscular disease. The high false positive probability in patients with no diseases can only be brought down by a comparatively extensive examination of the patients to exclude at least the most common diseases. Inspection of the remaining cases revealed three different problems:

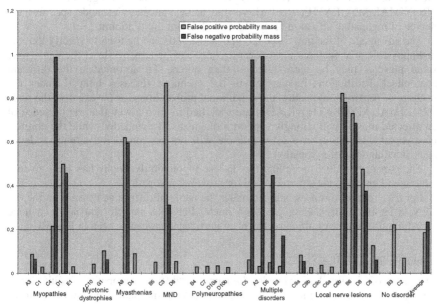

Fig. 1. Results for the 30 cases. The average false positive probability mass was 19% and the false negative probability mass was 23%.

1)   The structure of the CPN does not give sufficient freedom to specify different anatomical distributions of the diseases, for example the predominant affection of proximal muscles in patients with myopathy.

2)   The specification of the group of diseases labeled as diffuse neuropathy fails to reflect the correlation between the different pathophysiological changes caused by the different diseases in this group.

3)   The correlation between carpal tunnel syndrome on the left and right side needs to be modelled to agree with the high proportion of bilateral carpal tunnel syndromes.

The modifications of the structure of the CPN necessary to remedy these three problems are described below.

Specification of Anatomical Distributions

The restructuring of the CPN will be described using the specification of "proximal myopathy" as an example. In MUNIN, proximal myopathy is a group of diseases, containing for example Duchenne muscular dystrophy and facio-scapulo-humeral muscular dystrophy (FSH) and polymyositis. Although these two diseases share a general distribution with proximal muscles being more affected than distal muscles, there are details of the anatomical distribution that differ, as indicated by the name FSH. To be able to specify directly the degree of affection of different muscles, additional nodes were introduced in the CPN. For each muscle a node was introduced that specifies the degree of myopathic affection of that muscle. An example can be seen in Fig. 2, where the structure in Fig. 2A with direct links from PROXIMAL.MYOPATHY to the individual pathophysiological features for the muscles has been replaced (Fig. 2B) by a link that goes through the new node PROXIMAL.MYOPATHY.R.ADM. As the name indicates this node specifies the degree of myopathic affection of the right m. abductor digiti minimi.

The advantage of the new structure is that the node can be used to specify that the pathophysiological features must form a consistent pattern, while at the same time some muscles may be more affected than others. To accomodate the different anatomical distributions represented in the group of diseases lumped under the heading of proximal myopathy, the conditional probabilities for for example the node PROXIMAL.MYOPATHY.R.ADM are specified in such a way that the presence of an affected muscle will strongly support a diagnosis of myopathy, while the absence of myopathic affection in a given muscle will not be considered strong evidence against a diagnosis of myopathy.

The part of the CPN modelling the disease myotonic dystrophy has been given a structure identical to the structure used for proximal myopathy.

For the group of diseases, lumped under the name of diffuse neuropathy in the old CPN, a similar restructuring has been made. For each muscle and nerve, a node specifying the degree of affection has been introduced, as can be seen in Fig. 3B.

Remodelling of Diffuse Neuropathy

The group of diseases lumped under the name of "diffuse neuropathy" is quite large. It contains as diverse entities as for example polyneuro(no)pathies and motor neurone disease (ALS). To describe this broad range of affections, diffuse neuropathy was equipped with 5 attributes, describing:
1)   The severity (no, mild, moderate, severe)
2)   The anatomical distribution (distal, proximal, random)
3)   The type(motor, sensory, motor and sensory)
4)   The time course (acute, subacute, chronic, old) and
5)   The pathology (axonal, demyelinating, blocking)

In principle, these attributes are sufficient to describe the groups of diseases. For example, diabetic polyneuropathy could be described as a chronic, distal, sensory and motor, symmetric, axonal polyneuropathy.

Unfortunately, this description leaves room for diseases described as proximal, sensory, acute and axonal, which does not correspond to any known disease. This slack causes MUNIN to loose diagnostic accuracy, and we therefore decided to separate diffuse neuropathy into several better delineated groups of diseases. Out of those we only implemented two, axonal, sensory-motor polyneuropathy (POLYN) and motor neuron disease (MND), because the set of 30 test cases only had examples of those two groups of diseases. Eventually the remaining groups of diseases, such as Guillan-Barré, HMSN type I and pure sensory polyneuropathies will also have to be modeled.

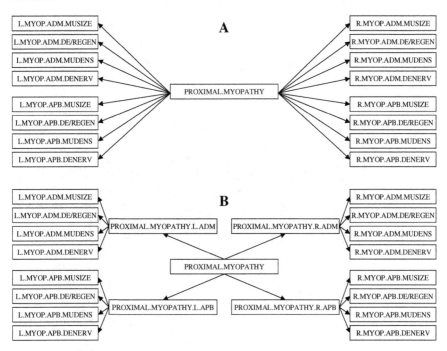

Fig. 2. A. The old model for proximal myopathy and the pathophysiological contributions in four of the six affected muscles. **B.** The new model for proximal myopathy, where a node has been added between the disease and the pathophysiological contributions in a muscle.

The resulting structure of the CPN is shown in Fig. 3B. As can be seen, POLYN and MND are represented separately, and the nodes mentioned in the section on specification of anatomical distributions have also been introduced. The effects of the two disease groups on spontaneous neural activity (NEUR-ACT) is specified separately, to make it possible to specify that fasciculations occur more frequently in MND than in polyneuropathies.

<u>Bilateral Carpal Tunnel Syndrome</u>

In the current version of MUNIN it is assumed that the population prevalence of carpal tunnel syndrome is 0.22% both on the left and the right side. When the FIDL-factor is set to YES, we can read from the CPN that the prevalence in the group of patients referred for EMG examination is 15% both on the left side and on the right side. On the other hand, if we have a patient, where a left sided carpal tunnel syndrome has been shown with very high probability, then due to the action of the

FIDL-factor, the old model will predict a 0.22% probability of finding a carpal tunnel syndrome on the right side. This is far from clinical reality, because carpal tunnel syndrome is quite often bilateral. This type of situation can be modelled by assuming that there is some common factor that gives the patient the disposition to develop carpal tunnel syndrome on both sides.

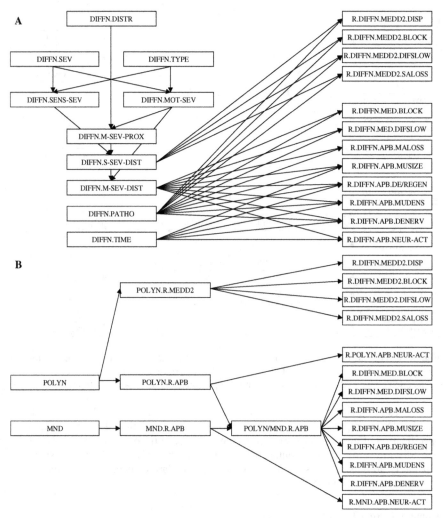

Fig. 3. A. The old model for diffuse neuropathy and the pathophysiological contributions in the sensory and motor median nerve and the abductor pollicis brevis muscle. **B.** The new model, where diffuse neuropathy has been replaced with polyneuropathy and motor neuron disease, and nodes have been added between the diseases and the pathophysiological contributions.

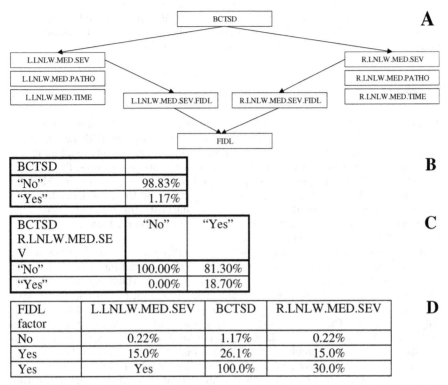

Fig. 4. A: Correlation between left and right median nerve lesions at wrist is modelled by introducing a new variable for bilateral carpal tunnel syndrome disposition (BCTSD). The prior probabilities for BCTSD are shown in B. The conditional probabilities for R.LNLW.MED.SEV are shown in C. The population prevalences for L.LNLW.MED, BCTSD and R.LNLW.MED are shown in the first row of D. The corresponding laboratory prevalences are shown in the second row. The probability of R.LNLW.MED and BCTSD, when we know that the patient has L.LNLW.MED is shown in the last row of D.

Fig. 4A shows the structure of such a CPN, where this common factor has been labelled Bilateral Carpal Tunnel Syndrome Disposition (BCTSD). The conditional probabilities in the CPN, shown in Fig. 4B and C have been adjusted, such that they respect the above mentioned prevalences of 0.22% and 15% respectively, but also so that the probability of a right sided carpal tunnel syndrome (R.LNLW.MED.SEV) is calculated to 30%, when the FIDL-factor has been set to YES and a left sided carpal tunnel syndrome has been established (L.LNLW.MED.SEV = YES) (Fig. 4D). This implies that in any patient where a carpal tunnel syndrome is present on one side, then it is justified to expect that there is a relatively high probability (30%) of also finding a carpal tunnel syndrome on the opposite side, even before the opposite side is examined at all.

Adjustments of Pathophysiology

The modifications of the CPN described above all involved structural changes in the CPN. In addition to these changes a number of minor modifications of the conditional probabilities in the CPN have been made for the pathophysiological nodes denervation, neuromuscular transmission, degeneration/regeneration, motor unit size, myotonia, fiber density, motor axon loss and diffuse slowing.

3 Results

To evaluate the remodelled diseases, we re-examined the 30 previously evaluated cases. Compared to the "silver standard" diagnoses the revised MUNIN had the main silver standard diagnosis as the diagnosis with the highest probability in all 30 cases, with the exception of case C6b. Due to the cases with multiple diseases, the 30 cases had 34 silver standard diagnoses. Using 50% probability as the cut-off point, MUNIN had diagnosed 32 out of the 34 diseases, (failing in C5 and C6b) and had added two diseases, not included in the silver standard diagnosis (in D4 and C6b). This corresponds to an observed sensitivity of 94% and an observed specificity also of 94% over the 30 cases in the case database.

If we consider the average false positive probability mass, we can see that it was reduced from 19% to 18%. The real benefit of the remodelling was seen in the reduction of the average false negative probability mass, which was reduced from 23% to 11%. The results for each case are shown in Fig. 5. MUNIN does not have problems in diagnosing myotonic dystrophy, motor neuron diseases and polyneuropathies. There are problems with some of the cases in the groups myopathies, myasthenias, multiple diseases and local nerve lesions. To gain insight into the nature of these problems, the 11 cases out of the 30, where either the false positive or the false negative probability masses exceeded the average were reviewed. The reviews of the three cases with the highest false positive or false negative probabilities, D4, C5 and C6 given below.

Case D4 is a patient with small cell lung cancer, who has myasthenic syndrome. MUNIN correctly diagnosed the myasthenic syndrome. The large false positive probability mass (92%) is due to a strong belief in polyneuropathy. Although the department submitting the case had not diagnosed a polyneuropathy in this patient, we believe that the patient actually does have a polyneuropathy. The sensory nerve conduction velocities were slightly reduced and the amplitudes of the sensory responses were low borderline values. We believe that the patient may have a sensory polyneuropathy, and therefore MUNIN's diagnosis is correct.

Case C5 is a patient with diabetic polyneuropathy and according to the silver standard diagnosis also an ulnar nerve lesion at elbow on the left side. The large false negative probability is due to a low belief in the ulnar nerve lesion. MUNIN fails to diagnose the ulnar lesion because the polyneuropathy to some extent explains the reduced conduction velocity of the ulnar nerve at the elbow and thus reduces the probability of an ulnar nerve lesion. The conduction velocity of the ulnar nerve in the forearm segment is 44 m/s and the conduction velocity across the elbow is 36 m/s. The ulnar abnormality at the elbow is thus neurophysiologically relatively mild. The available findings leave room for uncertainty about the diagnosis and it is not clear from those findings that the ulnar elbow lesion in silver standard diagnosis can be considered as established with certainty.

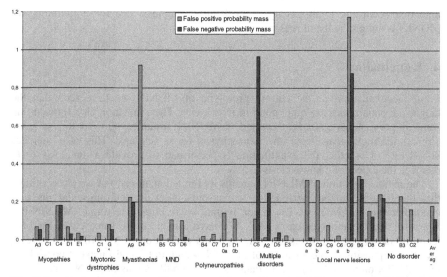

Fig. 5. Results for the 30 cases. The average false positive probability mass was 18% and the false negative probability mass was 11%.

Case C6 is a patient with a median nerve lesion at the elbow following an elbow luxation. On the first visit, case C6a, MUNIN diagnoses the lesion correctly. C6b is the follow-up study, which shows excellent recovery. However, it is not anymore possible to localize the lesion accurately. On the follow up the conduction block and conduction velocity in the median nerve at the elbow have improved and MUNIN is no longer able to localize the lesion. MUNIN has a 12% belief in a median nerve lesion at the elbow and assumes that the missing sensory nerve action potential and neurogenic EMG findings in the thenar muscles are due to a carpal tunnel syndrome with a 88% probability. In this case the purpose of the follow-up study was only to make sure the nerve lesion is regenerating as expected, and the findings from the follow-up study do not in their own right make it possible to determine that the lesion is located at the elbow. In other words, the mistake made by MUNIN is not due to incorrect interpretation of the findings, but due to the fact that MUNIN is not aware that C6b is a follow-up of C6a.

Table 2. Observations concerning the 11 cases, where either the false positive or the false negative probability masses exceeded the average, according to the reason.

Reason for false pos. and neg. prob. mass	C4	A9	D4	C5	A2	C9a	C9b	C6b	B6	C8	B3
Limited patient examination	X	X							X		X
Findings leave room for uncertainty				X	X				X		
Silver standard diagnosis questionable			X	X							
Monitoring – not differential diagnosis						X	X	X			

Table 2 summarizes our observations concerning the 11 cases with either false positive or false negative probabilities exceeding the average. For each case the reason(s) for the false negative or positive probabilities are given. It is interesting to note that according to this analysis, inadequate diagnosis due to shortcomings of MUNIN is not on the list of reasons.

4 Conclusion

From the evaluation of the current prototype of MUNIN we have seen that the diagnostic capabilities are quite good in most cases. The evaluation also showed that some improvements must be expected if MUNIN could be allowed to use other clinical findings, apart from the neurophysiological findings. This also includes knowledge of whether the examination is performed to provide a diagnosis or to describe the extent of a known lesion.

The major limitation of MUNIN remains its limited anatomy, but we are confident that the system can be expanded to cover most relevant neuromuscular diseases encountered in an EMG lab. The major limitation wrt. clinical testing of MUNIN has been the small number of cases (30). We have also used the same cases for both learning and testing purposes. A more rigorous evaluation of MUNIN will have to await an expansion of the anatomy of MUNIN, which in turn will make it possible to test MUNIN on a much larger case database. The modifications of MUNIN presented here is one of the last steps before this can be achieved.

References

1. Andreassen S, Jensen FV, Andersen SK, Falck B, Kjærulff U, Woldbye M, Sørensen AR, Rosenfalck A and Jensen F 1989. MUNIN - an expert EMG assistant. In: Computer-aided electromyography and expert systems, ed. JE Desmedt. Elsevier, Amsterdam, pp. 255-277.
2. Andreassen S, Jensen FV and Olesen KG 1991. Medical expert systems based on causal probabilistic networks. *International Journal of Biomedical Computing* 28: 1-30.
3. Andreassen S, Falck B and Olesen KG 1992. Diagnostic function of the microhuman prototype of the expert system - MUNIN. *Electroencephalography and Clinical Neurophysiology* 85: 143-157.
4. Andreassen S, Rosenfalck A, Falck B, Olesen KG and Andersen SK 1996. Evaluation of the diagnostic performance of the expert EMG assistant MUNIN. *Electroencephalography and Clinical Neurophysiology* 101: 129-144.
5. Jensen FV 1996. An introduction to Bayesian networks. UCL Press.
6. Olesen KG, Kjærulff U, Jensen F, Jensen FV, Falck B, Andreassen S and Andersen SK 1989. A MUNIN network for the median nerve - a case study on loops. *Applied Artificial Intelligence* 3: 385-403.
7. Olesen KG and Andreassen S 1996. A heuristic method for diagnosing multiple diseases in complex medical domains modelled by causal probabilistic networks. In: Medical Informatics Europe '96, eds. J Brender et al. IOS Press, pp. 614-618.
8. Pearl J 1988. Probabilistic reasoning in intelligent systems. Morgan Kaufmann.
9. Suojanen M, Olesen KG and Andreassen S 1997. A method for diagnosing in large medical expert systems based on causal probabilistic networks. In: Lecture Notes in Artificial Intelligence 1211, Proceedings of the 6th Conference on Artificial Intelligence in Medicine Europe (AIME'97), eds. E Keravnou et al. Springer, pp. 285-295.
10. Suojanen M, Andreassen S and Olesen KG 1999. The EMG diagnosis - an interpretation based on partial information. *Medical Engineering & Physics* 21: 517-523.
11. Suojanen M, Andreassen S and Olesen KG 2001. A Method for Diagnosing Multiple Diseases in MUNIN. *IEEE Transactions on Biomedical Engineering*. In press.

Extended Bayesian Regression Models: A Symbiotic Application of Belief Networks and Multilayer Perceptrons for the Classification of Ovarian Tumors

Peter Antal[1], Geert Fannes[1], Bart De Moor[1], Joos Vandewalle[1], Y. Moreau[1], and Dirk Timmerman[2]

[1] Electrical Eng. Dept. ESAT/SISTA, Katholieke Universiteit Leuven,
Kasteelpark Arenberg 10, B-3001 Heverlee (Leuven), Belgium
[2] Department of Obstetrics and Gynecology, University Hospitals Leuven,
Herestraat 49, B-3000 Leuven, Belgium

Abstract. We describe a methodology based on a dual Belief Network-Multilayer Perceptron representation to build Bayesian classifiers. This methodology combines efficiently the prior domain knowledge and statistical data. We overview how this Bayesian methodology is able (1) to define constructively a valuable "informative" prior for black-box models, (2) to provide uncertainty information with predictions and (3) to handle missing values based on an auxiliary domain model. We assume that the prior domain model is formalized as a Belief Network (since this representation is a practical solution to acquiring prior domain knowledge) while we use black-box models (such as Multilayer Perceptrons) for learning to utilize the statistical data. In a medical task of predicting the malignancy of ovarian masses we demonstrate these two symbiotic applications of Belief Network models and summarize the practical advantages of the Bayesian approach.

1 Introduction

The Bayesian approach is becoming more attractive for the machine learning community because it can cope with the valuable subjective prior information in a principled way and it provides more detailed information for decision support. These properties are particularly attractive in medical applications, since detailed uncertainty information can be vital in a medical decision and frequently abundant prior domain knowledge is available beside the statistical data. The appearance of powerful stochastic algorithms further helped the wider application of the Bayesian approach, since more complex models became manageable in a Bayesian way. However, the Bayesian application of such efficient black-box models is hindered by the fact that the domain knowledge cannot be formulated directly in terms of such models (i.e., as a prior probability distribution over its parametrization). To solve this problem, we used Belief Networks to formalize the prior knowledge in a Bayesian way [3] and suggested an algorithm based on

S. Quaglini, P. Barahona, and S. Andreassen (Eds.): AIME 2001, LNAI 2101, pp. 177–187, 2001.

Belief Networks to derive *informative* priors for black-box regression models [2]. Since the constructed Belief Network is a complete probabilistic domain model, it can be attached to regression models as an auxiliary model to handle missing values frequently occurring in a medical context [1]. The derived *informative* prior and the probabilistic auxiliary domain model can be important elements for the successful application of black-box regression models (for a related overview on knowledge-based neurocomputing, see [5]. In the paper we summarize these methods retrospectively from a unified perspective and compare the performance of these extended black-box regression models with Belief Network models in a real-life medical problem.

The paper is organized as follows: Section 2 reviews the Bayesian approach in classification problems. Section 3 recapitulates the medical problem which will serve as a test case, introduces the data and defines relevant performance measures. In Section 4 we discuss the applied Bayesian models, particularly the derived *informative* prior distributions and the missing value management. In Section 5 we describe shortly the algorithms used to approximate the Bayesian performance measures. Section 6 presents the performance of the models and the comparison of the models in the Bayesian framework. In Section 7 we summarize the advantages of Bayesianism in this classification problem and the proposed *informative* priors.

2   Classification in the Bayesian Context

Starting with a prior distribution expressing the initial beliefs concerning the parameter values of the model, we can use the observations to transform this into the posterior distribution for the model parameters expressing the beliefs after observing the data. Using this posterior distribution over the model parameters, useful random variables can be defined for functions depending on the model parameters, like predictions and error measures.

In a binary classification task this rationale means the following. We are primarily interested in the correct classification of an observation $\boldsymbol{x} \in \mathbb{R}^l$. This can be achieved by constructing a *binary decision function* $g(\boldsymbol{x}, \boldsymbol{\omega}) \in \{0, 1\}$ where $\boldsymbol{\omega} \in \Theta$ are the model parameters. A more informative predictive model provides not only a class label, but also the *class probabilities*, though it is a more complex task both from a statistical and computational point of view. As a further step in improving the decision support, *uncertainty information* can be provided for the class probabilities, for example the posterior distribution of class probabilities in the Bayesian framework. In this paper we follow the Bayesian approach to solve the classification problem for two main reasons: to incorporate prior background information in a general and principled way and to provide detailed information with clear semantics for decision support. Therefore we use a *probabilistic regression* model $P(T = 1|\boldsymbol{x}, \boldsymbol{\omega}) = f(\boldsymbol{x}, \boldsymbol{\omega}) \in [0, 1]$ with model parameters $\boldsymbol{\omega} \in \Theta$ and a prior distribution $p_{\boldsymbol{\Omega}}(.)$ over Θ. We assume a supervised learning scheme, that is the existence of a labeled training set $\underline{\boldsymbol{d}} = \{\boldsymbol{x}_k, t_k\}_{k=1}^n$, $(\boldsymbol{x}_k, t_k) \in \mathbb{R}^l \times \{0, 1\}$, where $\boldsymbol{x}$ is a real valued l-dimensional input vector and t is the corresponding class label. In the paper we use capitals for random variables, bold indicates a vector and an underline indicates a matrix.

Using the observed data $\underline{d}$ and applying Bayes' rule, the prior distribution can be transformed to the posterior distribution

$$p_{\Omega}(\boldsymbol{\omega}|\underline{d}) = \frac{p_T(t_1, \ldots, t_n|\boldsymbol{\omega}, \boldsymbol{x}_1, \ldots, \boldsymbol{x}_n)p_{\Omega}(\boldsymbol{\omega}|\boldsymbol{x}_1, \ldots, \boldsymbol{x}_n)}{p_{\underline{D}}(\underline{d})} \propto L(\boldsymbol{\omega}|\underline{d})p_{\Omega}(\boldsymbol{\omega})$$

where $L(\boldsymbol{\omega}|\underline{d})$ denotes the probability of the data given the parameters.

Once we have this posterior distribution for the model parameters, we can define random variables related to predictions, performance, etc. In classification problems for example, we are interested, for a given $\boldsymbol{x}$, in the random variable $f(\boldsymbol{x}, \boldsymbol{\Omega})$ where $\boldsymbol{\Omega}$ is a random parameter vector. In this way we have uncertainty information about the predicted class probability.

We can simplify this result to scalar values for the class probabilities $P(T = 1|\boldsymbol{x}, \underline{d})$. The optimal step back depends on the cost function attached to the reported scalar value. Assuming the L_2 loss function, the optimal strategy is to report the expectation of the class probability in the posterior parameter probability space $f(\boldsymbol{x}) := E_{\boldsymbol{\Omega}|\underline{d}}[f(\boldsymbol{x}, \boldsymbol{\omega})]$. A further simplification is to discretize this scalar value using some user specified threshold λ, deriving a binary decision function

$$g_{\lambda}(\boldsymbol{x}) := \begin{cases} 1 \text{ if } E_{\boldsymbol{\Omega}|\underline{d}}[f(\boldsymbol{x}, \boldsymbol{\omega})] \geq \lambda \\ 0 \text{ else.} \end{cases}$$

These three distinct levels ($f(\boldsymbol{x}, \boldsymbol{\Omega})$, $f(\boldsymbol{x})$ and $g_{\lambda}(\boldsymbol{x})$) provide diminishing possibilities for decision support. This is illustrated by the increasing information provided by the class labels, class probabilities and distributions of class probabilities, though the burdening statistical and computational complexity should be considered too.

3 Classification of Ovarian Masses

Ovarian malignancies represent the greatest challenge among gynaecologic cancers. A reliable preoperative prediction in terms of benign and malignant ovarian tumors would be of considerable help to clinicians selecting an appropriate treatment. There are two sources of information to construct such predictive models: prior knowledge and data.

The available relevant medical literature and expert knowledge is abundant and very diverse (for an overview, see [7]. In addition to the prior background information, data were collected prospectively from 300 consecutive patients who were referred to a single institution (University Hospitals Leuven, Belgium) from August 1994 until June 1997. The data collection protocol ensure that the patients had an apparent persistent extrauterine pelvic mass and excludes other causes that may have similar symptoms such as infection or pregnancy, so the primary aim is differentiation between benign and malignant masses (for a detailed description, see [7]. Univariate statistics of data set are presented in Table 1.

Table 1. Univariate statistics for the ovarian cancer data set.

	Age	Parity	CA 125	Color score	RI
$\widehat{E}[.|Benign]$	47.77	1.50	110.34	1.98	0.12
$\widehat{E}[.|Malignant]$	58.62	1.57	1222.299	3.20	0.41
$Std[.|Benign]$	15.60	1.40	976.56	0.84	0.77
$Std[.|Malignant]$	15.18	1.73	3779.64	0.95	0.46

Standard statistical studies indicate that a multi-modal approach – the combination of various types of variables – is necessary for the discrimination between benign and malignant tumors. Therefore Logistic Regression models, Multilayer Perceptrons and Belief Networks were previously applied [7, 3]. These models predicted the scalar class probabilities and they were developed and tested in the classical statistical framework.

A natural step to provide more detailed information for medical decision support is to apply the Bayesian approach to provide the distribution of class probabilities. We can use the classical statistical performance measures for the evaluation of the models in the Bayesian framework, since any performance measure is a function of the model parameters (for fixed observations/test data). These performance measures then become random variables which provide more information than a point estimate.

Because in the medical literature the Receiver Operator Characteristics (ROC) curve was advocated to assess and compare the performance of probabilistic classifiers, we use three performance measures: the misclassification rate $MR(\Omega, \underline{d})$, the ROC curve $ROC(., \Omega, \underline{d})$ and the area under the ROC curve $AUC(\Omega, \underline{d})$ (for the definition and interpretations of the ROC curve, see [8]. Finally, we computed the Bayes factors [9] to compare the models in a Bayesian way.

4   Applied Bayesian Models

In the paper a Multilayer Perceptron (MLP) and a Belief Network (BN) model are discussed. For each model we define and investigate two types of prior distribution: *informative* and *non-informative* priors, depending on the amount of incorporated prior background knowledge. Additionally, an auxiliary probabilistic domain model is introduced for the MLP models, which are not capable of coping with incomplete input samples. This auxiliary probabilistic domain model is not updated by the observed samples and is only used for coping with missing input values in the original data set[1].

---

[1] Note that the BN missing value mechanism is fundamentally different from this in two important respects: first, the mechanism is immediately provided since a BN model defines a joint probability distribution, second the prior distributions for Belief

4.1   Belief Network Models

A Belief Network model defines a joint probability distribution over the domain variables. It is a probabilistic *white-box* model, since it consists of a graph model about the conditional independencies of the domain variables and a quantitative part specifying the conditional probabilities for the domain variables. The prior knowledge available from experts and the literature can be directly represented in an *informative* prior distribution for this model using the following technique: Assuming that the parameter independence holds, we use the Dirichlet family to represent the prior distribution [4]. Using a Dirichlet distribution, an expert can express his belief in parametrizations, instead of giving only a point estimation for the parameters. The *non-informative* distribution for Belief Networks is a uniform distribution corresponding to the Dirichlet distribution with all hyperparameters equal to one.

We tried to build Belief Networks to formalize the available prior knowledge from expert and literature in three different ways [3]. In the first phase we experimented with "biological" models in which various causal models of the disease are incorporated. The specification of the structure was relatively easy, but the quantification was not possible from the literature, nor from the expert and we had a too small data set to quantify additionally introduced hidden variables. In the second phase we built "expert" models that reflect the expert's experience. The qualitative dependence-independency structure specification was again relatively easy. However the results were too biased because the medical expert participating in the project previously worked with the same collected data, so his estimates were largely based on the data set. In the third phase we built "heterogeneous" models containing biological models of the underlying mechanism quantifiable by the literature, parts quantified by a medical expert and parts quantified by previously published studies. The graphical structure of the Belief Network model is shown on the left side of Fig. 1.

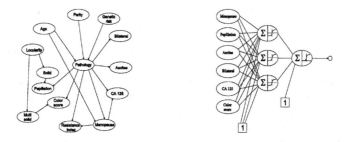

Fig. 1. The BN and MLP model structures.

Network models (and therefore the underlying mechanism to cope with the missing values) is updated by the data.

It is worth to note from a computational point of view that all the variables are discrete in this model class. Because of the extensive and complex usage of the prior knowledge we used a strict documentation method to track the route of the prior information from studies into the model. Conversion formulas were constructed to compile the raw prior knowledge to be compatible with the conditions of the model and the format of the Bayesian network.

Since a Bayesian network model is inherently capable of performing inference for incomplete cases, there is no additional technique for handling missing values. Consequently, we evaluate two Belief Network models: the same structure with *informative* and *non-informative* prior distribution.

4.2   Multilayer Perceptron Models

These probabilistic regression models are defined over a continuous input space specifying an input-output mapping which can be interpreted as a conditional probability $P(T = 1|\boldsymbol{x}, \boldsymbol{\omega}) = f(\boldsymbol{x}, \boldsymbol{\omega})$.

The MLP model structure used in the paper is shown on the right of Fig. 1 (for data preprocessing details, input and MLP structure selection, see [7, 2].

Since the Multilayer Perceptron (MLP) model is a *black-box* model, it is not possible to specify directly a prior distribution incorporating the available prior knowledge in a general way. To solve this problem we use the Belief Network models as a tool to acquire and represent the prior domain knowledge. The *informative* prior distribution for the BN is then transformed into a so called *informative* prior distribution for the MLP parameters.

Omitting the technical details, it is possible to define a mapping $\mathcal{T} : \Theta^{BN} \rightarrow \Theta$ that transforms a prior distribution $p_{\Omega^{BN}}(.)$ over the Belief Network parameter space to a prior probability distribution $p_{\Omega}(.)$ over the black-box model parameter space[2]: a black-box regression model $f(\boldsymbol{x}, \boldsymbol{\omega})$ is used for approximating the conditional distribution of the output class $P(T = 1|\boldsymbol{x}, \boldsymbol{\omega}^{BN})$ conditioned on the input $\boldsymbol{x}$, which is defined by the Belief Network. Thus we can define a mapping from every Belief Network parametrization $\boldsymbol{\omega}^{BN} \in \Theta^{BN}$ to the "best" approximating regression model parametrization $\boldsymbol{\omega} \in \Theta$.

The main steps for the application of this technique in the case of Multilayer Perceptron are the following (see [2] for details):

1a. Generate Belief Network parametrizations $\{\boldsymbol{\omega}_1^{BN}, \ldots, \boldsymbol{\omega}_l^{BN}\}$ from the Dirichlet distribution by standard methods.

1b. Generate block of prior samples $\{\underline{\boldsymbol{d}}_1^p, \ldots, \underline{\boldsymbol{d}}_l^p\}$ from each parametrization. It is advantageous to use the prior probabilistic domain model to compute $P(T = 1|\boldsymbol{x}, \boldsymbol{\omega}^{BN})$ for each sample instead of Bernouilli generated class labels according to this probability.

2. Train a Multilayer Preceptron for each block of samples resulting in a block of MLP parametrizations $\{\boldsymbol{\omega}_1, \ldots, \boldsymbol{\omega}_l\}$ (we applied the scaled conjugate gradient algorithm [11].

---

[2] For simplicity, only the Belief Network notations are differentiated with a BN superscript and we use the intact notation for the black-box MLP models.

3. Estimate the transformed distribution $p_\Omega(.)$ from the generated MLP parametrization $\{\omega_1, \ldots, \omega_l\}$ with a mixture of Gaussians.

The *non-informative* prior for the MLP model is a non-restrictive, complexity based prior $\mathcal{N}(0, \sigma^2 I)$ (cfr. weight decay for neural networks in the classical framework).

As mentioned previously, an auxiliary probabilistic domain model for the MLP models is introduced, which is represented by a Belief Network[3]. We use the prior Belief Network described earlier with its most probable a priori parametrization and assume a fixed data collection procedure with the *ignorable* condition [10]. In this case $P(\boldsymbol{X}^{miss}|\boldsymbol{X}^{obs}, T, \boldsymbol{Z}, \text{BN})$ gives the distribution of the missing values (for details see [1]) where $\boldsymbol{Z}$ are those variables that occur in the data set and in the attached auxiliary domain model, but not in the MLP model. It means that the auxiliary Belief Network model provides a theoretically optimal solution to use incomplete samples for learning and inference. Using these assumptions it can be shown [1] that the posterior and inference for such an extended regression model can be written as follows with $\boldsymbol{\mathcal{I}}$ a binary random vector, where $\mathcal{I}_i$ denotes the observed or missing status of the ith variable.

$$p_\Omega(\omega|t, \underline{x}^{obs}, \underline{z}, \boldsymbol{\mathcal{I}}, \text{BN}) = \int \ldots \int p_\Omega(\omega|t, \underline{x}^{obs}, \underline{x}^{miss}) \prod_{i=1}^{n} dP(x_i^{miss}|t_i, x_i^{obs}, z_i, \text{BN})$$

$$P(T = 1|x^{obs}, z, \boldsymbol{\mathcal{I}}, \omega) = \int f(x, \omega) dP(x^{miss}|x^{obs}, z)$$

5   Inference Algorithms

The target random variables to be estimated are hierarchical: the inference $P(T = 1|\boldsymbol{\Omega}, x^{obs}, z, \underline{d})$ and the performance related $AUC(\boldsymbol{\Omega}, \underline{d}), MR(\boldsymbol{\Omega}, \underline{d})$.

In the case of Belief Network prediction we sample the posterior distribution $p_\Omega(\omega|\underline{d})$ by direct sampling from the updated Dirichlet (see [6]) and compute the conditional probabilities of malignancy for the drawn parametrizations by an exact inference algorithm using a join tree (see [4]). Based on these predictions the corresponding AUC and MR values can be computed.

In the case of MLP prediction, at first we sample the unknown input variables conditioned on all the known variables using the auxiliary probabilistic BN model (i.e., according to $P(\boldsymbol{X}^{miss}|\boldsymbol{X}^{obs}, T, \boldsymbol{Z}, \text{BN})$). Then we sample from the posterior distribution based on the completed data set $p_\Omega(\omega|t, \underline{x}^{obs}, \underline{x}^{miss})$ by the Hybrid Monte Carlo method [13, 12]. Finally we compute the predictions and the corresponding AUC and MR values for the drawn parametrization on the test set by averaging over the missing input variables sampling $P(\boldsymbol{X}^{miss}|\boldsymbol{X}^{obs}, \boldsymbol{Z}, \text{BN})$.

---

[3] Note that the applied Belief Network is discrete valued, so we use additional probabilistic models for transformation between discrete and continuous values.

6 Results

We report results for the four models described in Section 4.1 using the algorithms summarized in Section 5. We partitioned the data set described in Section 3 randomly to a test (30%) and training (70%) set, the reported results are based on the test set. This was repeated 50 times to eliminate dependency on separation. The model classes are denoted as follows: Multilayer Perceptron model with *informative* prior (MLP-I) and with *non-informative* (MLP-N) and Belief Network model with *informative* prior (BN-I) and with *non-informative* prior (BN-N). The performance of the models are shown in Table 2. Note that most of the outliers for models with *non-informative* prior are omitted to focus on the most interesting region. Figure 2 shows the more detailed effect of the prior for varying sample size.

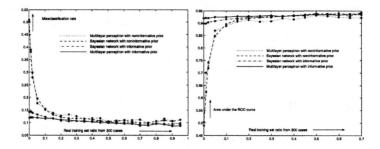

Fig. 2. Learning curves of MLP-N, MLP-I, BN-N, and BN-I models.

The Bayes-factors against the less probable model class (BN-N) are 1.29 (MLP-N), 1.45 (MLP-I) and 1.19 (BN-I) assuming uniform prior probabilities for the model classes[4].

7 Discussion

As can be seen from Table 2 the Belief Network models have the best performance, which is the consequence of the larger number of input variables (a more extensive comparison including Logistic Regression models can be found in [2]). Using the same input set as for the MLP models, the performance lags behind the performance of the MLP models, as Figure 2 shows (for details please see [2]).

---

[4] To eliminate the effect of the sample size we take the nth root of the likelihoods where $n = 300$ is the size of the sample (i.e., we estimate $\int_\Theta \sqrt[n]{\frac{P(\underline{d}|\omega,\,M=.)}{P(\underline{d}|BN-N)}}\,dP_\Omega(\omega)$ by the Monte Carlo method).

Table 2. The distributions of the area under the ROC curve, of the misclassification rates and the corresponding means and variances.

E[.]/Var[.]	MR	ROC
MLP-N	0.1019/0.0007	0.9361/0.0006
MLP-I	0.0964/0.0010	0.9362/0.0010
BN-N	0.0980/0.0008	0.9485/0.0006
BN-I	0.0944/0.0006	0.9371/0.0006

Figure 2 illustrates clearly the subtle advantages of the Bayesian incorporation of prior domain knowledge through *informative* priors: it has a large advantageous effect in the small sample region ($[0-0.4]$) and it has no restrictive effect in the large sample range.

The Bayes factors indicate that the posterior probability of MLP model with informative priors is the highest, but the Bayesian model comparison needs further investigation, such as the selection of appropriate priors for the models.

Beside numerical comparison, we performed a manual evaluation of the predictions. The application of the Bayesian approach, particularly for the MLP models, shows that when the model misclassifies a sample, the distribution of the predicted class probability is widespread. Therefore the introduction of an "uncertain" label can have important consequences on performances and thus on medical decision support. A further interesting medical result that all the models are regularly "uncertain" for a well-determined subset of patients, which suggests that the currently used input features are not enough to achieve reliable classification for these patients.

8   Conclusions

In the paper the applicability of complex regression models, Multilayer Perceptron models, in the Bayesian context was examined. We summarized a technique that derives informative prior distributions for such black-box models and overviewed the application of Belief Networks as auxiliary probabilistic models to handle incomplete cases for probabilistic regression models. We performed a retrospective analysis to predict malignancy in ovarian masses in which various Bayesian models were investigated: Multilayer Perceptron and Belief Network models. We reported standard performance measures in the Bayesian framework, investigated the usability of the more detailed predictions of Bayesian models and compared the models in the Bayesian framework.

Currently we are investigating a hybrid Belief Network model composed of a prior Belief Network and a probabilistic regression model, where we treat the prior Belief Network (including the auxiliary model) and a probabilistic regression model together in the Bayesian framework.

Acknowledgements. Joos Vandewalle is Full Professor at the K.U.Leuven. Bart De Moor is Full Professor at the K.U.Leuven. Sabine Van Huffel is a senior research associate with the F.W.O. (Fund for Scientific Research-Flanders). Peter Antal is a Research Assistant with the K.U.Leuven. Geert Fannes is a Research Assistant with the F.W.O. Vlaanderen. This work was carried out at the ESAT laboratory and supported by grants and projects from the Flemish Government: Concerted Research Action GOA-MEFISTO-666 (Mathematical Engineering for Information and Communication Systems Technology) and F.W.O. project G.0262.97: Learning and Optimization: an Interdisciplinary Approach and the F.W.O. Research Communities: ICCoS (Identification and Control of Complex Systems) and Advanced Numerical Methods for Mathematical Modelling and Bilaterale Wetenschappelijke en Technologische Samenwerking Flanders-Hungary, BIL2000/19; from National Fund for Scientific Research (OTKA) under contract number T030586; from National Fund for Scientific Research (OTKA) under contract number F-030763; from the Belgian State, Prime Minister's Office-Federal Office for Sci., Tech. and Cult. Affairs-Interuniversity Poles of Attraction Programme (IUAP P4-02 (1997-2001): Modeling, Identification and Control of Complex Systems. The scientific responsibility is assumed by its authors; from the European Community TMR Programme, Networks, project CHRX-CT97-0160; from the Brite Euram Programme, Thematic Network BRRT-CT97-5040 'Niconet'; from the IDO/99/03 project (K.U.Leuven) "Predictive computer models for medical classification problems using patient data and expert knowledge", of the FWO grants G.0326.98 and G.0360.98, the FWO project G.0200.00.

References

1. P. Antal, G. Fannes, S. Van Huffel, B. De Moor, J. Vandewalle, and Dirk Timmerman, *Bayesian predictive models for ovarian cancer classification: evaluation of logistic regresseion, multi-layer perceptron and belief network models in the bayesian context,* Proceedings of the Tenth Belgian-Dutch Conference on Machine Learning, BENELEARN 2000, 2000, pp. 125–132.
2. P. Antal, G. Fannes, H. Verrelst, B. De Moor, and J. Vandewalle, *Incorporation of prior knowledge in black-box models: Comparison of transformation methods from bayesian network to multilayer perceptrons,* Workshop on Fusion of Domain Knowledge with Data for Decision Support, 16th UAI Conf., 2000, pp. 42–48.
3. P. Antal, H. Verrelst, D. Timmerman, Y. Moreau, S. Van Huffel, B. De Moor, and I. Vergote, *Bayesian networks in ovarian cancer diagnosis: Potential and limitations,* Proc. of the 13th IEEE Symp. on Comp.-Based Med.Sys., 2000, Houston, pp. 103–109.
4. E. Castillo, J.M. Guttiérrez, and A.S. Hadi, *Expert systems and probabilistic network models,* Springer, 1997.
5. J. Cloete and J.M. Zurada, *Knowledge-based neurocomputing,* MIT Press, 2000.
6. D.J. Spiegelhalter et al., *Bayesian analysis in expert systems,* Statistical Science **8** (1993), no. 3, 219–283.
7. D. Timmerman et al., *Artificial neural network models for the pre-operative discrimination between malignant and benign adnexal masses,* Ultrasound Obstet. Gynecol. **13** (1999), 17–25.

8. J.A. Hanley et al., *The meaning and use of the area under receiver operating characteristic (roc) curve,* Radiology **143** (1982), 29–36.
9. J.M. Bernardo et al., *Bayesian theory,* Wiley & Sons, 1995.
10. A. Gelman, J.B. Carlin, H.S. Stern., and D.B. Rubin, *Bayesian data analysis,* Chapman & Hall, 1995.
11. M.F. Moller, *A scaled conjugate gradient algorithm for fast supervised learning,* Neural Networks **6** (1993), 525–533.
12. P. Müller and R.D. Insua, *Issues in bayesian analysis of neural network models,* Neural Computation **10** (1998), 571–592.
13. R.M. Neal, *Bayesian learning for neural networks,* Springer, 1996.

The Effects of Disregarding Test Characteristics in Probabilistic Networks

Linda C. van der Gaag, C.L.M. Witteman, Silja Renooij, and
M. Egmont-Petersen

Institute of Information and Computing Sciences, Utrecht University,
P.O. Box 80.089, 3508 TB Utrecht, The Netherlands
{linda,cilia,silja,michael}@cs.uu.nl

Abstract. In most medical disciplines, the results from diagnostic tests
are not unequivocal. To capture the uncertainties in test results, the
notions of sensitivity and specificity of diagnostic tests have been introduced. Although the importance of taking these test characteristics into
account in medical reasoning is stressed throughout the literature, they
are often not modelled explicitly in real-life probabilistic networks. In
this paper, we study the effects that disregarding the characteristics of
diagnostic tests can have on the performance of a probabilistic network.
We feel that the effects that we observed in a real-life network for the
staging of oesophageal cancer, are likely to be found in networks for other
applications in medicine as well.

1 Introduction

Since their introduction, probabilistic networks have become increasingly popular in medical decision support. A probabilistic network is a statistical model
comprised of a graphical structure and an associated set of probabilities [1].
The graphical structure models the statistical variables that are relevant in the
field of application, along with the influential relationships between them; the
strengths of the relationships are captured by conditional probabilities. Probabilistic networks have a number of methodological advantages compared to other
types of statistical model used in medical reasoning. Probabilistic networks can
for example adequately deal with data from patients in whom only a subset of
the relevant variables have been observed.

Medical reasoning with a probabilistic network amounts to entering a patient's symptoms and test results into the network. The network then computes
the most likely diagnosis for the patient, or another outcome of interest. In most
medical disciplines, a patient's symptoms and test results are not unequivocal.
As an example, we consider an X-ray of a patient's chest to establish the presence or absence of lung cancer. A physician interpreting the X-ray may easily
overlook a small tumour and falsely state a negative result. On the other hand,
the physician may state a false positive result based on a phantom image. The
uncertainties in a test's results are captured by the *sensitivity* and *specificity*
characteristics of the test. The sensitivity of a test is defined as the probability

S. Quaglini, P. Barahona, and S. Andreassen (Eds.): AIME 2001, LNAI 2101, pp. 188–198, 2001.

that a positive test result is found in a patient who actually has the disease. The test's specificity is the probability that the test yields a negative result for a patient without the disease. The notions of sensitivity and specificity are well-known in the field of medical decision making; textbooks in fact stress the importance of taking test characteristics into account in medical reasoning in order to avoid misdiagnosis [2,3].

Probabilistic networks allow for modelling test characteristics by distinguishing between variables that represent test results on the one hand and variables that model the (generally unobservable) truth on the other hand, and thus provide the means for dealing with the uncertainties in test results. In many real-life probabilistic networks, however, the sensitivity and specificity characteristics of tests are not explicitly modelled, not even in medical disciplines where these characteristics are readily available. Building a probabilistic network is a hard and time-consuming task and, in our experience, incorporating test characteristics contributes significantly to its difficulty. The main obstacle is not so much in capturing the characteristics themselves but rather in obtaining the probabilities for the variables that model the true values. We feel that this observation explains the absence of test characteristics from many real-life networks.

In this paper, we investigate the effects that disregarding the sensitivity and specificity characteristics of diagnostic tests can have on the performance of a probabilistic network. To this end, we study a real-life network for the staging of oesophageal cancer. We compare the performance of the complete network that captures full test characteristics, with the performance of a reduced network from which these characteristics have been removed. We feel that the various effects that we observe in the performance of these networks are likely to be found for probabilistic networks for other applications in medicine as well.

In Sect. 2, we briefly introduce our probabilistic network for the staging of oesophageal cancer. In Sect. 3, we present the design of our study. In Sect. 4, we describe the results from evaluations of the complete network and of the reduced network, using real-life patient data; these results are discussed in depth in Sect. 5. The paper ends with our concluding observations in Sect. 6.

2   The Oesophagus Network

The *oesophagus network* for the staging of oesophageal cancer has been constructed with the help of two experts in gastrointestinal oncology from the Netherlands Cancer Institute, Antoni van Leeuwenhoekhuis [4]. The network describes the presentation characteristics of an oesophageal tumour, such as its location in the oesophagus, and its histological type, length, and macroscopic shape. In addition, the network describes the pathophysiological process underlying the tumour's invasion into the oesophageal wall and adjacent organs. It further describes the process of metastasis. The depth of invasion and the extent of metastasis are summarised in the tumour's *stage*; this stage can be either I, IIA, IIB, III, IVA, or IVB, in the order of advanced disease. The oesophagus network includes 42 variables, for which almost 1000 probabilities have been specified by our experts. The network is depicted in Fig. 1, which also shows the prior probabilities computed per variable.

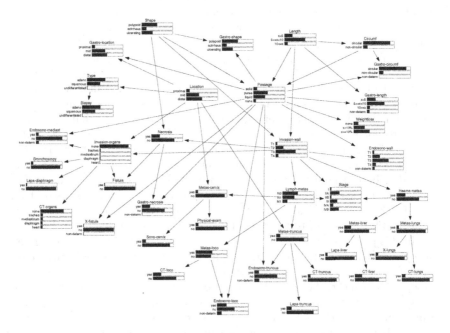

Fig. 1. The oesophagus network.

To establish the stage of a patient's oesophageal tumour, typically a number of diagnostic tests are performed, ranging from multiple biopsies of the tumour to a CT-scan of the patient's chest. The network includes 23 variables to model test results. The sensitivity and specificity characteristics of the tests are captured by the associated conditional probabilities. As an example, Fig. 2(b) shows the probabilities of the results of an X-ray of a patient's chest, given the actual presence or absence of lung metastases: the X-ray is stated to have a sensitivity of 0.85 and a specificity of 0.98. The diagnostic tests included in the oesophagus network differ considerably with respect to their sensitivity and specificity characteristics, that is, not every test result obtained for a patient is equally reliable.

3   The Study

To study the effects of disregarding the sensitivity and specificity characteristics of diagnostic tests, we compare the performance of the oesophagus network described in the previous section with that of a reduced network from which the 23 variables representing test results have been removed. We refer to the former as

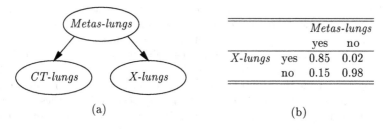

		Metas-lungs	
		yes	no
X-lungs	yes	0.85	0.02
	no	0.15	0.98

(a)   (b)

Fig. 2. A fragment of the oesophagus network (a) and some associated probabilities (b).

the *complete network* and to the latter as the *reduced network*. The performance of the two networks is compared using real-life patient data. For each patient, the most likely stage, given the available symptoms and test results, is computed from the two networks; the computed stages are then compared with the stage recorded in the data.

In the complete oesophagus network, test results are entered as values for the appropriate variables. For example, if a gastroscopic examination of a patient's oesophagus reveals a tumour length of less than 5 centimeters, this result is entered for the variable *Gastro-length*. From the reduced network, however, the variables modelling test results have been removed. As a consequence, no distinction can be made between a test result and the true value. Test results are therefore entered as if they were true values. For example, the result mentioned above is entered for the variable *Length* which models the true tumour length.

For variables for which a *single* test is performed, such as the variable *Length*, test results can be entered unambiguously into the reduced network. For several variables, however, two or more tests are available. For example, to establish the presence or absence of metastases in a patient's lungs, an X-ray or a CT-scan can be made, as indicated in Fig. 2(a). The results from such multiple tests can be conflicting, that is, it is possible that different results are yielded by the CT-scan and the X-ray. In case of such conflicting test results, we have to decide which result to enter. A range of different strategies can be designed for this purpose:

- a result is picked randomly (the *random-test strategy*);
- a result from a more reliable test is preferred over a less reliable result (the *reliable-test strategy*);
- a positive result is preferred over a negative one (the *positive-test strategy*).

The *reliable-test strategy* is closest to the reasoning strategy exhibited by the complete network: it takes the sensitivity and specificity of the various tests into account, even though these characteristics are not explicitly modelled. The *positive-test strategy*, on the other hand, seems to be the closest to the reasoning behaviour of the gastroenterologists who helped in the network's construction and collected the data. In our study, we therefore focus on these two strategies.

We would like to note that, in case of conflicting test results, the complete oesophagus network takes *all* results into account: it weighs the uncertainties involved and combines the results into an overall uncertain value. The network is said to exhibit *compensatory* reasoning behaviour. By removing the variables that represent test results, we have shifted part of this compensatory behaviour to outside the network. Our strategies for entering test results are *non-compensatory* as they do not weigh and combine results. With these strategies, the reduced network exhibits a reasoning behaviour that is *non-compensatory* to at least some extent.

In our study, we use data from the medical records of 156 patients from the Antoni van Leeuwenhoekhuis in the Netherlands diagnosed with oesophageal cancer. For these patients an average number of 12.9 test results are available, ranging from 6 to 19 results per patient.

4   The Results

The results from our study are summarised in Fig. 3. The matrix shown in Fig. 3(a) describes the results from the evaluation of the complete oesophagus network. The numbers on the diagonal of the matrix are the numbers of patients per stage, for whom the network yields the same stage as the one recorded in the data. Because, unfortunately, a *gold standard* for the staging of oesophageal cancer is wanting, we take the stages entered into the patients' medical records for our 'silver' standard of validity. The matrix then reveals that the network computes the correct stage for 110 patients, yielding a percentage correct of 71%, with a 95% confidence interval of (63.4%,77.7%).

The matrices shown in Fig. 3(b) and 3(c) describe the results from evaluating the reduced network, with the reliable-test strategy and the positive-test strategy, respectively. In contrast with the complete oesophagus network, the reduced network is not able to establish a stage for every patient from our data collection: for some patients, entering their data results in an inconsistency and an *error* is generated. The matrix from Fig. 3(b) reveals that the reduced network with the reliable-test strategy computes the correct stage for 66% of the patients, with a 95% confidence interval of (58.6%,73.5%); the data of 22 patients, or 14%, cannot be processed. With the positive-test strategy, the reduced network computes the correct stage for 76% of the patients, with a 95% confidence interval of (68.9%,82.4%); the data of 8 patients, or 5%, result in an error.

Fig. 3(d), to conclude, describes the difference in performance of the reduced network with the reliable-test strategy and with the positive-test strategy, respectively, for the patients for whom neither of the strategies results in an error. As all discrepancies occur below the diagonal of the matrix, it is readily seen that the positive-test strategy tends to result in higher stages being concluded than the reliable-test strategy.

		complete network						
		I	IIA	IIB	III	IVA	IVB	error
	I	**2**	0	0	0	0	0	0
	IIA	0	**37**	0	1	0	0	0
data	IIB	0	2	**0**	2	0	0	0
	III	1	17	0	**28**	0	1	0
	IVA	1	1	0	9	**28**	0	0
	IVB	0	1	0	6	4	**15**	0

(a)

		network, reliable test						
		I	IIA	IIB	III	IVA	IVB	error
	I	**1**	0	0	0	0	1	0
	IIA	0	**38**	0	0	0	0	0
data	IIB	0	2	**0**	2	0	0	0
	III	0	11	0	**29**	0	1	6
	IVA	0	2	0	4	**18**	0	15
	IVB	0	2	0	2	4	**17**	1

(b)

		network, positive test						
		I	IIA	IIB	III	IVA	IVB	error
	I	**1**	0	0	0	0	1	0
	IIA	0	**38**	0	0	0	0	0
data	IIB	0	2	**0**	2	0	0	0
	III	0	9	0	**33**	1	2	2
	IVA	0	1	0	4	**29**	0	5
	IVB	0	0	0	4	4	**17**	1

(c)

		network, reliable test					
		I	IIA	IIB	III	IVA	IVB
	I	**1**	0	0	0	0	0
	IIA	0	**50**	0	0	0	0
network,	IIB	0	0	**0**	0	0	0
positive	III	0	3	0	**36**	0	0
test	IVA	0	2	0	0	**22**	0
	IVB	0	0	0	1	0	**19**

(d)

Fig. 3. The performance of the complete network (a), of the reduced network with the *reliable-test* (b) and *positive-test strategies* (c), and a comparison of the latter two (d).

5   The Effects

In comparing the performance of the complete oesophagus network with that of the reduced network using the reliable-test and positive-test strategies, we observe several effects that can be attributed to test characteristics. These effects are discussed in Sect. 5.1 through 5.3; Sect. 5.4 addresses the overall effect.

5.1   The Effect of the Graphical Structure

The graphical structure of a probabilistic network portrays the influential relationships between its variables. More formally, the structure captures probabilistic dependences and independences [1]. Two variables A and B are *independent* given a set of observations if, on every trail between A and B, there is a variable Y for which one of the following conditions holds:

- Y is observed and on the trail there is at least one arc emanating from Y;
- Y has two incoming arcs on the trail and neither Y nor any of its descendants in the graphical structure is observed.

As the set of observed variables changes, so will the set of dependences and independences that are read from a network's graphical structure. For example, in Fig. 1, the variables *Shape* and *Length* are independent, yet become dependent if a value for *Passage* is entered. On the other hand, the variables *Gastro-length* and *Stage* are dependent, indicating that entering the test result of a gastroscopic examination of a patient's oesophagus with respect to tumour length, will affect the probabilities of the various stages. If the value of *Invasion-wall* would be known, however, entering the test result would no longer have this effect, because *Gastro-length* and *Stage* would then have become independent.

Since a patient's test results are entered for different variables in the complete oesophagus network and in the reduced network, different dependences and independences are taken into account in the networks' computations. To illustrate this observation, we consider the test results and symptoms of a specific patient:

Biopsy = adeno   *Gastro-circumf* = circular   *Gastro-length* = $5 \leq x \leq 10$
Passage = puree   *Gastro-shape* = polypoid   *Gastro-location* = distal
                    Gastro-necrosis = no

When these data are entered into the complete network, each test result and symptom affects the probabilities of the various possible stages for the patient's tumour: the variable *Stage* is dependent of every variable mentioned. Furthermore, four extra *dependences* arise that cause additional interaction effects of the test results and symptoms on the probabilities for the variable *Stage*. For the reduced network, the patient's data are interpreted as

Type = adeno   *Circumf* = circular   *Length* = $5 \leq x \leq 10$
Passage = puree   *Shape* = polypoid   *Location* = distal
                    Necrosis = no

When these values are entered, some new *independences* arise: the variable *Stage* has become independent of the variables *Type* and *Circumf*. As a consequence, the results from the biopsies of the tumour and from the gastroscopic examination of the tumour's circumference are no longer taken into account in the computation of the most likely stage. Furthermore, compared with the complete network, only two of the additional dependences arise, as a result of which fewer interaction effects of the data are captured.

In the complete oesophagus network, a maximum of 23 test results and two symptoms can be entered. Regardless of which test results and symptoms are available, the probabilities for the variable *Stage* depend on each of them; the only exception occurs when a value for the variable *Passage* renders the variable *Stage* independent of *Weightloss*. In the reduced network, a maximum of 15 values can be entered. Entering these values may give rise to new independences, causing a number of test results and symptoms to be disregarded in the computations. For our data collection, between 25% and 45% of the test results and symptoms per patient are thus disregarded.

5.2   The Effect of the Non-compensatory Strategies

The complete oesophagus network takes the uncertainties in a patient's test results into account in its reasoning behaviour. The network exhibits compensatory behaviour in the sense that it carefully weighs the uncertainties involved. For the reduced network, we have shifted part of this compensatory behaviour to outside the network. Since our strategies for entering test results are basically non-compensatory, the reduced network exhibits a reasoning strategy that is non-compensatory to at least some extent.

The way that people, including expert physicians, deal with uncertainties is studied in the field of cognitive science. Various studies have revealed that people interpret probabilistic information differently than probability theory prescribes. People, in fact, exhibit non-compensatory reasoning behaviour. As an example, we briefly review a study by D.M. Eddy [5], pertaining to the diagnosis of breast cancer. In the study, physicians were presented with the following information: the sensitivity of a mammography equals 0.90 and its specificity is 0.80. They were also told that one out of every 10 patients with similar complaints as a particular patient, indeed had breast cancer. The physicians were then asked to assess the probability that this patient, given a positive test result, had cancer. Many physicians in the study judged the probability to be 0.90; most others gave a probability over 0.50. However, when the requested probability is correctly calculated from the information presented, the result is 0.33, a much lower probability. The physicians who gave high probabilities apparently confused the conditional probability expressing sensitivity with its inverse: they thought that the probability of cancer given a positive test result must be equal to the probability of a positive test result given cancer. This confusion of the sensitivity of a test for the predictive value of a positive test result is often observed in cognitive studies. In practice, physicians tend to assume that diagnostic tests are quite sensitive and specific, and interpret a result as an unequivocal *yes* or *no*. They in fact prefer to act as if everything were deterministic [6].

Interpreting test results as true values can cause highly unlikely combinations of results to become truly conflicting. To illustrate this observation, we consider the test results that are mentioned in a particular patient's medical record. The record states *CT-organs* = none, indicating that on the CT-scan of the patient's chest no invasion of the tumour into adjacent organs is visible. For the patient is also stated *X-fistula* = yes, indicating that the X-ray shows an open connection between the oesophagus and the trachea. When these test results are entered into the complete oesophagus network, it weighs the uncertainties involved and combines them into an uncertain assessment for the variable *Invasion-organs*, which models the true invasion of the tumour beyond the oesophageal wall. In the reduced network, the test results are entered as *Invasion-organs* = none and *Fistula* = yes, regardless of the strategy used. Since a fistula can occur only if the oesophageal tumour has invaded the trachea, the two values constitute an inconsistency and an error is generated. While the complete network is able to handle highly unlikely combinations of test results by its compensatory reasoning behaviour, the reduced network, with its non-compensatory strategies, is not.

5.3   The Effect of Preferring Positive Test Results

Physicians are trained to save lives and, as a consequence, are *loss aversive* [7], that is, they will generally try to avoid losing a patient's life. Moreover, physicians have been found to look upon an omission, such as abstaining from surgery, which results in a serious condition, as less bad than performing an intervention which leads to the same condition. In the field of oesophageal cancer, for example, we have observed our gastroenterologists, when assessing the stage of a patient's tumour, to go by a positive result, even if another related test was yet available or had yielded a negative result: they seem to prefer to base their decisions on the positive result in order to be 'better safe than sorry'. This observation coincides with the *confirmation bias* that is often observed in cognitive studies [8]. Positive information tends to get more attention than negative information; in fact, negative information is simply neglected when positive information is available. We feel that these biases arise from decision considerations and should not be taken into account in probabilistic reasoning.

The positive-test strategy used with the reduced oesophagus network complies with the confirmation bias described above and closely resembles our expert gastroenterologists' interpretation of patient data. The results from Sect. 4 indicate that the reduced network with this strategy computes the correct stage for a larger number of patients than the complete network and than the reduced network with the reliable-test strategy. From this observation, we cannot simply conclude that the reduced network with the positive-test strategy performs best. We recall that in the absence of a gold standard for the staging of oesophageal cancer, we have taken the stages from the patients' medical records for our silver standard of validity. This standard, although the best available, is known to be imperfect: the data entered by the gastroenterologists reflect their biases. Since we are comparing against an admittedly imperfect standard, one network may perform better than another while in fact it could be worse. This phenomenon is well-documented in the field of medical decision making [2]. Based upon this observation, we feel that from the evaluation results described in Sect. 4, we can only conclude that the reduced network with the positive-test strategy best fits the data.

5.4   The Overall Effect

The results from our study, as presented in Sect. 4, show that the reduced network using the reliable-test strategy computes the correct stage for 66% of the patients from our data collection; the complete network yields a percentage correct of 71% and the reduced network with the positive-test strategy results in 76% of the patients being correctly classified. Although only moderately significant, we would like to comment on these differences. The difference in performance between the complete network and the reduced network with the reliable-test strategy can be explained from the effect of the graphical structure and from the effect of using a non-compensatory strategy for entering test results. We feel that these effects basically constitute the overall effect of disregarding test characteristics. These effects come into play also for the reduced network with the positive-test strategy. The overall effect of disregarding the characteristics of diagnostic tests, however, is now dominated by the effect of the strategy used because it closely matches the biases in the data.

6   Conclusions

We have investigated the effects that disregarding the sensitivity and specificity characteristics of diagnostic tests can have on the performance of a probabilistic network. To this end, we have compared the performance of a *complete network* for the staging of oesophageal cancer including full test characteristics, with that of a *reduced network* from which these characteristics have been removed. In the reduced network, test results are entered as if they were true values. For entering conflicting test results, we have introduced the *reliable-test* and *positive-test strategies*.

In our study of the oesophagus network, we have observed various effects of disregarding test characteristics that are likely to be found in most applications of probabilistic networks in medicine. We have found that the strategy for entering test results highly influences the reduced network's performance. Also, while the reliable-test strategy should perform better because it more closely resembles correct probabilistic reasoning, it is the positive-test strategy that gives the better result. We have attributed this paradoxical observation to the use of an imperfect standard of validity. We have further found that entering test results as true values results in a large number of errors for real-life patient data. Since a probabilistic network should be able to handle the data of real patients, such errors are highly unwished-for. If many errors are generated, the value of a network for clinical practice rapidly decreases. Based upon our observations, we believe that for most applications in medicine the characteristics of diagnostic tests should be explicitly modelled in a probabilistic network.

Acknowledgements. This research has been (partly) supported by the Netherlands Computer Science Research Foundation with financial support from the Netherlands Organisation for Scientific Research (NWO). We are most grateful to Babs Taal and Berthe Aleman from the Netherlands Cancer Institute, Antoni van Leeuwenhoekhuis, who spent much time and effort in the construction of the oesophagus network.

References

1. F.V. Jensen (1996). *An Introduction to Bayesian Networks*. London: UCL Press.
2. R.H. Fletcher, S.W. Fletcher, E.H. Wagner (1996). *Clinical Epidemiology. The Essentials*, 3rd ed. Baltimore: Williams & Wilkins.
3. D. von Winterfeldt, W. Edwards (1986). *Decision Analysis and Behavioral Research*. New York: Cambridge University Press.
4. L.C. van der Gaag, S. Renooij, C.L.M. Witteman, B.M.P. Aleman, B.G. Taal (2001). Probabilities for a probabilistic network: A case-study in oesophageal carcinoma, submitted for publication.
5. D.M. Eddy (1982). Probabilistic reasoning in clinical medicine: Problems and opportunities. In: D. Kahneman, P. Slovic, A. Tversky (editors). *Judgment Under Uncertainty: Heuristics and Biases*. Cambridge, UK: Cambridge University Press.

6. J. Baron (1994). *Thinking and Deciding*, 2nd ed. Cambridge, UK: Cambridge University Press.
7. D. Kahneman, A. Tversky (1979). Prospect theory: An analysis of decision under risk. *Econometrica*, vol. 47, pp. 263 – 291.
8. J.St.B.T. Evans, D.E. Over (1996). *Rationality and Reasoning*. Hove, UK: Psychology Press.

Knowledge Acquisition and Automated Generation of Bayesian Networks for a Medical Dialogue and Advisory System

Joachim Horn[1], Thomas Birkhölzer[2], Oliver Hogl[3], Marco Pellegrino[1], Ruxandra Lupas Scheiterer[1], Kai-Uwe Schmidt[4], and Volker Tresp[1]

[1] Siemens AG, Corporate Technology
Information and Communications
CT IC 4, D–81730 Munich, Germany
[2] Siemens AG, Medical Solutions
Software Components and Workstations
MED SW S, D–91050 Erlangen, Germany
[3] Bavarian Research Center for Knowledge–Based Systems
Knowledge Acquisition Group
Am Weichselgarten 9, D–91058 Erlangen, Germany
[4] Siemens AG, Medical Solutions
MED GT 2, D–91050 Erlangen, Germany

1 Introduction

Probabilistic models such as Bayesian networks [6] are well suited for medical decision support and are the basis of many successful applications [1,3,4,8,9,10]. Bayesian networks provide a rigorous and efficient framework for inference, i.e. for calculating the probability of each stochastic variable given a set of observations. However, knowledge acquisition and generation of the network are still demanding tasks when large medical domains have to be modelled.

Here, a novel approach for knowledge acquisition and generation of the network is presented. The approach was developed as part of the HealthMan® project [2]. First, the knowledge is collected and put into a structured representation using a software tool (MedKnow) tailored for the medical domain. MedKnow allows the expert to specify diseases and findings, their interconnections, and specific marginal and conditional probabilities. Next, another tool (Knowledge-Compiler) generates the Bayesian network using the structured knowledge. The resulting network can be used by the HealthMan® Dialogue and Advisory System.

2 Knowledge Acquisition Using MedKnow

There were two main goals in developing MedKnow: First, MedKnow allows medical experts to formulate their medical knowledge, without requiring intimate knowledge of Bayesian networks or probability theory. Second, MedKnow makes

S. Quaglini, P. Barahona, and S. Andreassen (Eds.): AIME 2001, LNAI 2101, pp. 199–202, 2001.
© Springer-Verlag Berlin Heidelberg 2001

sure that the acquired knowledge is complete such that the Bayesian network can be generated automatically.

MedKnow uses two classes of stochastic variables: diseases and findings. A finding may play the role of a symptom or the role of an enhancing or inhibiting factor of a disease. An example of knowledge representation using MedKnow is shown in figure 1. In the left part of the window, all defined diseases and findings are listed. In the main part of the window, the selected disease or finding is presented. Here, the medical domain of infections is modeled, and the disease 'measles' is selected.

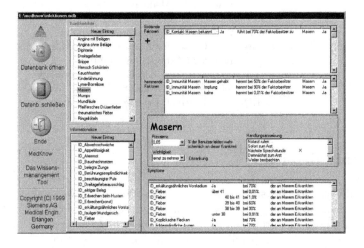

Fig. 1. Specification of measles using MedKnow

The upper part of the main window shows the enhancing and inhibiting factors of the disease, here contact to infected persons and immunity. Furthermore, conditional probabilities have to be specified to quantify the effect of the enhancing and inhibiting factors. The central part of the main window shows the selected disease, its marginal probability, and additional information used in HealthMan®, e.g. the urgency to see a doctor. The lower part of the main window shows the symptoms of the disease together with the conditional probability that the disease will cause the symptom.

A similar display is presented when a finding has been selected.

3   Automated Generation of Bayesian Networks Using KnowledgeCompiler

Generating the Bayesian network using the acquired knowledge can be divided into two subtasks: generating the graph and calculating the conditional probability tables.

Generating the graph is straightforward: each disease and finding is represented by a node and additional nodes are created for – separately – collecting enhancing and inhibiting factors of each single disease. Directed edges are drawn from diseases to the respective symptoms, from enhancing factors to the respective collecting nodes, from inhibiting factors to the respective collecting nodes, and from collecting nodes to the respective diseases. Figure 2 shows the graph of the Bayesian Network for infections generated by KnowledgeCompiler.

Calculation of the conditional probability tables of the Bayesian network is based on the probabilities specified and the type of gate selected by the medical expert. For findings, the expert may choose between gates like NoisyOR [6], NoisyMAX, and NoisyELENI [7]. Diseases are modelled as an enhance–inhibit–gate [5].

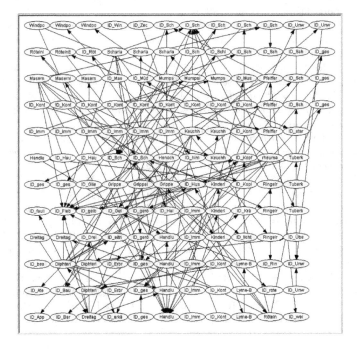

Fig. 2. Bayesian Network for infections generated by KnowledgeCompiler

4   Conclusions

An approach for knowledge acquisition and automated generation of Bayesian networks has been presented. First, the knowledge is acquired using the software tool MedKnow that allows the expert to specify diseases and findings, their interconnections, and specific marginal and conditional probabilities. Next, the software tool KnowledgeCompiler generates the Bayesian network in HUGIN format [6] using the acquired knowledge. The probabilities specified by the expert get transformed into the conditional probability tables according to [5,7]. The resulting Bayesian network can then be used by the HealthMan® Dialogue and Advisory System.

References

1. S. Andreassen, M. Woldbye, B. Falck, S. K. Andersen: "MUNIN – A Causal Probabilistic Network for Interpretation of Electromyographic Findings". *Proceedings of the Tenth International Joint Conference on Artificial Intelligence*, Milan, Italy, August 1987, pp. 366–372.
2. T. Birkhölzer, M. Haft, R. Hofmann, J. Horn, M. Pellegrino, V. Tresp: "Intelligent Communication in Medical Care". *Proceedings of the Joint European Conference on Artificial Intelligence in Medicine and Medical Decision Making (AIMDM 99)*, Aalborg, Denmark, June 1999, p. 4.
3. D. E. Heckerman, E. J. Horvitz, B. N. Nathwani: "Toward Normative Expert Systems: Part I. The Pathfinder Project". *Methods of Information in Medicine*, Vol. 31, 1992, pp. 90–105.
4. D. E. Heckerman, B. N. Nathwani: "Toward Normative Expert Systems: Part II. Probability–Based Representations for Efficient Knowledge Acquisition and Inference". *Methods of Information in Medicine*, Vol. 31, 1992, pp. 106–116.
5. J. Horn: *HealthMan Bayesian Network Description: Enhancing and Inhibiting Factors of Diseases.* Siemens AG, ZT IK 4, Internal Report, 1999.
6. F. V. Jensen: *An Introduction to Bayesian Networks.* UCL Press, 1996.
7. R. Lupas Scheiterer: *HealthMan Bayesian Network Description: Disease to Symptom Layer.* Siemens AG, ZT IK 4, Internal Report, 1999.
8. B. Middleton, M. A. Shwe, D. E. Heckerman, M. Henrion, E. J. Horvitz, H. P. Lehmann, G. F. Cooper: "Probabilistic Diagnosis Using a Reformulation of the INTERNIST–1/QMR Knowledge Base. II. Evaluation of Diagnostic Performance". *Methods of Information in Medicine*, Vol. 30, 1991, pp. 256–267.
9. K. G. Olesen, U. Kjaerulff, F. Jensen, F. V. Jensen, B. Flack, S. Andreassen, S. K. Andersen: "A MUNIN Network for the Median Nerve – A Case Study on Loops". *Applied Artificial Intelligence*, Vol. 3, 1989, pp. 385–403.
10. M. A. Shwe, B. Middleton, D. E. Heckerman, M. Henrion, E. J. Horvitz, H. P. Lehmann, G. F. Cooper: "Probabilistic Diagnosis Using a Reformulation of the INTERNIST–1/QMR Knowledge Base. I. The Probabilistic Model and Inference Algorithms". *Methods of Information in Medicine*, Vol. 30, 1991, pp. 241–250.

Educational Tool for Diabetic Patients Based on Causal Probabilistic Networks

M. Elena Hernando, Enrique J. Gómez, and F. del Pozo

Grupo de Bioingeniería y Telemedicina, Universidad Politécnica de Madrid, Spain
elena@gbt.tfo.upm.es

Abstract. EduDIABNET is an educational tool based on a physiological model that allows simulation and interpretation of the effect of therapeutic actions on the 24-hour blood glucose profile. The system aims to help patients to better their understanding of diabetes self-management and to provide health care professionals with an additional tool to complement the patient education. The physiological model is qualitative and is represented by a quantitative Causal Probabilistic Network. The system enables users to set model variables choosing from a group of qualitative options and presents qualitative results. The user interface has been developed using real-world graphical metaphors to hide the complexity of the physiological model and to increase system usability.

1 Introduction

Diabetes Mellitus is a chronic disease where the process of care is complex and requires the patient to take an active role. The daily management of diabetes mellitus implies that the patient has to be able to react in a proper manner under any situation that can appear during his/her daily life. For this reason, patient education is crucial and has become one of the keys to success in diabetes care. In 1989, the Saint Vincent declaration established education and training as one of the specific goals to be improved in diabetes care [1]. The use of Information Technologies can support many of the aspects included in patient education [2] covering topics such as the use of metabolic simulators, graphical representation and statistics of monitoring data, tools for diet management and advisors for day to day therapy adjustment. This paper presents an intelligent tool for diabetic patients education that makes use of a model for glucose metabolism for interpretation and simulation of common daily situations related to diabetes.

2 The Qualitative Model

The model used by EduDIABNET represents the physiological processes that are presented in diabetic patients. The model represents the day divided into four time

S. Quaglini, P. Barahona, and S. Andreassen (Eds.): AIME 2001, LNAI 2101, pp. 203–206, 2001.

intervals ('breakfast', 'lunch', 'dinner' and 'night' intervals). The inputs into the metabolic model are divided into two categories: self-monitoring patient data, that can be considered as the "symptoms" of the metabolic state (blood glucose and ketonuria measurements); and the "causes" affecting these measurements (insulin doses, meals, meal time and time span between insulin injections and their associated meals). The physiological parameters of this model are qualitative, this means that, for example, an intake is catalogued as "delayed" or "excessive in carbohydrate content" but no quantitative values in minutes or in grams are managed. The relations between the model parameters were obtained from experts and were represented with a qualitative Causal Probabilistic Network (CPN) [3]. The probability tables were obtained from expert knowledge and were refined using real cases. The CPN-model was previously developed and evaluated as the core of DIABNET [4], a decision support system for therapy planning that integrated the CPN-model in a hybrid architecture where the qualitative results were later on converted into quantitative insulin dose modifications adapted to the patient characteristics. The DIABNET system was evaluated with real patients [5] demonstrating the suitability of the qualitative CPN-model for therapy planning. One reason that makes a qualitative model suitable in the education process is that the knowledge used by professionals is also expressed to patients in qualitative terms, as for example: "If a main intake is delayed, then it is possible that it will produce ketonuria and a low blood glucose measurement". In addition, the choice of CPNs facilitates the model reutilization mainly because it supports both diagnostic and predictive reasoning. The previous characteristics greatly benefit any educational tool aiming to implement interpretation and simulation of data.

3   The EduDIABNET System

The EduDIABNET application allows the users to enter cases and to interactively get the interpretation and/or the simulation of them obtained from the internal model. The intended users of the system are mainly diabetic patients that want to improve their knowledge of the illness and also professional users (physicians and nurses) that use the system during training sessions to show the patients the interaction between variables in a visual manner. EduDIABNET runs on a PC with Windows 95 or later and has been implemented using Borland Delphi™ for the user interface and Visual C for the management of the model, integrating the C libraries of HUGIN™. The user tasks supported by EduDIABNET are the following ones:

• **Simulation/interpretation of cases:** The user interface allows the user to fix a set of parameters to simulate and/or interpret the daily blood glucose profile, including both blood glucose measurements and patient actions that can affect the metabolic state. These parameters are linked directly to the upper (causes) and lower (effects) nodes of the CPN qualitative model. Users can enter any combination of parameters to get the propagation of their values into the rest of the model variables and the results are visualized in the graphical interface.

• **Case management:** Users can create and store their own cases and can load examples predefined by physicians. Each case example is defined by a set of parameters that define the case and a text that explains the situation represented by it to aid the patient's understanding. Once the example is loaded the patient can modify any of the model parameters to perform further simulations.

• **Set up of normoglycemia patient-specific ranges**: Due to the differences of normoglycemic ranges across patients, EduDIABNET allows to enter both qualitative and quantitative BG values and to configure the system with their own normoglycemia ranges to translate numeric values into qualitative ones (normal, high, very high, low).

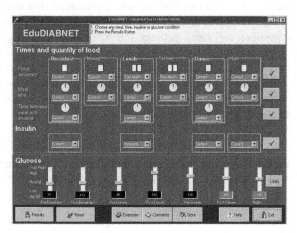

Fig. 1. Interpretation of blood glucose.

The main difficulty when developing an educational tool is to achieve that: 1) the information is displayed in user friendly manner; and 2) the user interaction with the system to enter information is easy and comfortable. To get a user interface (UI) of high usability we designed it following a complete Human Computer Interaction methodology [6]. EduDIABNET UI uses real-world graphical metaphors to hide the complexity of the physiological model and some graphical objects have been implemented to increase system usability, helping users to better their understanding and management of the information required and presented. The IU shows the parameters grouped in intervals associated to the main daily meals; users enter information by selecting one item from a pre-written list and, after that, a graphical icon is displayed on the screen to better understand the nature of data entered. The UI has an implicit horizontal time axe whereby all the parameters are presented on the screen according to the temporal moment they happen or are measured (see Figure 1).

4   Conclusions

EduDIABNET contributes to improve patient education combining the simulation of therapeutic decisions with the interpretation of how these actions influence the metabolic control. The availability of a qualitative model of the physiological process of blood glucose metabolism allows its use for performing different reasoning processes. In our case, such a model has been used with two different purposes: for therapy planning, in the DIABNET system, performing the interpretation of the patient state deviation; and for patient education, in the EduDIABNET system, allowing the simulation and interpretation of non-real cases. The main difficulty in implementing an educational tool is presentation of the information to users in an understandable manner and having a user-friendly interface. The possibility of using pre-recorded cases aids the education process and allows the health care professionals to present to patients those situations that are more representative in their own diabetes type. Nowadays, the availability and penetration of non expensive telecommunication links makes it possible to offer patients integrated telemonitoring and telecare services remotely managed by a health care organization [7]. Patient education must be another important pillar to be integrated into the diabetes care services. The current state of this work is the integration of the qualitative model into the DIABTel telemedicine service [8] and the European Union M2DM Project [9] for the provision of automatic data analysis, alarm generation and advice on therapy adjustment for diabetic patients.

Acknowledgements. This work has been partially funded by the European Project M2DM (IST-1999-10315) and the Spanish Research Council (TEL2001-x-CE and CM-9-0130-1999).

References

1. WHO/IDF EUROPE. Diabetes Care and research in Europe. The Saint Vincent declaration. Diabetic Medicine, 7, (1990).360.
2. Lehmann E.D. y Deutsch T. "Application of computers in diabetes care - a review. II. Computers for decision support and education". Medical Informatics 20 (1995) 303-329
3. Pearl, J. Probabilistic reasoning in intelligent systems: networks of plausible inference. San Mateo, California: Morgan Kaufmann (1988)
4. Hernando, M.E., Gómez, E.J., Del Pozo, F. y Corcoy, R. DIABNET: A qualitative model-based advisory system for therapy planning in gestational diabetes. Medical Informatics 21 (1996) 359-374.
5. Hernando, M.E., Gómez, E.J., Corcoy, R.and del Pozo, F. Evaluation of DIABNET, a decision support system for therapy planning in gestational diabetes. Computers Methods and Programs in Biomedicine 62 (2000) 235-248
6. Gómez, E.J., Quiles, J.A., Sanz, M.F. and Del Pozo, F. A User-Centered Cooperative Information System for Medical Imaging Diagnosis, Journal of the American Society for Information Science 49 (1998) 810-816.
7. M. E. Hernando, E. J. Gomez , A. Garcia y F. del Pozo A multi-access server for the virtual management of diabetes. In Proceedings: ESEM 99 (Fifth conference of the European Society for Engineering and Medicine), Barcelona (1999) 309-310.
8. Gómez, E.J., Del Pozo, F. and Hernando, M.E. Telemedicine for Diabetes Care: the DIABTel approach towards diabetes telecare. Medical Informatics 21 (1996) 283-296.
9. M2DM: multi-access services for the management of diabetes mellitus. EU Project. IST-1999-10315.

NasoNet, Joining Bayesian Networks, and Time to Model Nasopharyngeal Cancer Spread

Severino F. Galán[1], Francisco Aguado[2], Francisco J. Díez[1], and José Mira[1]

[1] Dpto. de Inteligencia Artificial, Facultad de Ciencias de la UNED, Paseo Senda del Rey 9,
28040 Madrid, Spain
{seve, fjdiez, jmira}@dia.uned.es
[2] Servicio de Oncología Radioterápica, Hospital Clínico Universitario San Carlos,
28040 Madrid, Spain
faguado@cgcom.org

Abstract. Cancer spread is a non-deterministic dynamic process. As a consequence, the design of an assistant system for the diagnosis and prognosis of the extent of a cancer should be based on a representation method which deals with both uncertainty and time. The ultimate goal is to know the stage of development reached by a cancer in the patient, previously to selecting the appropriate treatment. A *network of probabilistic events in discrete time* (NPEDT) is a type of temporal Bayesian network that permits to model the causal mechanisms associated with the time evolution of a process. The present work describes NasoNet, a system which applies the formalism of NPEDTs to the case of nasopharyngeal cancer. We have made use of *temporal noisy gates* to model the dynamic causal interactions that take place in the domain. The methodology we describe is sufficiently general to be applied to any other type of cancer.

1 Introduction

The diagnosis and prognosis of the extent of a cancer are tasks full of uncertainty. This is due, on the one hand, to the deeply non-deterministic nature of this disease and, on the other hand, to the incomplete, imprecise, or erroneous information that the oncologist may obtain. This situation is even more complicated in the case of nasopharyngeal cancer, since nasopharynx is a hidden and difficult to enter cavity located in the highest part of the pharynx. Therefore, early detection of a malignant nasopharyngeal tumor is not usual.

Bayesian networks [13] are a probability-based knowledge representation method, appropriate for the modeling of causal processes with uncertainty, such as those determining the evolution of a cancerous disease. A Bayesian network is an acyclic directed graph whose nodes represent random variables and links define probabilistic dependence relations between variables. These relations are quantified by associating a conditional probability table to each node. Each conditional probability table contains the probabilities of the values of a node given all the possible configurations of values of its parents. For root nodes, only its a priori probability is needed. Bayesian networks permit to specify dependence and independence relations in a natural way through the network topology. Diagnosis or prediction with Bayesian

S. Quaglini, P. Barahona, and S. Andreassen (Eds.): AIME 2001, LNAI 2101, pp. 207–216, 2001.

networks consists in fixing the values of the observed variables and computing the posterior probabilities of some of the unobserved variables.

Time is a fundamental factor in cancer since it usually determines the stage of the disease and, consequently, the type of treatment to be applied. Modeling the process that begins with the arising of a malignant tumor and ends with the appearance of several typical symptoms, metastasis, or affected lymph nodes, requires to represent the causal mechanisms that control this process over time. Some of the most widespread methods for modeling dynamic processes with uncertainty in medical domains [2, 1, 14, 11, 10] are based on the formalism of *dynamic Bayesian networks* [4, 8, 12, 3] or their extension *dynamic influence diagrams* [16]. These formalisms have the disadvantage of leading to complex networks, since time is discretized and a node is created for each random variable associated to each time instant. Usually, a copy of a static network is generated for each time point and links are established between nodes in adjacent static networks. In this way, Markovian processes can be modeled so that the future is conditionally independent of the past given the present.

A *network of probabilistic events in discrete time* (NPEDT) [7] is a temporal Bayesian network that leads to less complex networks than those obtained through the formalism of dynamic Bayesian networks, for domains involving temporal fault diagnosis and prediction. Under this formalism, time is discretized, nodes are associated to events, and each value of a node represents the occurrence of an event at a particular instant. The improvement in complexity is a consequence of restricting to one the number of possible occurrences over time for each event. Reversible processes can be represented through multiple events. The links in the network represent temporal causal mechanisms between neighboring nodes. Therefore, each conditional probability table expresses the most probable delays between parent events and the corresponding child event. Two major advantages of a NPEDT are that this model is not restricted to Markovian processes, and that we can make use of different *temporal noisy gates* [6, 7] that facilitate knowledge acquisition and representation. The process of cancer spread, previously to applying the appropriate treatment, is formed by a set of irreversible events. Each of these events can be represented by a node in a NPEDT. In this work, we show the application of the NPEDT approach to the modeling of nasopharyngeal cancer evolution. The network assists the clinician in the diagnosis and prognosis of the extent of this disease.

2   Nasopharyngeal Cancer

The nasopharynx is the highest part of the pharynx, which receives the air breathed through the nose. The nasopharyngeal cavity has a cuboidal shape: the lateral walls are formed by the Eustachian tube and the fossa of Rosenmuller, anteriorly are the posterior choanae and nasal cavity, the roof has the base of the skull above, the posterior boundary is formed by the muscles of the posterior pharyngeal wall, and inferiorly are the upper surface of the soft palate and the posterior pharyngeal wall.

The patient profile we are interested in corresponds to those patients coming from the Dept. of Otorhinolaryngology of a hospital, who are admitted to the Dept. of

Radiation Oncology; specifically, our work has been carried out in collaboration with oncologists from San Carlos University Clinical Hospital at Madrid.

A cancer of the nasopharynx [15, 9] arises as a malignant primary tumor localized on one of the nasopharyngeal walls. Primary tumors on lateral walls are the most frequent, whereas those on anterior and posterior walls are less probable. As time goes by, an initial primary tumor may either infiltrate the adjacent tissue (infiltrating tumor) or grow in volume inside the nasopharynx (vegetating tumor). Accordingly, any part surrounding the nasopharynx, or even any nasopharyngeal wall, may be affected by the tumor growth. Generally, vegetating tumors may obstruct the ducts connecting the nasopharynx to some of its surrounding parts: nasal cavity, ear, or soft palate. Infiltrating tumors may reach parts of vital importance, like the base of the skull, the cranial nerves... Infiltrating tumors in the nasopharynx are more invasive than vegetating ones, although the latter require a shorter period of time to spread. The usual symptoms of nasopharyngeal cancer are dysfunctions associated with breathing, speech, vision, hearing, and the sense of smell, among others. It is therefore crucial to detect the disease at early stages; otherwise, consequences could be irreversible to the patient. As in any other kind of cancer, there exists the possibility of regional (lymph node involvement) or distant metastases. The appearance of nasopharyngeal hemorrhage or infection also constitutes evidence of cancer.

3   Overview of NasoNet

3.1   Description of the Model

NasoNet is a NPEDT that models the process of progression of a nasopharyngeal cancer. The final model assists the oncologists in the diagnosis and prognosis of the extent of this type of cancer in a patient. A primary tumor on any of the naso-pharyngeal walls may spread and invade adjacent parts. It may also provoke distant metastases, and hemorrhage or infection in the nasopharynx. The previous processes are characterized by the occurrence of a series of events. These events —before treatment is applied— are generally irreversible, and causally interrelated. For example, a primary vegetating tumor on the anterior wall of the nasopharynx may occupy the nasal fossae and produce anosmia (loss of the sense of smell); a primary infiltrating tumor on the superior wall of the nasopharynx may spread to the right lateral wall, then to the cavernous sinus, later invade the right inner ear, and finally produce symptoms like tinnitus (ringing in the ears), autophony (resonance of one's voice), hypoacusis (diminished acuteness of hearing)..., associated to abnormalities in the ear. In NasoNet, these events and all of those causally related to the spread of a nasopharyngeal cancer are represented as nodes in the Bayesian network.

If we had decided not to represent time explicitly in the Bayesian network, each random event variable could take on the values *present* or *absent*; accordingly, we would have only needed binary random variables. On the contrary, as the causal processes we are modeling are not instantaneous and there is uncertainty as to their occurrence, we need to explicitly represent time. To that end, we consider the instant the primary tumor appears as our initial or reference instant, and we define the occurrence time of any other event with respect to the mentioned initial instant. We suppose there is only one primary tumor, which is a reasonable hypothesis. In our domain, the temporal range of interest are the three years following the primary tumor appearance, according to our experts opinion. We divide this period into trimesters. Each event represented in the network has its own typical period of occurrence. All these different periods are within the three-year term we have selected as our time horizon. As an example, lung metastasis may arise during the second or third year, and abnormal cervical lymph nodes may appear during the first semester.

Given an event node E with its occurrence period divided into trimesters, the random variable associated to E can take on the values $\{e[a], ..., e[b], e[never]\}$ where a, $b \in \{1, ..., 12\}$ and $a \leq b$. $E = e[j]$, with $j \in \{a, ..., b\}$, means that event E has taken place in the j-th trimester after the appearance of the primary tumor, and $E = e[never]$ means that E does not take place —or that take place at $t = \infty$—. For example, $Anosmia = anosmia[3]$ expresses the appearance of anosmia during the third trimester. As each random variable can take on a set of exclusive values, each event associated to a variable can occur only once over time. This condition is satisfied in our domain, since the processes involved, previously to treatment, are irreversible. (Reversible processes could be represented by multiple events.) The current version of NasoNet contains 15 nodes associated to tumors confined to the nasopharynx, 23 nodes representing tumors spread to nasopharyngeal surrounding sites, 4 nodes symbolizing distant metastases, 4 nodes related to abnormal lymph nodes, 11 nodes expressing nasopharyngeal hemorrhages or infections, and 50 nodes referring to symptoms or syndromes. The root nodes in the network correspond to events related to the appearance of primary infiltrating or vegetating tumors on each wall of the nasopharynx. As we assume there is at most one primary tumor, the probabilities of the root nodes should sum up to 1. To that end, we introduce an additional parent node for the previous root nodes. The leaf nodes represent the appearance of different symptoms or syndromes. Finally, the intermediate nodes are events related to the spread of the tumor to adjacent parts to the nasopharynx, infections, metastases...

NasoNet models the evolution of a nasopharyngeal cancer so that each arc represents a causal relation between one parent event and one child event. For instance, in Fig. 1, the appearance of infection in the nasopharynx may produce rhinorrhea (excessive mucous secretion from the nose). If these causal relations were static, we could apply the noisy OR-gate [13] to model the interactions between an effect and its causes. In the noisy OR model, each cause acts independently of the remaining causes to produce a determined effect. This independence of causal interaction is satisfied in our domain. As the causal relations in our domain are not instantaneous and, furthermore, the nodes in the network correspond to temporal events, we use the temporal noisy OR-gate [6, 7] as a model of causal interaction.

The temporal noisy OR-gate represents the case in which the effect is present as soon as one of its causes provokes it to be present. According to Fig. 1, if a primary vegetating tumor on the right lateral wall provoked the appearance of nasopharyngeal infection at trimester i, and a primary infiltrating tumor provoked the same infection at trimester j, with $i \neq j$, then the event „appearance of infection in the nasopharynx" would be considered to occur at trimester $\min(i, j)$.

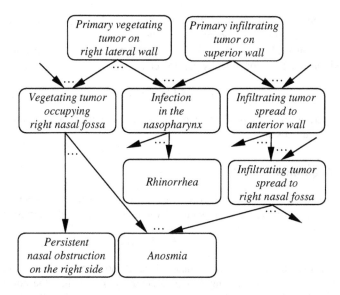

Fig. 1. Part of the Bayesian network modeling the evolution of a cancer of the nasopharynx

Let us consider a family of nodes with n causes X_1, ..., X_n and one effect Y. In principle, each of these event nodes may take place at any of trimesters $\{1, ..., 12\}$. In the temporal noisy OR-model, for each cause it is necessary to specify the parameters:

$$c_{y[k]}^{x_i[j_i]} \quad i \in \{1,...,n\}, j_i \in \{1,...,12\} \cup \{never\}, k \in \{1,...,12\} . \tag{1}$$

Each parameter is defined as the probability of Y being true at k, given that X_i is true at j_i and the rest of causes are absent. The conditional probability table for Y can be computed as follows (see Fig. 2 for a family with two causes):

$$P(y[k] \mid x_1[j_1],...,x_n[j_n]) = \sum_{\bar{k} \mid \min \bar{k}=k} \prod_i c_{y[k_i]}^{x_i[j_i]} \quad k, j_1,...,j_n \in \{1,...,12\} \cup \{never\} . \tag{2}$$

	$c_{y[1]}^{x_1[a]}{=}0.1$	$c_{y[2]}^{x_1[a]}{=}0.2$	$\cdots$	$c_{y[12]}^{x_1[a]}{=}0.1$	$c_{y[never]}^{x_1[a]}{=}0.2$	$P(y[k] \mid x_1[a], x_2[b])$
$c_{y[1]}^{x_2[b]}{=}0.1$	0.01	0.02	$\cdots$	0.01	0.02	$\rightarrow y[1], 0.12$
$c_{y[2]}^{x_2[b]}{=}0.2$	0.02	0.04	$\cdots$	0.02	0.04	$\rightarrow y[2], 0.18$
$\vdots$	$\vdots$	$\vdots$	$\ddots$	$\vdots$	$\vdots$	$\vdots$
$c_{y[12]}^{x_2[b]}{=}0.3$	0.03	0.06	$\cdots$	0.03	0.06	$\rightarrow y[12], 0.1$
$c_{y[never]}^{x_2[b]}{=}0.1$	0.01	0.02	$\cdots$	0.01	0.02	$\rightarrow y[never], 0.02$

Fig. 2. Temporal noisy OR-gate for two causes ($n{=}2$) and one effect

By ordering temporal indices from past to future $(1 < 2 < \ldots < 12 < never)$, just as illustrated in Fig. 2, a temporal noisy OR-gate leads to a noisy MIN-gate [5].

If there are non-explicit causes of Y in the model, they can be grouped together and represented through a vector of leaky parameters:

$$c^{*}_{y[k]} \quad k \in \{1,\ldots,12\} . \tag{3}$$

Each leaky parameter is the probability of the effect Y occurring at k, given that all the explicit causes are absent.

3.2 Data Acquisition

In principle, each arc making part of a temporal noisy OR-gate in NasoNet requires $(12 + 1) \cdot 12 = 156$ independent parameters. Among these parameters, those satisfying

$$c^{x_i[j_i=never]}_{y[k]} \quad k \in \{1,\ldots,12\} \tag{4}$$

are zero because the effect cannot take place if none of its causes is present. Furthermore, among the remaining 144 parameters, if $j_i > k$ then the corresponding parameter is zero because the effect cannot precede the cause. Finally, the remaining 78 independent parameters can be reduced to 12, since in our domain it is reasonable to assume *time invariance*:

$$c^{x_i[j_i+\Delta t]}_{y[k+\Delta t]} = c^{x_i[j_i]}_{y[k]} \quad \forall j_i, k, j_i + \Delta t, k + \Delta t \quad \{1,\ldots,12\} . \tag{5}$$

In summary, computing the conditional probability table associated to a family of nodes in NasoNet requires solely the specification of one parameter for each possible delay between cause and effect. The questions that the knowledge engineer has to ask the oncologists are:

Given that X_i takes place at a certain trimester, which is the probability that its effect Y occurs at the same trimester, if the rest of its causes are absent? And what is the probability that Y occurs at the next trimester? And so on.

It was difficult for the oncologists to answer the questions above. They argued that the answers depend on the cause event occurring in the early or late trimester. However, they felt more confident when answering the following questions:

Given that X_i takes place at a certain instant, which is the probability that its effect Y occurs at the next trimester, if the rest of its causes are absent? And what is the probability that Y occurs at the next's next trimester? And so on.

Let the parameters from the latter questions above be:

$$\tilde{c}^{X_i}_{Y}(\Delta t) \quad \Delta t \quad \{1,\ldots,12\} . \tag{6}$$

The following equality can be established between the two types of parameters we have[1]:

---

[1] The proof is omitted because of the lack of space.

$$c_{y[j_i+\Delta t]}^{x_i[j_i]} = \frac{\tilde{c}_Y^{X_i}(\Delta t)}{2} + \frac{\tilde{c}_Y^{X_i}(\Delta t + 1)}{2} \ . \tag{7}$$

In this way, we can compute the conditional probability tables in the network from the knowledge provided by the medical expert.

3.3 Example

Oncologists make use of the following information sources: the patient's medical history, the visual examination of the nasopharynx, and the result of different complementary tests. A finding involves determining the occurrence of an event represented by means of a node in NasoNet and establishing the time it occurred. NasoNet assists in determining, from the available findings, both posterior probabilities and occurrence times for the rest of events in the network. In order to simplify the example, we will suppose that our aim is twofold: firstly, we want to know whether the primary tumor is vegetating or infiltrating and, secondly, we are interested in finding out the wall where the primary tumor is located. Note that we are assuming there is at most one primary tumor in the patient.

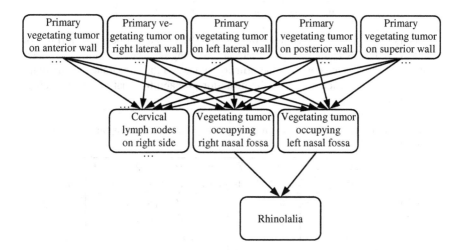

Fig. 3. Subnetwork of NasoNet

Consider the portion of NasoNet shown in Fig. 3. Any primary vegetating tumor may grow in volume inside the nasopharyngeal cavity and occupy the nasal fossae. This may produce rhinolalia (nasal voice produced by an alteration in the nasal fossae resonance). The appearance of a primary vegetating tumor may also provoke abnormal cervical lymph nodes on the right side. The parameters of the network in Fig. 3 are shown in Table 1.

Table 1. Parameters of the network in Fig. 3

X_i	Y	$\tilde{c}_Y^{X_i}(\Delta t)$
Pvtaw	Vtornf	0.225 for $\Delta t \in \{1,...,4\}$
Pvtaw	Vtolnf	0.225 for $\Delta t \in \{1,...,4\}$
Pvtaw	Clnrs	0.27 for $\Delta t=1$, 0.13 for $\Delta t=2$
Pvtrlw	Vtornf	0.175 for $\Delta t \in \{3,...,6\}$
Pvtrlw	Vtolnf	0.05 for $\Delta t \in \{3,...,6\}$
Pvtrlw	Clnrs	0.27 for $\Delta t=1$, 0.13 for $\Delta t=2$
Pvtllw	Vtornf	0.05 for $\Delta t \in \{3,...,6\}$
Pvtllw	Vtolnf	0.175 for $\Delta t \in \{3,...,6\}$
Pvtllw	Clnrs	0.14 for $\Delta t=1$, 0.07 for $\Delta t=2$
Pvtpw	Vtornf	0.00625 for $\Delta t \in \{5,...,12\}$
Pvtpw	Vtolnf	0.00625 for $\Delta t \in \{5,...,12\}$
Pvtpw	Clnrs	0.27 for $\Delta t=1$, 0.13 for $\Delta t=2$
Pvtsw	Vtornf	0.175 for $\Delta t \in \{3,...,6\}$
Pvtsw	Vtolnf	0.175 for $\Delta t \in \{3,...,6\}$
Pvtsw	Clnrs	0.27 for $\Delta t=1$, 0.13 for $\Delta t=2$
Vtornf	Rhinolalia	0.2, *instantaneous*
Vtolnf	Rhinolalia	0.2, *instantaneous*

Doctors know from the anamnesis that on 9/20/99 the patient began suffering from rhinolalia. With this unique finding, there are as many possible scenarios as possible delays between the appearance of the primary tumor and the appearance of rhinolalia, 12 in this case. For each scenario, the posterior probabilities that appear in Table 2 can be obtained in NasoNet.

Table 2. Posterior probabilities for primary vegetating tumors with temporal localization for each scenario

	sc1	...	sc6	sc7	sc8	sc9	sc10	sc11	sc12
	rhino[12]	...	rhino[7]	rhino[6]	rhino[5]	rhino[4]	rhino[3]	rhino[2]	rhino[1]
Pvtaw	0	...	0	0	0	0.022	0.0401	1	1
Pvtrlw	0	...	0	0.4059	0.3817	0.364	0.3434	0	0
Pvtllw	0	...	0	0.4072	0.386	0.3629	0.3477	0	0
Pvtpw	1	...	1	0.0089	0.0088	0	0	0	0
Pvtsw	0	...	0	0.1778	0.2233	0.2509	0.2686	0	0

9/20/96   12/20/96   12/20/97   3/20/98   6/20/98   9/20/98   12/20/98   3/20/99   6/20/99

On 12/30/99, the patient detects neck nodes on the right side and is received in the Dept. of Radiation Oncology, where oncologists establish by palpation the presence of abnormal cervical lymph nodes on the right side. Since the presence of abnormal cervical lymph nodes can only occur during the next semester to the appearance of the primary tumor (see Table 1), only one scenario is possible: *rhinolalia*[1], *clnrs*[2], and primary tumor appearance between 6/30/99 and 9/20/99. The posterior probabilities obtained from this scenario show that the evidence can exclusively be explained by a primary tumor on the anterior wall. This is a valuable result that permits a better interpretation of the information obtained from subsequent complementary tests.

3.4 Construction of NasoNet

NasoNet has been implemented in GeNIe, a development environment for building graphical decision-theoretic models. GeNIe was developed at the Decision Systems Laboratory of the University of Pittsburgh.

As a previous step towards the final construction of NasoNet, we developed an atemporal Bayesian network in which each node represents the occurrence or not of a certain event. The graph of this network is the same as that of NasoNet and the type of causal interactions for each family of nodes is modeled through the noisy OR-gate. The atemporal network consists of 276 arcs with multiple loops. Once introduced prior and conditional probabilities, evidence propagation from clustering algorithms took about one second. We have evaluated the atemporal network from typical cases presented by the oncologists, covering a wide range of possibilities in the evolution of the disease. Moreover, several clinical histories were randomly selected and contrasted with the results given by the network for each case. The results were satisfactory.

The introduction of an explicit representation of time prompted the use of both multivalued variables and the temporal noisy OR model. The average number of values each variable in the network could take on increased to 9.6. The complexity of the temporal network prevented us from performing evidence propagation through exact algorithms. This fact became evident once we had introduced an explicit representation of time to nearly the third part of nodes in the atemporal network. However, stochastic simulation algorithms permit to obtain acceptable approximate results in a few minutes. Due to limitations of time, we have only evaluated the atemporal version of NasoNet.

4 Conclusions

We have presented NasoNet, a temporal Bayesian network for the diagnosis and prognosis of the extent of a nasopharyngeal cancer. Cancer spread is a process full of uncertainty, in which time must be taken into account. NasoNet makes use of the *temporal noisy OR-gate* to model the different dynamic causal interactions that take place during cancer spread. NasoNet constitutes the first system to apply the approach of *network of probabilistic events in discrete time* (NPEDT) to a real-world domain. This approach offers important advantages over other kinds of temporal Bayesian networks as to the representation and management of irreversible processes, like those occurring during cancer spread, previously to applying the appropriate treatment.

Several issues regarding knowledge acquisition, knowledge representation, inference, and verification of the system have been discussed. Testing of clinical cases is the main task to be carried out in the future, in order to perform a thorough eval-uation of the system. Another future task is to extend NasoNet to cope with cancer evolution after treatment.

Acknowledgements. This research was supported by the Spanish CICYT, under grants TIC97-0604 and TIC-97-1135-C04-04.

References

1. Andreassen, S., Hovorka, R., Benn, J., Olesen, K.G., Carson, E.R.: A model-based approach to insulin adjustment. In: *Proceedings of the Third Conference on Artificial Intelligence in Medicine*, 239-248, Maastrich, The Netherlands, 1991. Springer-Verlag.
2. Dagum, P., Galper, A.: Forecasting sleep apnea with dynamic network models. In: *Proceedings of the 9th Conference on Artificial Intelligence*, 64-71, Washington D.C., 1993. Morgan Kaufmann, San Francisco, CA.
3. Dagum, P., Galper, A., Horvitz, E.: Dynamic network models for forecasting. In: *Proceedings of the 8th Conference on Uncertainty in Artificial Intelligence*, 41-48, Stanford University, 1992. Morgan Kaufmann, San Francisco, CA.
4. Dean, T., Kanazawa, K.: A model for reasoning about persistence and causation. *Computational Intelligence* 5, 142-150, 1989.
5. Díez, F.J.: Parameter adjustment in Bayes networks. The generalized noisy OR-gate. In: *Proceedings of the 9th Conference on Uncertainty in Artificial Intelligence*, 99-105, Washington D.C., 1993. Morgan Kaufmann, San Francisco, CA.
6. Galán, S.F., Díez, F.J.: Modelling dynamic causal interactions with Bayesian networks: temporal noisy gates. In: *Working Notes of CaNew'2000, 2nd International Workshop on Bayesian and Causal Networks*, 1-5, ECAI-2000, Berlin (Germany).
7. Galán, S.F., Díez, F.J.: Networks of probabilistic events in discrete time. Submitted to *International Journal of Approximate Reasoning*.
8. Kjærulff, U.: A computational scheme for reasoning in dynamic probabilistic networks. In: *Proceedings of the 8th Conference on Uncertainty in Artificial Intelligence*, 121-129, Stanford University, 1992. Morgan Kaufmann, San Francisco, CA.
9. Lee, A., Foo, W., Law, S., Poon, Y.F., O, S.K., Tung, S.Y., Sze, W.M., Chappell, R., Lau, W.H., Ho, J.: Staging of nasopharyngeal carcinoma: From Ho's to the new UICC system. *International Journal of Cancer*, Vol. 84, Issue 2, 179-187, 1999.
10. Leong, T.: Multiple perspective dynamic decision making. *Artificial Intelligence*, 105(1-2): 209-261, 1998.
11. Magni, P., Bellazzi, R.: DT-Planner: an environment for managing dynamic decision problems. *Computer Methods and Programs in Biomedicine*, 54: 183-200, 1997.
12. Nicholson, A.E., Brady, J.M.: Sensor validation using dynamic belief networks. In: *Proceedings of the 8th Conference on Uncertainty in Artificial Intelligence*, 207-214, Stanford University, 1992. Morgan Kaufmann, San Francisco, CA.
13. Pearl, J.: *Probabilistic Reasoning in Intelligent Systems: Networks of Plausible Inference.* Morgan Kaufmann, San Mateo, CA, 1988. Revised second printing, 1991.
14. Provan, G.M., Clarke, J.R.: Dynamic network construction and updating techniques for the diagnosis of acute abdominal pain. *IEEE Transactions on Pattern Analysis and Machine Intelligence*, 15 (3): 299-307, 1993.
15. Schantz, S.P., Harrison, L.B., Forastiere, A.A.: Tumors of the nasal cavity and paranasal sinuses, nasopharynx, oral cavity, and oropharynx. In: *Cancer: Principles and Practice of Oncology* (V. T. DeVita Jr, S. Hellman, and S. A. Rosenberg, Eds.), Lippincott-Raven Publishers, Philadelphia, 741-801, 1997.
16. Tatman, J.A., Shachter, R.D.: Dynamic programming and influence diagrams. *IEEE Transactions on Systems, Man, and Cybernetics*, 20 (2): 365-379, 1990.

Using Time-Oriented Data Abstraction Methods to Optimize Oxygen Supply for Neonates

Andreas Seyfang[1], Silvia Miksch[1], Werner Horn[2], Michael S. Urschitz[3,4],
Christian Popow[4], and Christian F. Poets[3]

[1] Institute of Software Technology, University of Technology, Vienna, Austria
seyfang@ifs.tuwien.ac.at
[2] Department of Medical Cybernetics and Artificial Intelligence, University of
Vienna, and Austrian Research Institute for Artificial Intelligence, Austria
[3] Department of Neonatology and Pediatric Pulmonology, School of Medicine,
Hannover, Germany
[4] Department of Pediatrics, University of Vienna, Austria

Abstract. Therapy management needs sophisticated patient monitoring and therapy planning, especially in high-frequency domains, like Neonatal Intensive Care Units (NICUs), where complex data sets are collected every second. An elegant method to tackle this problem is the use of time-oriented, skeletal plans. *Asgaard* is a framework for the representation, visualization, and execution of such plans. These plans work on qualitative abstracted time-oriented data which closely resemble the concepts used by experienced clinicians.

This papers presents the data abstraction unit of the *Asgaard* system. It provides a range of connectable data abstraction methods bridging the gap between the raw data collected by monitoring devices and the abstract concepts used in therapeutic plans. The usability of this data abstraction unit is demonstrated by the implementation of a controller for the automated optimization of the fraction of inspired oxygen (FiO_2). The use of the time-oriented data abstraction methods results in safe and smooth adjustment actions of our controller in a neonatal care setting.

1 Introduction

Most Intensive Care Units (ICUs) are well equipped with modern devices for patient monitoring. On-line recording of patient data and storage in computer-based patient records (CPR) and patient data management systems (PDMS) become common place in today's ICUs. Still, the workload of the clinical staff prevents the optimal utilization of these measurements since it limits the number of adjustments during daily routine. To ease a particular part of that workload we have developed a system that helps the medical staff in automatically providing the necessary oxygen supply to newborn infants within the optimal range.

Previous experience [6,10] shows that patient monitoring may be improved by using therapy management strategies, e.g., by using a data abstraction unit for processing the raw monitoring data. This unit must be integrated into a larger

S. Quaglini, P. Barahona, and S. Andreassen (Eds.): AIME 2001, LNAI 2101, pp. 217–226, 2001.

system that supports therapy planning and the execution of clinical protocols. In this paper we describe temporal data-abstraction methods and their application to control the adjustment of the fraction of inspired oxygen (FiO_2) based on continuously recorded pulsoximeter derived arterial oxygen saturation (SpO_2) monitoring data. The system is part of the Asgaard framework [9] which supports the application of time-oriented, skeletal plans in the medical domain.

1.1   FiO$_2$ Controller

The oxygen delivery to a premature or sick newborn infant must be adjusted very closely in order to grant adequate tissue oxygenation while minimizing possible toxic effects of supplying oxygen.

Correct FiO_2 settings are achieved by manual adjusting the FiO_2 according to the oxygen saturation readings from pulsoximetry, transcutaneous and invasive blood gas measurements. In some patients this requires frequent adjustments within short intervals. In order to reduce the cumbersome frequent alarms and FiO_2 adjustments, we often notice generous SpO_2 limits resulting in an oversupply of oxygen. We therefore consider manual adjustments of the FiO_2 not as an optimal solution.

The aim of our project is to develop a continuously operating automated FiO_2 controller for optimizing the oxygen delivery to newborn infants. The automated FiO_2 controller will adjust the FiO_2 settings based on the continuous transcutaneous SpO_2 measurements. During each control cycle, data are read from the pulsoximeter, validated, and in case preset SpO_2 limits are exceeded or fall short of, the FiO_2 is adjusted accordingly.

A similar approach is the fuzzy logic assisted controller developed by Sun et al. [11]. However, the functionality of this fuzzy controller has the important disadvantage that it resulted in an huge number of FiO_2 changes. This could lead to disturbances of the immature respiratory system of preterm infants and should be avoided.

The controller described in this paper uses temporal data abstraction. It accounts for stability of the data, recognizes trend, and applies qualitative reasoning similar to that performed by clinicians.

1.2   Temporal Data Abstraction

Data abstraction derives meaningful information (seen as abstractions) from raw data able to support specific knowledge-based problem-solving activities. Temporal data abstraction methods represent an important subgroup where the processed data are temporal [5].

Common methods of intelligent data analysis are time-series analysis, control theory, and probabilistic or fuzzy classifiers [2]. These approaches have a lot of shortcomings, which lead to applying knowledge-based techniques to derive qualitative values or patterns of current and past situations of a patient. The RÉSUMÉ project [10] performs temporal abstraction of time-stamped data without predefined trends. The system is based on a knowledge-based temporal-abstraction method. Larizza et al. [4] have developed methods to detect predefined courses in a time series. Complex abstraction allows one to detect specific temporal relationships between intervals. Bellazzi et al. [1] utilize Bayesian techniques to extract overall trends from cyclic data in the field of diabetes.

All these approaches are dealing mostly with low-frequency data, i.e., only few data items per day have to be processed. On the contrary, in the ICU we receive a set of data items every second. This results in the problems of oscillating data, frequently shifting contexts, repeating patterns of states and events as well as different expectations of the development of parameters.

Promising approaches for high-frequency data are the Time Series Workbench [3] which approximates data curves through a series of line-segments and VIE-VENT [6]. The temporal abstraction module of VIE-VENT focuses on the high-frequency domain of artificial ventilation of newborn infants. VIE-VENT incorporates fixed, but context-dependent temporal data abstraction schemata. It uses an epsilon region to reduce frequent qualitative changes when oscillations occur around borders of qualitative regions. However, none of these two methods offer the flexibility of a general data abstraction unit which provides methods for stable processing even on changing signal quality.

To overcome limitations observed in previous approaches, namely to arrive at a system combining temporal data abstraction with the execution of skeletal, time-oriented plans representing clinical treatment plans, the *Asgaard* framework was developed.

In the following section we describe the data abstraction methods of the Asgaard system. Their use in a practical application—the FiO_2 controller—is demonstrated in Section 3. This is followed by notes on the evaluation and concluding remarks.

2   Data Abstraction in Asgaard

In this section we first give an overview of those parts of Asgaard dealing with plan execution and data abstraction followed by a description of the data abstraction unit in greater detail.

2.1   Introduction to Asgaard

The Asgaard framework [9] outlines task-specific problem-solving methods to support both design and execution of skeletal plans. This project tries to build a bridge between the medical approaches and the planning approaches, addressing the demands of the medical staff on the one side and applying rich plan management on the other side. For the representation of plans, a time-oriented, intention-based, skeletal plan-representation language, called Asbru, was developed [8]. Asbru is used to define skeletal plans which are instantiated during plan execution. Figure 1 shows those parts of the Asgaard framework which deal with the execution of plans including the data abstraction unit:

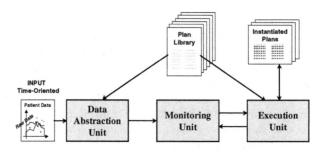

Fig. 1. Runtime Modules of Asgaard.

- Data Abstraction Unit: The data abstraction unit receives the data from the input sources and processes it through a set of abstraction methods described in the next section.
- Monitoring Unit: The monitoring unit receives a list of parameter propositions (i.e., parts of conditions) which are relevant for future plan-state transitions from the execution unit and compares it to the high-level abstractions delivered by the data abstraction unit. If it detects a match, it informs the execution unit which performs the resulting state transitions.
- Execution Unit: The execution unit handles the state transitions of the plans. It instantiates plans from the plan library and governs their life-cycle according to the state of the world as reported by the monitoring unit.

2.2   The Data Abstraction Unit

Asgaard implements 15 classes of abstraction methods which can be connected to each other on instantiation. Their instances are configured in the domain definition of the plan library. We distinguish the following classes (written in *italics*).

- A *raw data interface* performs error checking on data directly coming from the input sources.
- *Numeric calculations* are based on parameters and constants and comprise elementary arithmetic functions.
- *Logical combinations* are applied on Boolean parameters. Like the other abstractions, they can cope with undefined values.
- The *spread* [7] is used to smooth noisy raw data. We slide a time window of constant width over the curve in small steps. For each position of the time window, we calculate a linear regression of the valid data points within the window. On the center of the line we plot the adapted standard error. Connecting the ends of each bar with those of its neighbors yields a band (called *spread*). It vertically follows the average of the curve. The width shows the uncertainty involved in its calculation. The smaller the spread, the better the quality of the curve.

- Based on the spread, a set of abstractions are derived: *slope, standard deviation, standard error, center,* and *end point* (of the regression line), and *time to alarm* (intersection of the elongation of the regression line with a defined threshold value).
- Quantitative abstractions based on raw data are *change rate* and *average*. In contrast to the spread, they are calculated in the conventional way which is more suitable for low-frequency data.
- *Qualitative abstractions* are based on context-sensitive transformations of quantitative parameters using context-sensitive transformation schemata based on the spread.
- *Logical dependency* definitions yield qualitative or quantitative abstractions based on a set of logical expressions.
- *Boolean parameters* are abstracted from logical expressions.

In practical applications, instances of the above classes are connected in a directed graph which fills the gap between the input sources and the monitoring unit. Each instance receives time-stamped data (one measurement at a time) from more basic instances of abstraction methods, refines the information to a higher level of abstraction and passes the result to other instances along the graph.

Both the connections between the abstraction methods and their parameters are defined in the domain definition of the Asbru plan-library.

3   The FiO$_2$ Controller – A Practical Example

In the following we describe an application of Asgaard's data abstraction capabilities to control the oxygen delivery to premature newborn infants. The aim of our controller is the optimization of oxygen supply through small adjustments at a moderate rate. It is designed for closed-loop operation which adjusts the FiO$_2$ by executing instantiated skeletal plans. For safety considerations, changes exceeding a limit of 10% are to be acknowledged by the medical staff. Adjustments result from an abstract view of the SpO$_2$ data stream.

3.1   Temporal Data Abstraction for the FiO$_2$ Controller

In this section we show how the instances of Asgaard's data abstraction methods are configured to form the controller necessary to meet the aims described above. The overall goal is to keep the SpO$_2$ in the range of normal values with minimum adjustments. We distinguish four modes of operation:

Normal operation: If none of the following exceptions described below occur, the adjustment based on the current abstractions from the SpO$_2$ readings is performed and wait mode is entered. If the SpO$_2$ is in the target region, no adjustment is performed.

Wait mode: After any change in the FiO_2 setting the system waits for five minutes (This parameter depends on the mode of ventilation.) before it takes another action based on the fact that it takes that long until the change in the FiO_2 setting shows an effect in the SpO_2 of the patient. This is implemented in the filter conditions of the plans [8] performing the adjustment. These plan details are not described in this paper.

Check mode: Since the signal from pulsoximetry is not valid all the time, a set of criteria is defined under which the system temporarily suspends its actions. They are detailed below. The system displays the check mode but no acknowledgment by the user is demanded since our system is not aimed at alarming but at optimization of the FiO_2 in standard situations.

Postpone mode: If the system should adjust the FiO_2, but most recent information seems to invalidate this action the adjustment is postponed until the short term observations match the intended action or another adjustment is considered which is in accordance with recent observations. The reasoning behind this is given below.

Figure 2 shows the instances of abstraction methods employed in our example and the connections between them. Figure 3 shows a retrospective analysis of a 45-minutes sequence of SpO_2 recording together with the output of the controller.

In the following we describe the instances of the abstraction methods used to form the FiO_2 controller.

Raw Data Selection and Validation. The interface to the data delivered by the pulsoximeter is defined in the specification of **raw-data**. It contains the low-level identification of the parameter SpO_2 and the range of values allowed.

Underlying Spreads. Two spreads [7] are fundamental for the abstraction process: the **state-spread** and the **trend-spread**. The **state-spread** is calculated from a time-window of five minutes as a basis of the qualitative **state** of the SpO_2, while the **trend-spread** is based on a one-minute time-window to include most recent development in the SpO_2 reading.

State and Trend. On the *center* of the **state-spread** the *qualitative abstraction* **state** of the SpO_2 is obtained. Five qualitative values are derived from the state: substantially above, above, normal range, below, and substantially below. They are the foundation of the adjustment values for the FiO_2. Based on the *slope* of the **trend-spread** the **trend** is abstracted. It knows whether SpO_2 is increasing, stable, or decreasing.

Check Mode. The credibility of a system heavily depends on its ability to recognize its limits. We therefore implemented in **check-mode** (an instance of *Boolean*) the following conditions under which the system signals that the situation is beyond its scope of operation:

 − If the *standard error* of the **state-spread** calculated for the previous five minutes exceeds a limit of 1.5, data are too unreliable to be a basis of further reasoning. Figure 3 shows two such periods. These are visualized by red/gray bars in line CHECK.

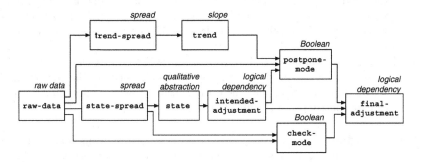

Fig. 2. Combination of abstraction methods used in the FiO$_2$ controller. The names of the **instances** of the abstraction methods are inside the boxes while their classes are given in *italics* on top of them.

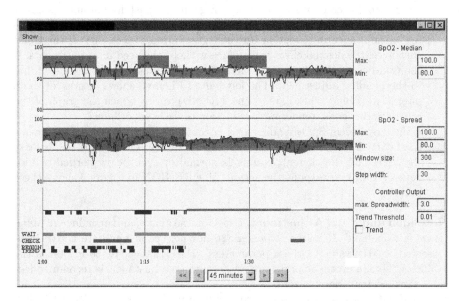

Fig. 3. Retrospective analysis of controller operation using recorded data. The top graph shows the qualitative values abstracted from the median of the SpO$_2$. The graph in the middle shows the **state-spread** and the qualitative values (**state**, displayed as horizontal bars) abstracted from it. Below we display the controller output (from top to bottom): The **intended-adjustment**: first decrease FiO$_2$ (in black) multiple times until 1:20, then the target region is reached (green/light gray bars); the periods of wait mode following each adjustment (gray); two periods of check mode (red/dark gray); and a series of short periods during which the value of **raw-data** contradicts the **intended-adjustment** (line REGION) or the **trend** dissuades from decreasing FiO$_2$ (line TREND), both in blue/black.

- If the input from the pulsoximeter (`raw-data`) is missing or invalid due to movements of the patient or the sensor, any change of the FiO_2 would not seem plausible, even if 95% of the data in the time window under consideration were valid.
- If the current reading of SpO_2 drops below 80% for more than four seconds, an acute hypoxy is occurring which will be signaled by the pulsoximeter. Since our system is aimed at the optimization of SpO_2 in normal situations, it cannot contribute to handling such emergencies.

Postpone Mode. In addition to the above reasons for pausing operation there are situations during normal operation in which it is not feasible to take the intended action since the current data contradicts the results of the analysis of the previous minutes. In the following situations the adjustment is postponed:

- If the trend observed for the last minute shows a change in the same direction which the adjustment tries to achieve, an additional change in the FiO_2 setting could lead to over-reactions. E.g., if the past five minutes suggest decreasing the oxygen supply but during the last minute SpO_2 was decreasing without such intervention, further observation is necessary. If the trend continues, the desired effect takes place without the need for adjustments. If the trend changes unfavorably, the FiO_2 setting must be changed according to the pending adjustment. The left half of Figure 3 shows a series of short intervals (as blue/black bars in line TREND) during which the graph of the raw data descends, rendering a reduction of FiO_2 superfluous.
- If the most recent SpO_2 reading grossly contradicts the intended adjustment, the latter is not issued. This is the case if the system intends to decrease the FiO_2 and the current reading is normal or even below normal or vice versa. Again we postpone the action. Line REGION in Figure 3 shows these periods.

Intended and Final Adjustment. Based on the `state`, an `intended-adjustment` is calculated. If neither `check-mode` nor `postpone-mode` are active (represented as true-value of these parameters), the `final-adjustment` takes the value of the `indented-adjustment`. Otherwise no adjustment is recommended, i.e., `final-adjustment` is zero.

Figure 3 shows a period from 1:00 to 1:20 during which decreasing the FiO_2 by 1% is intended, interleaved with one period of `check-mode` and a series of short periods during which either the `trend` or a mismatch of `state` and `raw-data` hint at postponing the adjustment. From 1:20 onwards the qualitative value of SpO_2 is in the target region and no adjustment is necessary as marked by the green/gray bar.

The output of the data abstraction—`final-adjustment`—is fed into the plan execution unit via the monitoring unit which performs the instantiation and execution of the plans (compare Figure 1). The plans refer to the `final-adjustment` in their filter conditions, i.e., an appropriate user-performed plan is started to realize the adjustment whenever necessary.

4 Limitations

The spread algorithm is suitable for high-frequency, noisy signals. It is not appropriate for low-frequency data nor for data which shows meaningful oscillations. However, the data-abstraction unit can handle low-frequency data using other modules.

The current implementation handles several measurements per second without problems. The absolute limit of performance depends on the complexity of the instantiated data-abstraction, the performance of the computer used, and the data format and transmission speed of the measuring device(s) connected to the serial port.

5 Evaluation and Further Work

We currently perform a three step evaluation process of the FiO_2 controller. In a first step, we compared the spread to median filtering. The spread leads to a more stable judgment of the patient's situation and therefore reduces the number of unnecessary adjustments of FiO_2 (see Fig. 3, top and middle graphs). We retrospectively evaluated recordings obtained from 10 patients. In a total of 126 hours (median 12, range 3–24) the adjustment based on the *spread* changed 148 times compared to 519 changes in the adjustment based on the median.

In a second step, we implemented the logic described above to derive adjustments of the FiO_2 setting. This proved to fully eliminate controversial adjustments.

In the next step the system will be evaluated online in a Neonatal Intensive Care Unit (NICU). The clinical study is designed to incorporate 13 premature infants, first 3 for tuning the parameters of the controller, the others to evaluate the performance. For safety reasons the system will run in open-loop mode. The necessary adjustments to the FiO_2 are displayed to the medical staff and set manually. In three consecutive 2-hours periods the neonates are managed by the ward staff, an expert giving special attention to ventilation management, and the open-loop controller. Comparison of performance will give insights to improvements in health-care offered by automated devices.

6 Conclusion

The work described in this paper shows that temporal data abstraction needs a complex intelligent toolset to provide complex solutions necessary in real-world applications such as optimizing the oxygen supply of premature neonates. The data abstraction facilities provided by the Asgaard system are powerful enough to implement such a system.

The design using formal data abstraction methods offers the flexibility to adapt the FiO_2 controller to different settings required by the various ventilation modes used in the NICU. The controller is flexible enough to be used with an incubator, in CPAP (continuous positive airways pressure) mode and with

226   A. Seyfang et al.

controlled ventilation. Future work will be devoted to fine-tune the parameters to various situations in the field of artificial ventilation of neonates.

Acknowledgments. This project is supported by "Fonds zur Förderung der wissenschaftlichen Forschung - FWF" (Austrian Science Foundation), P12797-INF. We appreciate the support given to the Austrian Research Institute of Artificial Intelligence (ÖFAI) by the Austrian Federal Ministry of Education, Science, and Culture.

References

1. R. Bellazzi, C. Larizza, P. Magni, S. Montani, and G. De Nicolao, 'Intelligent analysis of clinical time series by combining structural filtering and temporal abstractions', in *Artificial Intelligence in Medicine*, ed., Horn, W. et al., pp. 261–270, Berlin, (1999). Springer.
2. M. Berthold and D.J. Hand, *Intelligent Data Analysis: An Introduction*, Springer, Berlin, 1999.
3. J. Hunter and N. McIntosh, 'Knowledge-based event detection in complex time series data', in *Artificial Intelligence in Medicine*, ed., Horn, W. et al., pp. 271–280, Berlin, (1999). Springer.
4. C. Larizza, R. Bellazzi, and A. Riva, 'Temporal abstractions for diabetic patients management', in *Artificial Intelligence in Medicine*, ed., Keravnou E. et al., pp. 319–330, Berlin, (1997). Springer.
5. N. Lavrac, E. Keravnou, and B. Zupan, 'Intelligent data analaysis in medicine', in *Encyclopaedia of Computer Science and Technology*, ed., Kent, A. et al., volume 42, 113–157, Marcel Dekker, New York, Basel, (2000).
6. S. Miksch, W. Horn, C. Popow, and F. Paky, 'Utilizing temporal data abstraction for data validation and therapy planning for artificially ventilated newborn infants', *Artificial Intelligence in Medicine*, **8**(6), 543–576, (1996).
7. S. Miksch, A. Seyfang, W. Horn, and C. Popow, 'Abstracting steady qualitative descriptions over time from noisy, high-frequency data', in *Artificial Intelligence in Medicine*, ed., Horn, W. et al., pp. 281–290, Berlin, (1999). Springer.
8. A. Seyfang, R. Kosara, and S. Miksch, 'Asbru 7.2 reference manual', Technical Report Asgaard-TR-2000-3, Vienna University of Technology, Institute of Software Technology, (2000). available at
   http://www.ifs.tuwien.ac.at/asgaard/asbru/asbru_7_2_new/.
9. Y. Shahar, S. Miksch, and P. Johnson, 'The Asgaard Project: A task-specific framework for the application and critiquing of time-oriented clinical guidelines', *Artificial Intelligence in Medicine*, **14**, 29–51, (1998).
10. Y. Shahar and M. A. Musen, 'Knowledge-based temporal abstraction in clinical domains', *Artificial Intelligence in Medicine*, **8**(3), 267–298, (1996).
11. Y. Sun, I.S. Kohane, and A.R. Stark, 'Computer-assisted adjustment of inspired oxygen concentration improves control of oxygen saturation in newborn infants requiring mechanical ventilation', *Journal of Pediatrics*, **131**(5), 754–756, (1997).

Visual Definition of Temporal Clinical Abstractions: A User Interface Based on Novel Metaphors

Luca Chittaro and Carlo Combi

Department of Mathematics and Computer Science, University of Udine,
via delle Scienze 206, 33100 Udine, Italy
{chittaro, combi}@dimi.uniud.it

Abstract. In this paper, we describe a novel user interface for the visual definition of temporal abstractions based on a set of intuitive metaphors, which represent both temporal features and logical relations of abstractions.

1 Introduction

Visualizing and interactively exploring patient clinical information is a relevant need in the medical domain [1]. One of the problems that has attracted particular attention since the early '90s [4] has been the visualization of patient histories. Lifelines [5] is the most widely known visualization environment that deals with this problem. It displays facts as lines on a graphic time axis, according to their temporal location and extension; color and thickness are then used to represent categories and significance of facts. Subsequent proposals have basically followed the Lifelines approach, enriching it with additional elements. Although the proposals for visualizing medical histories deal with the representation of intervals and interval relations to some extent, they are not meant to facilitate the visual expression of more complex temporal relations such as those present in temporal abstractions [2].

In this paper, we describe a system for the visual definition of temporal abstractions by physicians with no special skills in computer science. The adopted metaphors were chosen by evaluating alternative designs on more than 30 physicians, strictly following the methods used in the field of Human-Computer Interaction, as described in [3].

2 Visual Definition of Temporal Abstractions

In defining abstractions, we distinguish two different kinds of information: temporal and logical. *Temporal* aspects concern the definition of temporal relations between the components (e.g., "headache before analgesics") and the definition of the interval associated to the abstraction (e.g., "3 days before the start of analgesics up to the end of analgesics"). *Logical* aspects specify how the components have to be considered in

S. Quaglini, P. Barahona, and S. Andreassen (Eds.): AIME 2001, LNAI 2101, pp. 227–230, 2001.

the definition of the abstraction (e.g., "analgesics AND headache", or "headache AND NOT analgesics").

The proposed user interface supports the definition process by allowing the user to: (i) easily set the relative temporal positions among components, (ii) define the temporal interval associated to the abstraction on the basis of the intervals of components, and (iii) logically relate the components through the standard connectives AND, OR, NOT, which can be combined to define more complex expressions.

The interface has been designed with the following features in mind: (i) use of simple graphical metaphors related to the physical world, (ii) visual separation of temporal and logical aspects into two different graphic windows, (iii) point-and-click selection of the components and the various graphic operators (the abstraction can be interactively defined without resorting to the keyboard), (iv) use of different colors to highlight different kinds of abstractions, (v) clear connection among graphic objects in the temporal and logical parts of a given abstraction.

2.1   Temporal Aspects: Displaying Intervals and Temporal Relations

Intervals for abstractions are visualized as paint strips. The temporal location of these strips can be specified in different ways (see Figure 1, part A):

☐ Paint strips can be represented plainly without any attached object (Figure 1, part A: strip *analgesics*). In this case, we want to represent intervals' ends that have a precisely set position with respect to other intervals. The commonsense reasoning motivating this choice is that "the end of a paint strip cannot move by itself".

☐ Alternatively, any end of a strip can be attached to a paint roller, connected to a weight by means of a wire. This notation expresses that the end of the interval can take different positions on the time axis: the roller can extend the end of the paint strip up to the wall, which stops the roller.

☐ Finally, a weight can be connected to more than one roller simultaneously to represent intervals' ends which can move keeping their relative position (Figure 1, part A: strips *antidepressants* and *corticosteroids*).

2.2   Logical Aspects: Displaying Expressions

To visualize and interactively compose logical expressions, each involved component is first graphically associated to a circle. Every circle is filled with the same color associated to the abstraction. Moreover, a numeric ID is used as an additional mean to relate a single abstraction to its two visual representations (one for its related temporal interval and one for the propositional part), as shown in the following section. The AND and the OR connectives are represented by elliptical areas, containing all the circles which have to be connected. The NOT operator is represented as a diagonal line which can be applied either to a circle or to an elliptical area. The edge of areas are either a continuous line or a dotted one, to distinguish between conjunctions and disjunctions, respectively. As an example, let us consider three different therapy-related abstractions *antidepressants*, *corticosteroids*, and *analgesics*, identified by IDs

3, 5, and 8, respectively. Part D of Figure 1 depicts the expression (*analgesics* AND (*corticosteroids* OR *antidepressants*)).

2.3   The User Interface

The user interface is organized into two parts: the first one is devoted to the visual specification of temporal relations among components, and the definition of the name and validity interval of the abstraction; the second one is devoted to the visual definition of the logical expression on the components. Figure 1 is a screenshot of the user interface during the definition of an abstraction involving three components.

In the first panel, displayed in the upper part of the screen (Figure 1, part A), the system displays the temporal intervals for the components, according to their relative positions, following the previously described metaphors. For a given abstraction, a label (e.g., *analgesics* in Figure 1) describing its propositional (atemporal) content is displayed at the beginning of the same line. The color of paint strips is related to the considered component. Insertion, modification, deletion, and connection of different graphic objects can be performed by switching among the different options either through the "Temporal" menu and its sub-items or through a suitable toolbar (Figure 1, element B). A scrollbar allows one to display different components, in case they cannot be displayed at the same time into the window. The lowest part of this panel (Figure 1, part C) is devoted to the definition of the features of the resulting abstraction: the user selects the color which has to be associated to the abstraction, inserts the name of the abstraction, and defines its temporal extent on the basis of the temporal extents of components. The endpoints of the interval associated to the abstraction can coincide with any of the endpoints of the components. These endpoints are displayed as vertical bars within the white strip in part C. When the extent is selected through the pointing device, the corresponding part of the strip assumes the chosen color. A further possibility is to add (subtract) some fixed time span to the chosen endpoints: e.g., with respect to the pattern in Figure 1, the user could define, through a dialog window, an abstraction interval starting three days before the start of analgesics. In this case, a small arrow (pointing to the left) would appear near the left endpoint of the abstraction interval.

The second panel (Figure 1, part D), allows one to define the logical expression. Abstractions are displayed as described in Section 2.2. Insertion, modification, and deletion of different graphic objects can be performed by switching among different options either in the "Logic" menu or through a toolbar (element E). As an example, in Figure 1, the OR between abstractions 3 and 5 is being selected, as highlighted by the dotted square containing the OR ellipsis. The same abstraction can appear more than once in the logical expression: this is graphically achieved by allowing to duplicate the circles associated to a specific ID. The expression under definition appears at the top of the panel in textual form using either IDs or abstraction labels. The two representations can be selected through a suitable button (element F).

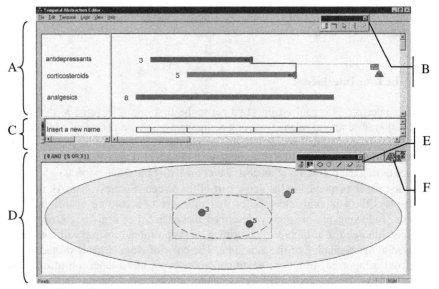

Fig. 1. The user interface for the visual definition of temporal abstractions.

Acknowledgements. This work was partially supported by MURST program COFIN 2000 ("Analysis, Information Visualization, and Visual Query in Databases for Clinical Monitoring"). We are grateful to Claudia Vicenzotto for her programming effort.

References

1. Chittaro, L. (ed.). (2001) Special Issue on Information Visualization in Medicine. *Artificial Intelligence in Medicine*, in press.
2. Combi, C., Chittaro, L. (1999) Abstraction on Clinical Data Sequences: an Object-Oriented Data Model and a Query Language Based on the Event Calculus. *Artificial Intelligence in Medicine*, 17(3): 271-301.
3. Combi, C., Chittaro, L. (2001) Representation of Temporal Intervals and Relations: Information Visualization Aspects and their Evaluation. *Proceedings Eighth International Symposium on Temporal Representation and Reasoning (TIME-01)*. Los Alamitos, IEEE Computer Society Press, in press.
4. Cousins, S.B., Kahn, G. (1991), The visual display of temporal information. *Artificial Intelligence in Medicine*, 3: 341-357.
5. Plaisant C, Mushlin R, Snyder A, Li J, Heller D, Shneiderman B. (1998) LifeLines: Using Visualization to Enhance Navigation and Analysis of Patient Records. *Proc. American Medical Informatics Association Annual Fall Symposium*. AMIA, 76-80.

Using Temporal Probabilistic Knowledge for Medical Decision Making

Nicolette de Bruijn[1], Peter Lucas[2], Karin Schurink[1], Marc Bonten[1], and Andy Hoepelman[1]

[1] Department of Internal Medicine, University Medical Centre Utrecht, Heidelberglaan 100, 3584 CX Utrecht, The Netherlands, {N.C.deBruijn,K.Schurink,M.J.M.Bonten,I.M.Hoepelman}@digd.azu.nl
[2] Department of Computing Science, University of Aberdeen, Aberdeen, AB24 3UE, Scotland, UK, plucas@csd.abdn.ac.uk

Abstract. Time plays an important role in medical decision making, as a patient's disease is a dynamic process that changes over time; medical doctors, therefore, have to deal with the temporal nature of these processes as well. However, it is not clear whether time is equally important in every aspect of medical decision making. This paper explores the role of time in the diagnosis and treatment of ventilator-associated pneumonia (VAP) in ICU patients. The aim of this study was to obtain insight into the advantages and limitations of dealing with time explicitly in the context of VAP.

1 Introduction

Both time and uncertainty play an important part in medical decision making. The signs and symptoms of a patient's disorder evolve, revealing the temporal evolution of the underlying disease process. As most medical decisions are made in the face of incomplete knowledge about the patient's disorder, uncertainty is also a central feature of medical decision making.

A typical clinical situation where the above holds is in the diagnosis and treatment of patients with infectious diseases in the intensive-care unit (ICU) of a hospital. The most important temporal pattern in the development of infectious diseases in hospital patients is the process of bacterial colonisation. As the normal defence mechanisms against pathogens are frequently compromised in ICU patients, high percentages of patients become infected. In addition, the high levels of antimicrobial resistance in ICUs render effective diagnosis and treatment even more crucial, but far less easy; in particular junior doctors may require some form of decision support in this respect.

We have developed a model of ventilator-associated pneumonia, VAP for short, which will be incorporated into a decision-support system, aimed at offering clinicians advice in the diagnosis and optimal antimicrobial treatment of VAP [1].

In this paper, we investigate the temporal reasoning capabilities of the model in the context of medical decision making, using data of a prospectively collected set of data of ICU patients.

S. Quaglini, P. Barahona, and S. Andreassen (Eds.): AIME 2001, LNAI 2101, pp. 231–234, 2001.

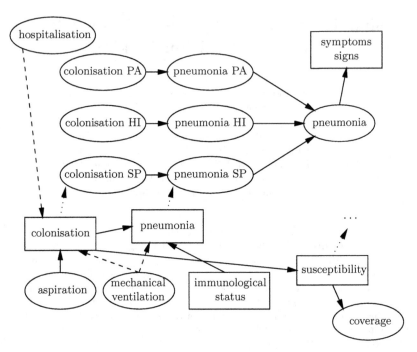

Fig. 1. Detailed structure of part of the Bayesian VAP model. Only three of the seven microorganisms included in the model are shown. Dotted arcs point to the actual topology of the probabilistic network; boxes stand for collections of similar vertices. Abbreviations: PA = Pseudomonas aeruginosa, HI = Haemophilus influenzae, SP = Streptococcus pneumoniae.

2   A Bayesian Model of Ventilator Associated Pneumonia

Knowledge of the process of colonisation by bacteria after the patient has entered the ICU is of major importance in determining the cause of a suspected or established pneumonia in the patient. The colonisation process is influenced by a number of interacting factors. Although the temporal nature of this process may be represented quite naturally as a Markov process, it was decided to use the less demanding, both in terms of required data and computational resources, representation of a Bayesian network $\mathcal{B} = (G, \mathrm{Pr})$, with acyclic directed graph G and factorised probability distribution Pr. A schema of the resulting Bayesian network model is shown in Fig. 1.

The temporal nature of VAP is modelled by the variables HOSPITALISATION, representing duration of stay in the ICU, and MECHANICAL VENTILATION, standing for the time the patient is on a mechanical ventilator. Furthermore, the occurrence of pneumonia follows colonisation in time. Pneumonia in turn will give rise to a number of signs and symptoms which can be observed, and are essential to diagnose the presence of pneumonia in the patient. The efficacy of antibiotic

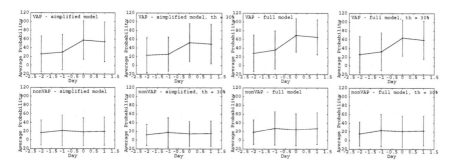

Fig. 2. Plot of the posterior probability (mean ± standard deviation) of pneumonia given symptoms and signs, and either without temporal information (four left-most plots) or including temporal information (four right-most plots). Top row: VAP patients; bottom row: patients without VAP.

treatment, and hence of treatment selection, depends on the pathogens by which the patient is likely to be infected.

For the signs and symptoms of VAP modelled in the network, it was assumed that most of these are conditionally independent given PNEUMONIA.

3   Temporal Reasoning under Uncertainty

3.1   Patients and Methods

A sample of data of 50 patients was selected from a prospective dataset with data of approximately 500 patients; only with 24 of these patients had the clinical diagnosis VAP been associated. The remaining 26 patients without VAP have been randomly selected from the dataset.

We used two models as vehicles of the study. In the first model, the variables HOSPITALISATION and MECHANICAL VENTILATION, shown in Fig. 1, were not instantiated, yielding results in which time was not explicitly taken into account. We refer to this model as the *simplified model*. The second model is the full Bayesian network, referred to in the following as the *full model*.

3.2   Diagnosis and Time

In the first study, the nature of the interaction between colonisation pattern and patient findings in diagnosing VAP was investigated, either or not using a 30% probability threshold on the individual colonisation variables; when less than 30%, the marginal probabilities were reset to 0, indicating that those pathogens could be ignored.

Fig. 2 summarises the results obtained for the patients with and without VAP. Clearly, for patients with VAP (top row), most of the temporal trends in the posterior probability $\Pr^*(pneumonia)$ appear to result directly from the signs and

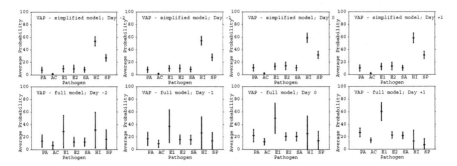

Fig. 3. Plot of average posterior probability (mean ± standard deviation) of colonisation by pathogens causing VAP in patients *with VAP*. Names of pathogens are abbreviated (e.g. PA is *Pseudomonas Aeruginosa*).

symptoms observed in the patients, which apparently dominated the influence of the colonisation process. Nevertheless, some influence from the colonisation model part can be recognised for VAP patients. No clear temporal pattern was discerned for non-VAP patients, confirming the conclusion that explicit temporal information is not of major importance for the purpose of diagnosis of VAP.

3.3 Treatment Selection and Time

A similar study of temporal trends was undertaken for the colonisation process, which yields essential information for treatment selection.

The top row of Fig. 3 summarises the effects of information regarding signs and symptoms when all available temporal information was omitted. Very similar plots were obtained for the patients without VAP, and these were therefore omitted. The bottom row of Fig. 3 indicates that temporal information is of significant importance in predicting the colonisation process in patients. A similar pattern was observed in patients without VAP.

4   Discussion

It was shown that the implicit temporal nature of signs and symptoms in patients will be of greater significance in diagnosing pneumonia in patients than the temporal model of bacterial colonisation. However, explicit temporal information appeared to be essential for predicting colonisation, the most important factor determining treatment selection.

References

1. P.J.F. Lucas, N.C. de Bruijn, K. Schurink, I.M. Hoepelman. A Probabilistic and decision-theoretic approach to the management of infectious disease at the ICU. *Artificial Intelligence in Medicine* 19(3) (2000) 251–279.

Temporal Issues in the Intelligent Interpretation of the Sleep Apnea Syndrome

M. Cabrero-Canosa, M. Castro-Pereiro, M. Graña-Ramos,
E. Hernandez-Pereira, and V. Moret-Bonillo

Laboratory for Research and Development in Artificial Intelligence (LIDIA),
Computer Science Dept., University of A Coruña, 15071 A Coruña, Spain.
civmoret@udc.es

Abstract. Automation of the medical diagnosis of the Sleep Apnea Syndrome
(SAS) requires an intelligent analysis of the pneumological and
neurophysiological signals of the patient that combines both
conventional and Artificial Intelligence techniques in order to
detect respiratory abnormalities and construct a hypnogram for the
patient, and a process of temporal fusion and correlation between
the signals for both a correct classification of the apneic events within a
sleep stage framework, and to explain the occurrence of abnormal sleep
patterns as a consequence of these events. In this article, the most important aspects of the analysis and information integration processes are
described and the preliminary validation results obtained are discussed.

1 Introduction

An Sleep Apnea Syndrome (SAS) automatic diagnostic system should carry out
two principal tasks, namely the classification of sleep stages and the detection
and classification of apneic respiratory events, on the basis, respectively, of neurophysiological and pneumological signals. Most of the systems developed to date
only solve very specific aspects of these two tasks, and none draw up a reasoned
interpretation of results or even a diagnosis. There is an evident need, in the
area of intelligent SAS diagnosis, for reliable and integrated decision support
systems that both permit correct interpretation of apneic episodes in the context of patient sleep stages and explain the patient sleep stage transitions within
the context of respiratory abnormalities. This is the approach that is incorporated into our system, which is defined as a computerised system for respiratory
analysis and sleep study, with a facility for data abstraction and symbolic manipulation that contextually correlates and integrates the information available
so as to arrive at a diagnostic conclusion as to the existence/non-existence of
SAS and its classification.

2 Material and Methods

Our system combines classical signal processing and Artificial Intelligence techniques in an intelligent approach to the implementation of the following tasks:

S. Quaglini, P. Barahona, and S. Andreassen (Eds.): AIME 2001, LNAI 2101, pp. 235–238, 2001.

(1) extraction of symbolic information from the most relevant features of the signals[1]; (2) definition of the temporal intervals having clinical significance; (3) detection of the apneic events in these intervals[2]; (4) temporal correlation of the information so as to confirm events; and finally (5) fusion and correlation of all the data in order to obtain a customised diagnosis. Data abstraction processes are applied in order to obtain a sequence of intervals of variable duration that are labelled symbolically on the basis of medical criteria. Subsequently, all the symbolic information obtained is correlated temporally and contextualised with dynamic variables (such as the position signal and the EMG), with static information (such as age, weight, height, etc), and finally, with information on the sleeping habits of the patient. The result is a set of real apneic events. A final phase involves the development of a customised diagnosis for the patient, determining the existence/non-existence and class of SAS.

After that the vertical abstraction of all the symbolic information generated previously is performed , with a view to: (a) confirming the respiratory irregularities detected as apneic events; (b) identifying the type of apneic event as an apnea or hypopnea, and finally, (c) classifying type in function of the behaviour of the respiratory effort (central, obstructive or mixed). Task execution is based on a production system having three islands of knowledge specific to the resolution of each of the previous tasks. The sequence of tasks corresponding to the correlation process (Figure 1) are described as follows:

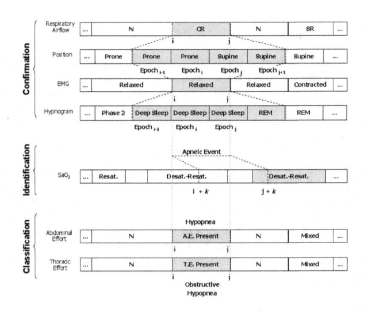

Fig. 1. Vertical abstraction from the preprocessed neurophysiological and pneumological signals

- **Confirmation.** The intervals marked in the respiratory airflow signal as manifesting reduction (CR label in Figure 1) represent hypothetical apneic events (apneas or hypopneas) that require confirmation.
- **Identification.** The apneic events confirmed in the previous phase can be classified as one of two kinds, depending on the extent of the reduction in the interval: apnea for a totally reduced label (TR), and hypopnea for a clearly reduced label (CR) when there is, in addition, a desaturation-resaturation pattern that commenced during or after the event[3].
- **Classification.** The classification phase checks the behaviour of the thoracic and abdominal effort signals during the interval of the apneic event in order to determine the type of the event[4].

As a result of this process, a set of apneic events is obtained that have been confirmed and classified by a combined correlation and interpretation of pneumological and neurophysiological information over time.

Once the existence of SAS has been confirmed, an Apnea/Hypopnea Index (AHI) is calculated for each kind of apneic event confirmed, and the syndrome is classified in function of the greatest value of the AHI. The outcome of this task is a diagnostic conclusion as to the existence/non-existence of the SAS.

3   Results and Conclusions

An independent and blind analysis of a total of 2819 minutes of polysomnographic recordings corresponding to 7 patients was carried out by our system and an expert collaborating in the design of the system. Pairs' measurements were made and the performance of the system was studied in terms of the identification and classification of events and the construction of the hypnogram[5]. Table 1 shows the results obtained for the validation of the system using *Sensitivity (Se)*, *Specificity (Sp)*, *Positive Predictive Value (PPV)*, *Negative Predictive Value (NPV)*, *Precision (P)*, and finally, the *Jaccard coefficient (J)* to measure performance.

A series of conclusions can be drawn from the results obtained, as follows:

Firstly, in the events identification category, for hypopneas the level of *false positives* is high, reflected in the low values for the *Positive Predictive Values* and the *Jaccard measurement*.

Secondly, in the classification of the central and mixed events, the unsatisfactory results for the *Sensitivity* and *Positive Predictive Value* and the high values for the *Sensitivity* and *Negative Predictive Value* can be explained by the fact that the majority of the 7 patients in the study population suffer from obstructive apneas, and the expert's classification is consequently conditioned by this knowledge.

Finally, the system obtained very satisfactory results in terms of sleep stage classification. In particular, it successfully differentiated between the wakefulness and REM phases, which happens to be the most frequent error in existing automated systems.

Table 1. Performance measurement for (a) apneic events detection and classification; (b) apnea/hypopnea identification and (c) sleep stage classification

		%Se	%Sp	%PPV	%NPV	%P	%J
Events	Apneas	80.0	82.7	90.5	66.7	80.8	73.8
Identification	Hypopneas	53.2	82.2	19.4	95.5	80.0	16.6
Classification	Obstructive	87.5	52.0	85.3	56.6	79.0	76.1
of Apneas &	Central	20.7	96.5	26.1	95.3	92.2	13.0
Hypopneas	Mixed	50.0	89.8	52.2	88.7	82.5	34.3
	Wakefulness	62.0	79.2	59.3	80.9	73.5	43.5
Sleep	Phase 1	43.9	81.4	19.4	93.4	77.9	15.6
Stages	Phase 2	25.4	89.8	31.1	86.9	79.9	16.3
Classification	Deep Sleep	47.7	94.4	77.4	81.7	80.9	41.9
	REM	66.8	93.9	63.5	94.7	90.2	48.3

Our conclusion, therefore, is that the system can be considered to perform satisfactorily, despite the discrepancies observed. Nevertheless, a more complete validation based on a larger data sample and the opinions of various experts in the field is required.

Acknowledgements. The authors wish to thank Dr. Antonio Martins Da Silva and INESC-N (Portugal), and Dr. Hector Verea Hernando and Dr. Maite Martin Egaña (Complejo Hospitalario Juan Canalejo, A Coruña, Spain) for their valuable suggestions in developing this project. This research has been financed by Xunta of Galicia (Project PGIDT99COM10503) and by CICYT (Project TIC-96-0590).

References

[1] O. Pacheco. *Sistema Assistido por Computador de Classificaçao do Electroencefalograma do Sono e Detecçao de Micro Despertares.* PhD thesis, Universidade de Aveiro, Portugal, 1996.
[2] T. Roth, T. P. Moyles, and R. F. Erlandson. A nonparametric statistical approach to breath segmentation. *IEEE Engineering in Medicine and Biology Society*, 330-331, 1989.
[3] F. Sériès, Y. Cormier, and J. La Forge. Role of lung volumes in nocturnal postapneic desaturation. *European Respiratory Journal*, 2:26–30, 1989.
[4] S. C. Mishoe. The diagnosis and treatment of sleep apnea syndrome. *Respiratory Care*, 32(2):183–201, 1987.
[5] V. Moret-Bonillo, E. Mosqueira-Rey, and A. Alonso-Betanzos. Information analysis and validation of intelligent monitoring systems in intensive care units. *IEEE Transactions on Information Technology in Biomedicine*, 1(2):87–99, 1997.

Generating Symbolic and Natural Language Partial Solutions for Inclusion in Medical Plans

S. Modgil and P. Hammond

Biomedical Informatics Unit, Eastman Dental Institute,
University College London.
{S.Modgil, P.Hammond}@eastman.ucl.ac.uk

Abstract. We describe the generation of partial solutions to Prolog queries posed during the design of medical treatment plans. Given a set of Prolog encoded safety principles, the queries request advise on plan revisions to conform with safety requirements. The user unfolds queries interactively, navigating a path through the solution search space by interacting with natural language representations of the Prolog terms. In this way, both symbolic and natural language representations of partial solutions can be generated. The former can be included in the plan, and the latter exported to a protocol document describing the plan. Hence, useful and informative partial solutions are still obtained despite incompleteness of the underlying knowledge base, which ordinarily would mean failure of a query. Furthermore, the user can avoid being overwhelmed by surplus solutions, and unfold to levels of detail suitable for different plans and their accompanying protocols.

1 Background and Introduction

Previously, generic principles concerned with safety and efficacy of plans were abstracted from an empirical analysis of chemotherapy plans [5]. Table 1 shows textual representations of the principles at a high level of abstraction. Expressed in rule-based form, the principles have been used as constraints in software for the run-time management of complex, hazardous procedures such as chemotherapy treatment [6]. Here, we are interested in their use as obligations when devising symbolic representations of new treatment plans for export to such software; specifically in advising how a plan should be further specified, or revised, to conform to the obligations. We also focus on assisting the production of a protocol document which describes the plan, its associated hazards and their management. Protocols are required when new treatment plans are under trial or about to be introduced into clinical practice, and permission is required from ethical or regulatory bodies. They are also referenced by clinicians managing patients.

Represented as Prolog rules, the safety principles can be specialised/ instantiated for inclusion in a plan and translation into useful natural language components of a protocol document. By way of illustration, the *prevention* principle can be represented as the following Prolog rule:

$$advise\_plan(\ Action,\ Plan,\ Prevention,\ ameliorate(Action,\ Effect)\ ) :- \qquad (1)$$

S. Quaglini, P. Barahona, and S. Andreassen (Eds.): AIME 2001, LNAI 2101, pp. 239–248, 2001.

Table 1. Generic safety principles

Exacerbation	Avoid exacerbating anticipated hazards	Monitoring	Monitor responses which herald hazardous situations
Diminution	Avoid undermining the benefits of essential actions	Efficacy	Ensure that overall plans are efficacious in pursuing stated objectives
Interaction	Ensure that an action does not interact with another action to cause harm	Sequencing	Order (essential) actions temporally for good effect and least harm
Reaction	React appropriately to ameliorate detected hazards	Critiquing	Critique proposal of certain hazardous actions even if they are well motivated
Warning	Warn about hazards due to incorrect execution of essential actions	Prevention	Prevent or ameliorate hazards before executing an essential action

> *part_of_plan(Action,Plan),*
>
> *effect(Action, Effect),*
>
> *hazardous(Effect),*
>
> *prevention(Action, Effect, Prevention).*

Suppose a treatment plan involves administration of the chemotherapeutic drug cisplatin. With all required information in the knowledge base, solving the query:

? advise_plan(admin(cisplatin), plan_1, Prevention, Reason).   (2)

would generate advice about associated hazards (*Reason*), and symbolic descriptions of preventative actions (*Prevention*) for inclusion in the plan. The corresponding textual form of the solution for inclusion in the protocol is:

Preventative actions:
- prior to administering cisplatin administer hydration regime: normal saline 1-2 litre
- after administering cisplatin administer hydration regime: normal saline 1-2 litre
are advised in plan 1 (administering cisplatin causes dehydration).   (3)

However, there are situations where such a naive animation of the principles is inadequate. On the one hand, evaluating a query on an incomplete knowledge base may result in failure to solve, ignoring the possibility of partial and informative solutions. For example, if no information about particular hydration schemes is present, then the query would fail and no advice at all would be forthcoming. This ignores derivation of a useful partial solution and the corresponding advice:

Preventative actions:
- administer a type of hydration regime prior to administering cisplatin
- administer a type of hydration regime after administering cisplatin
are advised in plan 1 (administering cisplatin causes dehydration).   (4)

On the other hand, there is potentially a vast amount of electronic drug information available, and if linked to the knowledge base could totally overwhelm the user with suggested solutions. More generally, clinicians often need to produce different versions of a protocol document for different regulatory situations, sometimes fully detailed and sometimes less so. What is required is for the user to have full control over query evaluation, enabling specialisation of principles to the required degree, and ignoring surplus solutions.

In this paper, we demonstrate a meta-interpeter that enables the user to specialise the safety principles in an interactive manner [7]. In a process known as "unfolding", the user generates and walks over the proof tree associated with the query requesting advice. Type extensions to the underlying Prolog system and other natural language translation facilities enable the user to interact with accessible textual versions of clauses rather than their Prolog formulations. The user selects individual goals to be resolved until the natural language version of the principle is at the right level of detail for inclusion in the protocol document. Should a goal fail due to incomplete knowledge, the user includes a symbolic representation of the partial solution (thus far obtained) in the plan, as well as the corresponding textual clause (e.g., (4)) in the protocol. Evaluation of the partial solution may be completed later when the knowledge base is updated.

The work described here forms part of the Design-A-Trial (DaT) project in which software is being developed to aid design of a clinical trial, generating a symbolic representation of the planned design (for export to software systems managing trials) as well as a textual protocol. The problem of incomplete knowledge is particularly pertinent given that trials often assess new and unusual combinations of drugs. Thus, DaT's knowledge base will often be deficient on some aspect of drug behaviour. Conversely, DaT will ultimately be linked to computerised medical databases so that tighter control on detail will be required.

The rest of the paper is organised as follows. In section 2 we describe the unfolding meta-interpreter and its control by the user. In section 3 we describe techniques used to generate natural language translations of Prolog rules. In particular, we motivate and describe implementation of a typed Prolog. Section 4 concludes with a discussion of related and future work.

2   User Interaction with the Unfolding Meta-interpreter

The unfolding meta-interpreter is a variation of the standard Prolog *demo* predicate [10], in which selection of goals and the clauses are made by the user.

$$unfold(stop,Rule). \hspace{8cm} (5)$$

$$unfold(continue,(Head :\text{-} Goals)) :\text{-}$$
$$\quad select\_goal(Head, Goals, Goal, RestGoals),$$
$$\quad select\_clause(Goal,(Goal :\text{-} Body)),$$
$$\quad add\_body(Body, RestGoals, NewGoals),$$
$$\quad next\_step(Choice),$$
$$\quad unfold(Choice,(Head :\text{-} NewGoals)).$$

Suppose a knowledge base containing (1) (*prevention* obligation) and the clauses:

$$part\_of\_plan(admin(cisplatin),plan\_1). \hspace{5cm} (6)$$
$$effect(admin(cisplatin),dehydration). \hspace{5.2cm} (7)$$
$$effect(admin(cisplatin),nephrotoxicity). \hspace{4.9cm} (8)$$
$$hazardous(dehydration). \hspace{6.5cm} (9)$$

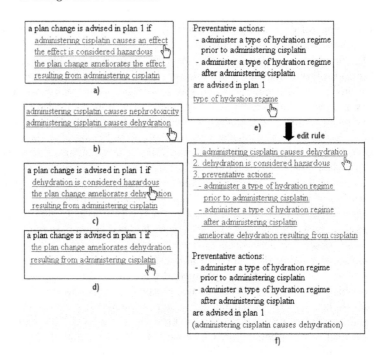

Fig. 1. User unfolding *prevention* principle

$$prevention(admin(cisplatin),dehydration, \qquad (10)$$
$$[pre(admin(cisplatin),hydration(Type,P)),post(admin(cisplatin),hydration(Type,P))]$$
$$:\text{-}\ hydration(Type,P).$$

The meta-interpreter and knowledge base are encoded in an Amzi Prolog [www. amzi. com] "logic server", which interfaces with a web-browser interface written in Visual Basic. To illustrate, suppose the user selects the *prevention* obligation for unfolding and the previously specified action 'administration of cisplatin'. Then, the first goal in the body of (1) is automatically unfolded, resulting in:

$$advise\_plan(admin(cisplatin),plan\_1,Prevention,ameliorate(admin(cisplatin),Effect))\ :\text{-}$$
$$effect(admin(cisplatin),\ Effect), \qquad (11)$$
$$hazardous(Effect),$$
$$prevention(admin(cisplatin),Effect,Prevention).$$

This rule and the goals in its body are translated to natural language forms, written to an HTML file, and displayed in a web-browser window (fig.1a). The user can now unfold the rule. Selecting the first goal[1], the matching clauses (7) and (8) are translated and displayed whereupon selection of (7) (following

---

[1] If a non ground negated goal is selected (i.e., the safeness condition is violated [10]) the user is advised (with explanatory text) to select another goal. For the sake of transparency, this option is preferred to disabling the selection of such goals.

unification) results in replacement of the goal in the body of (11) with the (empty) body of (7), resulting in clause (12):

advise_plan(admin(cisplatin),plan_1,Prevention,ameliorate(admin(cisplatin),dehydration)) :-   hazardous(dehydration),
prevention(admin(cisplatin),dehydration,Prevention).   (12)

The new rule and its body are translated and displayed (fig.1c). Since there is only one matching clause (9), selecting 'dehydration is considered hazardous' results in automatic unfolding to (fig.1d):

advise_plan(admin(cisplatin),plan_1,Prevention,ameliorate(admin(cisplatin),
dehydration)) :- prevention(admin(cisplatin), dehydration, Prevention).   (13)

Choosing the only available goal (fig.1d), there is only one available clause (10), and so automatic unfolding gives (fig.1e):

advise_plan(admin(cisplatin),plan_1,[pre(admin(cisplatin),hydration(Type,P)),   (14)
post(admin(cisplatin),hydration(Type,P))],ameliorate(admin(cisplatin),dehydration)):-
hydration(Type,P)).

Selecting 'type of hydration regime', the user is told that there are no clauses describing hydration regimes, and so opts to edit the partial solution thus far obtained. A history of the heads of clauses selected (including unique clauses not offered for selection) is shown. These can be included in parentheses after the textual rule (fig.1f). The resulting text can then be exported to the protocol. The results ((14)) of unfolding (effectively partial evaluation) can be included in the symbolic representation of the plan. Should the knowledge base be updated at a later date, the user has the option to attempt completion of evaluation and so avoid execution of the general principle. This is preferred on grounds of efficiency. Also, commitment to a subspace of possible solutions is maintained, the user having rejected solutions considered superfluous during unfolding.

We conclude with an example illustrating animation of the *exacerbation* principle (fig.2) specialised for actions of the kind *admin(Drug)*. The knowledge base for this example is shown below (*nsai* stands for *non steroidal anti-inflammatory agent*). Notice the typing information included (declaration of infix operators $\ll$, *or, and* and : is assumed) and atoms from a hierarchy of drug types labelling drug names and variables (to be described in section 3).

invalid(user_suggestion(admin(drug : Drug),Plan)) :-   (15)
part_of_plan(admin(drug : Drug2),Plan),
effect(admin(drug : Drug2),Effect),
hazardous(Effect),
exacerbation(admin(drug : Drug),admin(drug : Drug2),Effect).

part_of_plan(admin(drug : cisplatin),plan_1).   (16)
effect(admin(drug : cisplatin),nephrotoxicity).   (17)
effect(admin(drug : cisplatin),dehydration).   (18)
effect(admin(antibiotic : gentamicin),nephrotoxicity).   (19)
effect(admin(antibiotic : cephalosporin),nephrotoxicity).   (20)
hazardous(nephrotoxicity).   (21)
hazardous(dehydration).   (22)

$exacerbation(admin(antibiotic : X), admin(drug : cisplatin), nephrotoxicity) :-$ (23)
    $effect(admin(antibiotic : X), nephrotoxicity).$

$exacerbation(admin(steroid \ or \ nsai \ or \ aminoglycoside: X),$ (24)
    $admin(drug : cisplatin), nephrotoxicity).$

$steroid \ll drug. \ antibiotic \ll drug. \ aminoglycoside \ll drug. \ nsai \ll pain\_killer.$
$pain\_killer \ll drug.$

$nsai : aspirin. \ antibiotic : cephalosporin. \ antibiotic : gentamicin.$

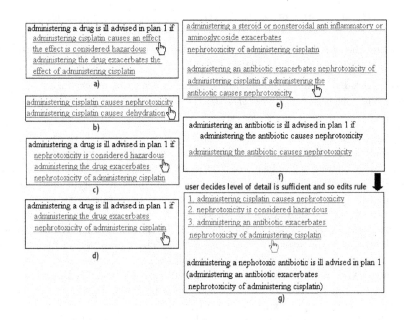

Fig. 2. User unfolding *exacerbation* principle

The *exacerbation* and *diminution* principles are typically animated as constraints during computerised enactment of a designed plan; e.g., vetoing adventitiously suggested treatments which exacerbate hazardous effects of an action in a plan. However, there are advantages to unfolding these two principles at design time. Inclusion of the final textual clause (fig.2g) in the protocol, demonstrates awareness of possible hazards that may arise during patient management. Also, the initial generic constraint has been partially evaluated, specialised to account for administration of cisplatin. Hence, the underlying:

$invalid(user\_suggestion(admin(antibiotic : X), plan\_1)) :-$ (25)
    $effect(admin(antibiotic : X), nephrotoxicity)$

can be included in the plan, and run as a specialised constraint deterring administration of nephrotoxic antibiotics during plan enactment.

3   Typing of Terms and Natural Language Translation

Our use of types affords more compact knowledge representation and improves natural language translation. In general, we use $\lambda : X$, where X is an atom (usually a specific drug, e.g., gentamicin) or a variable, and $\lambda = t_1 op_1 t_2 \ldots op_n t_n$, where for $i = 1 \ldots n, t_i$ is a drug type (e.g., antibiotic) and op_i is one of *or* or *and*. If $\lambda = t_i$ we say that λ is *atomic*. The type hierarchy is declared in the knowledge base using the transitive operator $\ll$, where $t_1 \ll t_2$ indicates that t_1 is a subtype of t_2 (e.g., *antibiotic* $\ll$ *drug*). The types of individual drugs are also declared in the knowledge base as *type : drug* (e.g., *antibiotic : gentamicin*).

We have extended the standard Prolog unification procedure [10]. Resolution of $p(TypeY : Y)$ with $p(TypeX : X)$ obtains $p(TypeZ : Z)$, where Z is the unifier of X and Y in the standard way, and $TypeZ$ is the *atomic* unification of *atomic* labels $TypeY$ and $TypeX$, informally described as follows:

Let Γ denote a set of type declarations $\{t_1 : x_1, \ldots, t_n : x_n\}$ and $\Sigma = \{t_1 \ll t_2, \ldots, t_m \ll t_n\}$ where Σ includes the transitive closure of $\ll$.

1. If either $TypeY$ and/or $TypeX$ is a variable, then $TypeZ$ is the unifier of $TypeY$ and $TypeX$ in the standard way, e.g., $p(Z : gentamicin)$ resolves with $p(antibiotic : X)$ obtaining $p(antibiotic : gentamicin)$.
2. If both $TypeY$ and $TypeX$ are atoms, then $TypeZ = TypeY$, iff
   a) $TypeY \ll TypeX \in \Sigma$, and
   b) if Y is a variable and X an atom (in which case $Z = X$), then either $TypeY : X \in \Gamma$, or there exists a $TypeQ$ such that $TypeQ \ll TypeY \in \Sigma$, and $TypeQ : X \in \Gamma$.

In the unfolding step in fig.2d, we have the underlying:

$$invalid(user\_suggestion(admin(drug : X), plan\_1)) :- \qquad (26)$$
$$exacerbation(admin(drug : X), admin(drug : cisplatin), nephrotoxicity).$$

Resolving the goal in the body of (26) with (23), then *admin(drug : X)* resolves with *admin(antibiotic : X)* obtaining *admin(antibiotic : X)*. To illustrate 2b), resolution of $p(drug : asprin)$ with $p(painkiller : X)$ to give $p(painkiller : asprin)$ proceeds because we have *nsai : asprin*, and *nsai* $\ll$ *painkiller*.

Typing facilitates more compact and elegant logical representation and natural language translation. For example, we have (23) rather than:

$$exacerbation(admin(X), admin(cisplatin), nephrotoxicity) :- \qquad (27)$$
$$effect(admin(X), nephrotoxicity),$$
$$antibiotic(X).$$

and the textual rule in fig.2f rather than the more cumbersome "administering **a drug** is ill... if administering the **drug** causes... and **the drug is an antibiotic**". For these reasons, we have also catered for *compound* type expressions. For example, the disjunction of types labelling X in (24), rather than *steroid(X) ; nsai(X) ; aminoglycoside(X)* in the body of (24) and the resultant need for backtracking to generate all solutions. The textual translation in fig.2e is more concise and elegant in comparison to "and the drug is a steroid or ...". We also allow conjunctions, so that we might have *p(drug : X) :- q(drug : X)* and *q(antibiotic and sulphonamide : X)*, resolving to give *p(antibiotic and sulphonamide : X) :- q(antibiotic and sulphonamide : X)*, rather than *p(X) :- q(X), drug(X)* and *q(X) :- antibiotic(X), sulphonamide(X)*. Use of conjunctions facilitates a form of sentence aggregation or *set formation* [12]; e.g., "It is an antibiotic and a sulphonamide" rather than "It is an antibiotic. It is a sulphonamide".

We describe how γ is given by the *complex* unification of α and β when resolving $p(\alpha : Y)$ with $p(\beta : X)$. Firstly, we describe **conjunct** unification:

c_1 *and* c_2 *and* ... *and* c_p is the **conjunct** unification of a_1 *and* a_2 *and* ... *and* a_n with b_1 *and* b_2 *and* ... *and* b_m (where all a_i and b_i are *atomic*), iff
for all pairs $(a_i, b_j) \in \{a_1, a_2, \ldots, a_n\} \times \{b_1, b_2, \ldots, b_m\}$, there exists an *atomic* unification c_k of a_i and b_j, in c_1 *and* c_2 *and* ... *and* c_p (i.e., $p = n \times m$).

α and β are initially rewritten in their *disjunctive normal forms* $\alpha' = a_1$ *or* ... *or* a_n and $\beta' = b_1$ *or* ... *or* b_m respectively (all of a_i and b_i are conjuncts of *atomic* types). Then γ is given by the **disjunct** unification of α' and β', where:

$\gamma = c_1$ *or* c_2 *or* ... *or* c_p is the **disjunct** unification of a_1 *or* a_2 *or* ... *or* a_n with b_1 *or* b_2 *or* ... *or* b_m, iff
for all $(a_i, b_j) \in \{a_1, a_2, \ldots, a_n\} \times \{b_1, b_2, \ldots, b_m\}$, if c_k is a *conjunct* unification of a_i and b_j, then c_k is in c_1 *or* c_2 *or* ... *or* c_p, and $p \geq 1$ (i.e., at least one disjunct in a_1 *or* a_2 *or* ... *or* a_n unifies with at least one disjunct in b_1 *or* b_2 *or* ... *or* b_m).

To illustrate, resolving the goal in the body of (26) with (24), then *steroid or nsai or aminoglycoside* is the *disjunct* unification of *drug* and *steroid or nsai or aminoglycoside*. If only *steroid* $\ll$ *drug* was declared in the knowledge base, then the *disjunct* unification would be *steroid*.

The "query the user" facility [13] is another technique for coping with incomplete knowledge bases. We have implemented this facility for type declaration and hierarchy information. For example, suppose a goal fails because *pain_killer : piroxicam* fails to unify with *nsai : X*. Then the user is informed, and may be prompted to add typing information such as *piroxicam* is a *nsai* drug. The goal is evaluated again. Note that the goal (unification) may still fail if *nsai* $\ll$ *pain_killer* is not present. Again the user is informed, and after inputting the required type hierarchy information, the goal is then evaluated successfully.

We conclude by describing some features of our natural language translation of clauses. We refer to the text in fig.2a generated from the underlying rule:

$$invalid(user\_suggestion(admin(drug : Drug),plan\_1)) :- \qquad (28)$$
$$effect(admin(drug : cisplatin),Effect),$$
$$hazardous(Effect),$$
$$exacerbation(admin(drug : Drug), admin(drug : cisplatin), Effect).$$

At the top level we have:

$$show\_clause(Clause, Text) :- label\_variables(Clause, LClause), \qquad (29)$$
$$clause\_read\_as(LClause, Text, []).$$

When translating variables (other than those denoting drugs), assignment of meaningful names is effected by *label_variables* referencing templates in the knowledge base. For example, "effect" is assigned to *Effect* in *effect(admin(drug : cisplatin),Effect)* in (28), by correlating the position of the variable *Effect* in the clause with the positioning of the name "effect" in the template *var_template (effect(admin(drug_type : drug),effect))*. Note that correlation is complicated when instantiations of a variable can be with terms of different types (space limitations preclude a more detailed account). Of course, reference to templates of the above kind is not always possible, so that for a goal such as *Effect \ = dehydration*, a previous assignment to the variable *Effect* is looked for (e.g., if this goal appeared after the first goal in the body of (28)). Finally, note that *label_variables* also annotates variables with a marker indicating how many times it has already been referenced. This enables choice between indefinite and definite articles.

Space limitations preclude an account of the definite clause grammar [10] which defines *clause_read_as*, and renders translation of the labelled clause. However, one feature to note is the reification of predicates; e.g., "nephrotoxic antibiotic" rather than "administering the antibiotic causes nephrotoxicity" in fig.2g.

4   Conclusions

Work related to ours includes [14] in which partially evaluated proof trees are used to generate *conditional* answers to cope with incomplete knowledge. Our work is also related to the study of *Intensional Answers (IAs)* to database queries [8]. One notion of *IAs* is that they are partial evaluations of a query. In [4] a method is proposed for intensional query answering based on program transformation using partial evaluation [9]. Our work can be viewed as applying such a method within a restricted domain and for a specific subclass of the programs considered in [4]. There are a number of generic approaches using typing in an inheritance hierarchy to help describe linguistic structures (e.g., [2]). In particular, [3] makes use of types in natural language translations of intensional answers to database queries. However, [3] considers only *atomic* and not *compound* types. More generally, note that since our approach provides a natural language interface to the meta- interpreter, the user has full control over navigation through the search space, unfolding to the required degree and ignoring uninteresting paths. This flexibility is missing from earlier work in which the generation of answers is pre-determined by the system designer. Of course, one drawback is that we sacrifice generality. Since our natural language generation procedures are essentially template based, our approach does not transfer to arbitrary domains.

In section 2, we referred to completing evaluation of partial solutions upon later updates to the knowledge base. If completion is effected during the management of patients on a designed plan, then the clinician (unlikely to be the same individual as the plan designer) is committed to those choices made by the plan designer at the time of unfolding. One possible solution is to restrict unfolding to invariant solutions [1], i.e., those based only on the intensional part of the database, without use of facts in the extensional part. However, one would need to weaken this restriction to exclude only medical facts, but allow solutions based on new facts introduced by the designer of the plan.

In future work we plan to consider more sophisticated natural language generation techniques such as sentence aggregation, use of referring expressions, and elimination of redundant phrases [12]. Also, at present our generation of natural language translations is very sensitive to the precise Prolog encoding of the medical obligations. A future research goal is the provision of a framework in which the encoding of medical expert knowledge conforms to pre-defined schema, and natural language translation is defined in relation to these more generic schema. Finally, evaluation of the unfolding meta-interpreter, in terms of its impact on protocol quality, will be conducted as part of the evaluation of the Design-a-Trial system in which the meta-interpreter has been integrated [11].

References

1. Cholvy L. Answering queries addressed to a rule base. In: Revue d'intelligence artificielle, 4(1), pp 79–98, 1990.
2. Erbach G. ProFIT: Prolog with Features, Inheritance, and Templates. In: Seventh Conference of the European Chapter of the Association for Computational Linguistics, pp 180-187, Dublin, 1995.
3. Gaasterland T., and Minker J. User needs and language generation issues in a cooperative answering system. In: ICLP Workshop on Advanced Logic Programming Tools and Formalisms for Language Processing, Paris, France, June, 1991.
4. Giacomo D. Intensional query answering by partial evaluation. In: Journal of Intelligent Information Systems, 3(7), pp 205-233, Kluwer Academic Publishers, 1996.
5. Hammond P., Harris AL., Das SK., and Wyatt JC. Safety and decision support in oncology. In: Methods of Information in Medicine, 33(4), pp 371-381,1994.
6. Hammond P., and Sergot MJ. Computer support for protocol-based treatment of cancer. In: Journal of Logic Programming, 26(2), pp 93-111, Feb 1996.
7. Hammond P., Sergot M.J., and Wyatt J.C. Safety reasoning in medical decision support. In: Artificial Intelligence in Medicine: Research Frontiers and Funding Opportunities. IEE. Digest No: 96/031, 1996.
8. Imielinski T. Intelligent Query Answering in Rule Based Systems. In: Foundations of Deductive Databases and Logic Programming, 1988 (ed. Minker T.,), Morgan Kaufman, Washington, D.C.
9. Lloyd J.W., and Shepherdson J.C. Partial evaluation in logic programming. In Journal of Logic Programming, 11(3&4), pp 217-242, 1991.
10. Nilsson U., and Matuszynski J. Logic, Programming and Prolog. John Wiley and Sons, 1990.
11. Potts H., Wyatt J., Modgil S., Hammond P., Altman D. Evaluating decision support systems with distinctive or complex output: solutions from the Design-a-Trial project. Submitted to 8th European conference on AI in Medicine, AIME'01. 2001.
12. Reiter E., and Dale R. Building Applied Natural Language Generation Systems. In: Journal of Natural-Language Engineering, (3), pp 57-87, 1997.
13. Sergot MJ. A Query-the-User facility for Logic Programming. In: Integrated Interactive Computer Systems, 1983 (eds. Degano and Sandewall); E. North Holland.
14. Wolstenholme DE., 1988. Saying "I don't know" and conditional answers. In: Research and Development in Expert Systems IV, 1988, (ed. Moralee, D.S.), pp 115-125. Cambridge University Press.

Using Part-of-Speech and Word-Sense Disambiguation for Boosting String-Edit Distance Spelling Correction

Patrick Ruch, Robert Baud, Antoine Geissbühler,
Christian Lovis, Anne-Marie Rassinoux, and Alain Rivière

Medical Informatics Division, University Hospital of Geneva
{ruch,baud,geissbuhler,lovis,rassinoux,riviere}@dim.hcuge.ch

Abstract. We report on the design of a system for correcting spelling errors resulting in non-existent words. The system aims at improving edition of medical reports. Unlike traditional systems, both semantic and syntactic contexts are considered here. The system is organized along three steps. The first module is based on a context independent string-to-string edit distance calculus. The second module, based on the morpho-syntactic context attempts to rank more relevantly the data set provided by the first module, finally a third contextual module processes words with the same part-of-speech by applying some contextual word-sense disambiguation. Modules 2 and 3 are using both hand written rules and data-driven Markovian matrices. A final evaluation shows a significant improvement compared to context-free spelling correction.

1 Introduction

The system we design aims at correcting errors resulting in non-existent words. The system is organized along three steps. The first module is based on a context independent string-to-string edit distance calculus (cf. [1] for a survey of the probabilistic models of pronunciation and spelling). The second module, based on the morpho-syntactic context, attempts to rank more relevantly the data set provided by the first module, finally a third contextual module processes words with the same POS (part-of-speech, also called morpho-syntactic category, i.e. *verb, noun, adjective...*) by applying contextual WS (word-sense, as for example *body part, temporal concept...*) disambiguation. A final evaluation shows a significant improvement compared to context-free spelling correction, at least at the level of the POS filtering.

On an applicative point-of-view, spelling-correction in medical patient records (as reported in [2], rates of misspelling in medical texts -up to 10%- are incomparable to misspellings rates in other corpora, such as newspaper samples) constitutes a critical issue, likely to result in dramatic side effects, as it has been extensively studied and reported in the medical literature ([3], [4]). These studies conclude that automated measures of similarities between medication names can form the basis of

S. Quaglini, P. Barahona, and S. Andreassen (Eds.): AIME 2001, LNAI 2101, pp. 249–257, 2001.

highly accurate, sensitive, and specific tests of the potential for errors with look-alike and sound-alike medication names.

1.1 Basic Typology

Spelling correction problems can be separated in two categories. The first category addresses the problem of correcting spelling that result in valid, though unintended words (as for example[1] in *a peace of cake*, where *piece* is misspelled) and also the problem of correcting particular word usage errors (such as *among* and *between*). The second category is concerned only with errors that result in words that cannot be found in a lexicon, and therefore cannot be detected by conventional spelling checkers such has the DEC-10 spell. While the first problem is sometimes referred as *context sensitive spelling correction*, with numerous studies (see [5][6][7]), as opposite to the second, referred implicitly *as context free spelling correction*, often perceived as a problem where progress can not be made[2] [8], some works show the importance of the context for improving accuracy of the second category too [9][10]. At this level, we suggest a new terminology for qualifying each category: we will call *word correction* the first category, and *character correction* the second, leaving the *context sensitivity/insensitivity* question opened for both correction types.

1.2 Morpho-Syntactic Filtering and Higher Level Linguistic Modules

While recent experiments on word correction application use more linguistic modules (mainly POS disambiguation tools as in [5]) for handling the context, we observe that character correction tools –even when they use the context- do not use comparable approaches, and instead rely on word language models ([9], [10]). The first specificity of our system consists in applying morpho-syntactic disambiguation to the character correction problem.

Working on a word correction problem, Golding and Shabes [5] introduce a method using POS trigrams to encode the context. Although this method greatly reduces the number of parameters compared to methods based on word trigrams[3], it empirically

---

[1] The experiment was conducted on French corpora, however when possible, examples are provided in English for sake of clarity.

[2] However, the problem is still very crucial for agglutinative languages [11], where the vocabulary can be hardly listed in an exhaustive manner. Although some authors [12] underlined the high compositionally of the medical language even for morphologically poor languages such as French and English, the French medical language will be considered exhaustively listed in a manageable size list of words (i.e. about 10^5 entries).

[3] POS n-grams represent the morpho-syntactic level, word n-grams represent the token level, and WS n-grams the semantic level, thus the phrase *we diagnosis* can be represented by 3 different models: *we diagnosis* (word level), *prop v[12]* (morpho-syntactic level), and *pers diap* (semantic level). The meaning of prop, v[12], pers, and diap is respectively: personal pro-

appeared to discriminate poorly when words in the confusion set have the same POS. In this last case, the method is coupled with a more traditional word model. Like them, we start filtering with a POS tagger, but then, instead of using an expensive word language module, we use a WS tagger for discriminating among candidates, which have the same POS. Here is located the second specificity of the approach.

1.3 Syntactic Correction

Another related promising way of research concerns syntactic correction. Syntactic correction addresses a) word order/presence, and b) agreement problems:

  a.   He wants play tennis *to*. / He wants to play tennis.
  b.   They pick*s* a piece of cake. / They pick a piece of cake.

Of course, character correction and word correction may be necessary for processing a correct syntactic correction, therefore in such systems, the usual processing is: first, a string edit module solves the character errors, and second a syntactic module looks for syntactic errors [13]. Here lies the third specificity of our approach as we apply syntactic constraints at the character correction level!

1.4 String-to-String Edit Distance

Our approach consists in using the surrounding context of the spelling error in order to rank more relevantly the well-spelled candidates. Another promising way of research attempts to improve the string edit distance module ([9] [14] [15]). This complementary improvements shall not be treated here: first, because it would go far beyond the scope of the paper, second because all these investigations require large amount of training data (as for example [15] worked with a 3 millions word corpus for speech recognition) that are often absent out of some very small set of domains and languages, and anyway absent in the French medical jargon. Section 2.1 provides more algorithmic information.

1.5 Balancing Act

The morpho-syntactic and semantic filtering can be seen has a winner-takes-all process, where only the most reliable part-of-speech candidates are given more weight, similarly to what occurs in a decision-list system. The taggers combine regular-like handcrafted constraints, and Hidden Markov models (for processing the remaining ambiguities) in order to select the most reliable part-of-speech or word-sense candidates. Unlike standard Bayesian approaches, however, such approach does not combine the log-likelihood of each classifier, but bases its classification solely on the most reliable piece of evidence identified in the target context. Perhaps surprisingly, this approach (similar to decision lists [16]) provides the same or even slightly better precision than the combination of evidence approach [17], however, its major advantage

---

noun, verb 1st and 2nd person, human being (UMLS T016), and diagnostic procedure (UMLS T060). POS tags attempt to follow the MULTEXT morpho-syntactic description.

is maybe to gather multiple heterogeneous classifiers, operating on non-independent source of evidence, in a unified and traceable framework. Thus, in the context of developing a spelling checker tailored for medical texts, using both symbolic constraints and data-driven source of evidence, together with facing sparse data issues, such architecture seems particularly well adapted.

This balanced architecture for disambiguation: rules and transition probabilities rather than log-likelihood combination constitutes the last originality of our character correction system. The rule-based part-of-speech tagger we used, as well as its HMM (Hidden Markov Model) component have been extensively described elsewhere ([18] and [19]), and shall not be presented here, instead we will present the application of the tool to the character correction task. The semantic filtering behaves along the same lines as the morpho-syntactic one, and has also been described in detail together with the 40 UMLS-based semantic types it uses ([20] and [21]).

2   Method

We first collected a set of misspelled words together with the left adjacent context (2 words), and got a total of 324 records. This set is split in two equivalent subsets, set A is used for tuning the system, while set B is kept as final test set. This collection step was fulfilled manually and semi-automatically, and will be the matter of a future report[4]. Here is an example of the misspelled words (in French):

Example 1. Records of the misspelled word database

key	Context2	Context1	Mispelled word	Well-formed word
77	évidence	un	oedéme	oedème
78	une	paroi	souilée	souillée
79	par	le	sphinter	sphincter

The lexical resources[5] we used are the following: a 90000 items list of well written tokens for the string-to-string edit distance module, a 30000 lexemes lexicon for the POS filtering [12], among this lexemes about 20% are provided with a semantic type (the semantic classes follow and extend the UMLS semantic network).

2.1   String-to-String Edit Distance Calculus

Modern spelling checkers[6] are usually based on a variant of the Levenshtein-Damereau distance. Most misspellings can be generated from correct spellings by a

---

[4] Corpora for spelling correction are rare in French. The misspelled word database we collected should become publicly available as additional package of the FRIDA project:
http://www.fltr.ucl.ac.be/fltr/germ/etan/cecl/Cecl-projects/Frida/frida.htm.

[5] All these resources allow a correction time of less than 200 ms. It is enough at interactive runtime, there is still scope for optimization strategies as described in [8].

[6] Alternative approaches include n-gram distances and similarity keys, cf. [23].

few simple rules. Damerau [22] indicates that 80 percent of all spelling errors are the result of:

a. transposition of two adjacent letters: he*ap*titis (err1)
b. insertion of one letter: hep*p*atitis (err2)
c. deletion of one letter: hepattis (err3)
d. replacement of one letter by another one: hepat*o*tis (err4)

In the standard model, each of these operations cost 1, i.e. the distance between err1, err2, err3, err4 and the word *hepatitis* is 1, while the distance between *hepatitis* and *heppatotis* is 2 (one replacement + one insertion). But more accurate models, where each operation might have an associated cost, depending on the left adjacent letter have been developed [14]. The error model we developed includes such refinements. Thus, if the default replacement operation has a one unit cost, some more probable replacements (a frequent confusion is for example the letter set {ï, i}) will be weighted less expensively. The cost matrix was trained manually by using regression tests on the set A. Indeed, considering the size of the set A, maximization-expectation methods were not applicable here [15].

2.2 Contextual Filtering

After processing by the edit distance module, each candidate word comes out with a score. This score expresses the distance between the candidate and the misspelled word. The two next modules are applied sequentially in order to get a more optimal ranking of the candidates.

It is important to notice that if one word within the candidate set is not provided with a POS tag, then the following filters (POS and WS) are not applied. Similarly, the WS filter is not applied if one of the candidates is provided without WS tag. This caution is important in order not to select a priori the words listed in our lexicon vs. words appearing in the 90000 items list.

2.2.1 Part-of-Speech Filtering

The goal of this module is to modify the edit-distance scoring by combining the morpho-syntactic information. Let us consider a misspelled word in context together with a short list of likely candidates. List 1 provides the list as returned by the MS-Word 2000 English spell checker, while List 2 shows what would be expected if MS-Word would use the left adjacent context (Fig. 1):

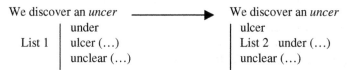

Fig. 1. Example of part-of-speech filtering

In this example, it is clear that list 2 provides a more accurate ranking than list 1 for the misspelled string *uncer*, if we consider the adjacent left context[7]: a determiner like *an* cannot be followed by a preposition like *under*.

The POS tagger attempts to attribute one part-of-speech (expressed by a tag) to every token. Thus, in the above example, and after a lexical access (Fig. 3) the tool provides the following choice (Fig. 2; the meaning of the POS tags is given first):

-prop: personal pronoun   -v[12]: verb first or second person
-d[s]: d[s] determiner singular   -nc[s]: common noun singular
-sp: preposition   -a: adjective

We   discover   an   *uncer*   ⟶   ulcer
prop v[12]   d[s] nc[s]

Fig. 2. POS disambiguation (after POS tagging)

We   discover   an   *uncer*
prop v[12]   d[s] sp   (under)
                         nc[s] (ulcer)
                         a   (unclear)

Fig. 3. POS lexical ambiguity (before POS tagging)

In the above figures, the candidate(s) with the tag *nc[s]* are factorized to get ranked closer to the misspelled word.

2.2.2 Word-Sense Filtering

There are traditionally two ways to process the semantic filtering: implicitly, for example when working with word language models, indeed, in such case both syntax and semantics are handled by word transition, or explicitly by using syntactic and semantic representation levels.

In the following example, the part-of-speech does not provides any discrimination rule between the candidates, as both have the same part-of-speech (*nc[s]*). However, the semantic left adjacent context can operate as a discriminator, indeed *until the* is to be followed by some temporal concept (*temp*), like for example *summer*, rather than by some human person (*pers*), which is the tag of *swimmer* (Fig. 4; the meaning odf the WS tags is given first):

-rtemp: temporal relations (UMLS T136)
-temp: temporal concept (UMLS T079)
-pers: human, person (UMLS T016)

---

[7] In this experiment, we rely exclusively on the left context has it is the only available context when spelling checker are working in user interaction. If the target application was batch then a wider context could have been used.

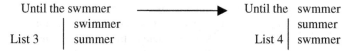

Until the swmmer			Until the	swmmer
	swimmer			summer
List 3	summer		List 4	swmmer

Fig. 4. Example of word-sense filtering[8]

When processing the above sentence, and after lexical access (Fig. 6), the word-sense tagger returns the following output (Fig. 5):

Until the   swmmer ➡ summer
.rtemp   temp

Fig. 5. WS disambiguation (after WS tagging)

Until the swmmer
rtemp   temp (summer)
     pers(swimmer)

Fig. 6. WS disambiguation (before WS tagging)

3 Results and Conclusion

Table 1 provides the result of the evaluation on the set B. The string-to-string edit distance is taken as a baseline for assessing the improvement brought by the POS filtering and the WS filtering (after POS filtering).

Five types of measures are provided: best candidate, when the well-formed token is provided at the top of the returned list; top-3, when the well-formed token appear within the three first items of the returned list; top-5, top-7 for respectively the five and seven first items; and top-20 when considering all the list of candidates.

Table 1. Results of the evaluation

	String-edit (%)	+ POS filtering (%)	+ WS filtering (%)
Best candidate	89.5	95.7	96.3
Top-3	96.9	98.1	98.1
Top-5	97.9	98.8	98.8
Top-7	98.1	98.8	98.8
Top-20[9]	98.8	98.8	98.8

In comparison to the string-edit output, results are quite encouraging for the POS filtering as the improvement considering the best candidate and the top-3 score is

---

[8] When applying WS tagging, stop words (determiner, auxiliary…) are removed, therefore the phrase *until the swmmer*, lexically tagged *rtemp def temp/pers* is processed as *rtemp temp/pers*, where the determiner *the* (tagged *def* as definite determiner) is removed.

[9] The best score is 98.8%, as 2 items of the 162 records in the set B were not listed in the 90000 words list: one is the concatenation of two words (*protectionplastique*), which are listed, while the other one was simply missing.

about 5-6%. Of course, filtering improvements (by improving the rules and the transition matrices) is still possible, as the rules were not designed to process huge ambiguity sets. This point constitutes an interesting challenge: thus, the remaining error rate for the best candidate score using the POS filter is largely caused by short misspellings: they contribute for 83% (5 misspellings) to the error rate (3.8%, i.e. 6 misspellings). For example, the misspelled word *raee* generates 16 candidates (with a given edit distance threshold): rasée, ratée, rayée, race, rade, rage, raie, rame, rare, rase, rate, ré, râle, rasé, rayé, ruée). Hopefully these short words account for a manageable fraction of the lexicon, therefore a possible improvement would be to develop special strategies for correcting short words: we could for example calculate a word language model that would include a set of examples tailored for these words. More generally, we should explore the use of a word-language model, which would bring a labor-cheap (but memory-consuming) way to improve the candidate selection.

On the opposite, the improvement provided by the WS module seems small (0.6% for a test set of 162 items) considering the best candidate score, and disappears at the level of the top-3 score. Many reasons can explain the bad results of the WS filtering. In a general way, WS disambiguation does not perform so well like POS disambiguation (about 96% vs. 98-99%, cf. [19] vs. [20]). But the probably major problem lies in the sparseness of the WS lexical resources compared to the POS lexical ones, indeed very often some of the candidate tokens where absent from the WS lexicon, so that the whole WS filtering was given up (as semantic resources are small for the task, it may have been worst to privilege tokens listed into the lexicon vs. tokens not occurring in the lexicon).

Similarly, the list of well-formed words could reach a better coverage, as about 2% of the set B are absent from this list.

Finally, all these results underline the lack of high coverage publicly available lexical resources (from fine grained semantic lexicons down to simple word frequency lists!) adapted to the medical domain (this statement is true for any European languages, except the English language, which is well-covered by the SPECIALIST lexicon).

References

1. Jurafsky D. and Martin J.H.: Speech and Language Processing, Prentice Hall. London.
2. Hersh W.R., Campbell E.M., Malveau S.E.: Assessing the feasibility of large-scale natural language processing in a corpus of ordinary medical records: a lexical analysis.. Proc AMIA Annu Fall Symp (United States), 1997, p580-4
3. Lilley L.L., Guancy R.: Sound-alike cephalosporins. How drugs with similar spellings and sounds can lead to serious errors. Am J Nurs (United States), Jun 1995, 95(6) p14
4. Lambert B.L.: Predicting look-alike and sound-alike medication errors. Am J Health Syst Pharm (United States), May 15 1997, 54(10) p1161-71
5. Golding A.R., Shabes Y.: Combining Trigram-based and Feature-based Methods for Context-Sensitive Spelling Correction. In Proc. of the 34th Annual Meeting of the ACL, Santa Cruz, (1996) p. 71-78.
6. Golding A.R., Roth D.: Applying Winnow to Context-Sensitive Spelling Correction. In Proc of ICML (1996): p 182-190.

7. Mangu L., and Brill E.: Automatic Rule Acquisition for Spelling Correction. In Proc. of ICML, (1997).
8. Peterson, JL.: Computer Programs for Detecting and Correcting Spelling Errors. Computer Practices, Communications of the ACM (1980), vol. 23, number 12.
9. Brill E. and Moore R.C.: An Improved Error Model for Noisy Channel Spelling Correction. Proc. of the 38th Annual Meeting of the ACL, Hong-Kong (2000) p. ?.
10. Mays E., Damereau F., Mercer R.L.: Context based spelling correction. Information Processing and Management, 27(5), (1991), p. 517-522.
11. Oflazer, K.: Error-tolerant Finite State Recognition with Applications to Morphological Analysis and Spelling Correction. Computational Linguistics (1996), 1-18. Association for Computational Linguistics Eds.
12. Baud R., Lovis C., Ruch P., Rassinoux A.-M.: A Toolset for Medicl Text Processing, in Medical Infobahn for Europe, Proc. of MIE'2000. A. Hasman, B. Blobel, J. Dudeck, R. Engelbrecht, G. Gell, H.-U. Prokosh (eds). IOS Press. (2000).
13. Courtin J., Dujardin D., Kowarski I., Genthial D., De Lima V.L.: Towards a complete detection/correction system. Proc. of the ICCICL, Penang, Malaysia. (1991), p. 158-173.
14. Church K.W., Gale W.A.: Probability scoring for spelling correction. In Stat. Comp. 1., (1991) p. 93-103.
15. Ristad E., and Yanilos P.: Learning String Edit Distance. Int. Conf. on Machine Learning, Morgan Kaufmann. (1997).
16. Rivest R.L.: Learning Decision Lists, in Machine Learning, 2, (1987) 229-246.
17. Yarowsky D.: Decision Lists for Lexical Ambiguity Resolution: Application to Accent Restoration in Spanish and French. In Proc. of ACL (1994), p. 88-95.
18. Ruch P., Baud R., Bouillon P., Rassinoux A.-M., Robert G.: Tagging medical text: a rule-based experiment, in Medical Infobahn for Europe, Proc. of MIE'2000. A. Hasman, B. Blobel, J. Dudeck, R. Engelbrecht, G. Gell, H.-U. Prokosh (eds). IOS Press. (2000).
19. Ruch P., Baud R., Bouillon P., Robert G.: Minimal Commitment and Full Lexical Disambiguation: Balancing Rules and Hidden Markov Models. In Proc. of CoNLL-2000 (ACL-SIGNLL). Lisbon. ACL (ed). (2000), p.111-115.
20. Ruch P., Baud R., Bouillon P., Rassinoux A.-M., Scherrer J.-R., MEDTAG: Tag-like Semantics for Medical Document Indexing. In Proc. of the AMIA'99 Annual Symposium. Washington. (1999).
21. Bouillon, P., Baud R., Robert G., Ruch P., Indexing by statistical tagging. In Proc. of the JADT'2000. Lausanne. (2000).
22. Damereau, F.J.: A technique for computer detection and correction of spelling errors. Commun. ACM, vol. 7, number 3. (1964)
23. Pollock J.J., Zamora A.: Automatic spelling correction in scientific and scholarly text. Computer Practices, Communications of the ACM (1984), vol. 27, number 4.

Semantic Interpretation of Medical Language – Quantitative Analysis and Qualitative Yield

Martin Romacker[1,2] and Udo Hahn[1]

[1] Text Knowledge Engineering Lab, CLIF Group, Freiburg University
[2] Department of Medical Informatics, Freiburg University Hospital
http://www.coling.uni-freiburg.de/

Abstract. We report on results from an empirical analysis of the semantic interpretation of medical free texts. Our approach to semantic interpretation is based on a lean collection of interpretation rules which are triggered by well-defined configurations in dependency graphs in order to compute a conceptual representation of the texts' contents. We evaluate the accuracy of semantic interpretation for three types of syntactic dependency patterns, viz. genitives, auxiliary and modal verb complexes, and prepositional phrases. Besides quantitive considerations, we focus on the heuristic guidance, as provided by patterns underlying the semantic interpretation of prepositional phrases, for monitoring the quality of the medical domain knowledge base.

1 Introduction

The automatic extraction of information from medical free texts can be considered as a rather restricted form of semantic interpretation, since only few, *a priori* selected knowledge templates have to be filled properly. This renders evaluation feasible, as the accuracy of interpretation can be measured by the degree of overlap between a human-supplied gold standard and the results achieved by the information extraction system under consideration [2]. Recent findings in the medical domain indicate that the performance of human experts and IE systems on such a task are on an equal par [4].

When it comes to the general case of the evaluation of the semantic interpretation performance of natural language systems, i.e., ones which lack the above-mentioned interpretation bias, the full range of understanding subtleties has to be accounted for, in principle at least. This creates a tremendous methodological problem, since it seems unlikely that a general consensus can be achieved what amounts to a canonical understanding of a document, even in technical or scientific domains.

Different suggestions have already been made how an appropriate evaluation framework for such a scenario should look like. Friedman & Hripcsak [1] emphasize the need for objective criteria for such an evaluation. Zweigenbaum *et al.* [11] demonstrate how the performance for such a knowledge acquisition task can be assessed by comparing the results of knowledge extraction by domain experts to those produced by a knowledge acquisition system. Following

S. Quaglini, P. Barahona, and S. Andreassen (Eds.): AIME 2001, LNAI 2101, pp. 258–267, 2001.
© Springer-Verlag Berlin Heidelberg 2001

on that work, we here propose to focus on the evaluation of the semantic interpretation of characteristic patterns of syntactic structures (such as genitives, modal verbs or auxiliaries and prepositional phrases) in order to evaluate the understanding accuracy of a text knowledge acquisition system. We claim that syntactic structures act as a filter by which the enormous diversity of linguistic and conceptual data that occur in the process of text understanding can be kept manageable, while we still retain a large variety of interpretation phenomena. The quantitative results we achieve will then be complemented by considerations how ontological knowledge can be extracted from such natural language data, as given by co-occurrence patterns [6].

2   A Framework for Semantic Interpretation

In this section, we briefly introduce the framework of the text understanding system MEDSYNDIKATE [3] in which semantic interpretation is performed [8]. Syntactic structures are represented in terms of dependency graphs. In a dependency graph, nodes represent words only, which are connected by labeled and directed edges called dependency relations. These dominance relations within a dependency graph capture head-modifier relations. For example, in the dependency graph for Sentence (1) the syntactic head *"wird"* *("is")* governs one of its modifiers, *"Lamina propria"*, by means of the *subject* relation (cf. Figure 1).

(1)   *Die Lamina propria der Schleimhaut wird vermehrt von Lymphozyten infiltriert.*
       [The lamina propria of the mucosa is increasingly infiltrated by lymphocytes.]

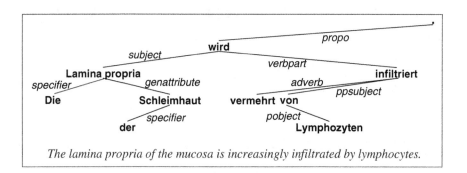

The lamina propria of the mucosa is increasingly infiltrated by lymphocytes.

Fig. 1. A Sample Dependency Graph (Sentence (1))

The word nodes of any dependency graph can be devided into two sets. Members of the first set are open-class content words, i.e., they have a concrete lexical meaning in the sense that they can be mapped to some corresponding entity in the world (for Sentence (1), we have *"Lamina propria"*, *"Schleimhaut"*

(*"mucosa"*), *"vermehrt"* (*"increasingly"*), *"Lymphozyten"* and *"infiltriert"* (*"infiltrated"*) in this category). Members of the second set are closed-class items which still contribute to the semantic interpretation of an utterance but their meaning is quite unspecific since they have no reasonable correlate in the given domain (e.g., *"Die/der"* (*"the"*), *"wird"* (*"is"*) and *"von"* (*"by"*)).

The semantic interpretation rests on well-defined configurational patterns within the dependency graph, so-called *semantically interpretable subgraphs* (cf. [8]). Such a subgraph is given by a connection of two content words via a number of edges without a third content word intervening on that path. Thus, two basic patterns can be distinguished. A *direct linkage* is encountered, if there is a single edge directly connecting two content words (e.g., *"Lamina propria"* – genattribute – *"Schleimhaut"*) — the path length is exactly one. When more than one connecting edge occurs between two content words, we speak of a *mediated linkage* (e.g., *"Lamina propria"* – subject – *"wird"* – verbpart – *"infiltriert"*). Note, e.g., that the subgraph made of *"Lamina propria"* and *"Lymphozyten"* does not form a minimal interpretable subgraph, since the (content word) node *"infiltriert"* intervenes on the connecting path (cf. Figure 1).

Whenever during the incremental analysis process a semantically interpretable subgraph is completed, a semantic interpretation process is triggered. It consists of a search for conceptual relations in the knowledge base between the conceptual correlates of the two content words in the minimal subgraph. The domain knowledge provided by the MEDSYNDIKATE system consists of an ontology which is expressed in terms of a KL-ONE-like knowledge representation system [10]. Restrictions which can be derived from dependency relations and the intervening lexical material within a semantically interpretable subgraph are integrated into the search to further constrain the search space for conceptual relations [8].

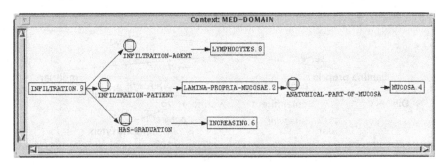

Fig. 2. Semantic Interpretation for the Dependency Graph of Sentence ((1))

The result of the semantic interpretation for Sentence (1) is depicted in Figure 2 in terms of graphical representation for conceptual structures. Sentence (1) contains four semantically interpretable subgraphs that are successively interpreted. For example, for the subgraph *"Lamina propria"* – genattribute – *'Schleimhaut"* containing LAMINA-PROPRIA-MUCOSAE.2 and MUCOSA.4 the relation ANATOMICAL-PART-OF-MUCOSA is computed. The subgraph *"Lamina propria"* – subject – *"wird"* – verbpart – *"infiltriert"* maps to INFILTRATION.9 INFILTRATION-PATIENT LAMINA-PROPRIA-MUCOSAE.2. In this subgraph semantic interpretation leads to a normalization of the passive construction at the conceptual level. As a final result, four conceptual relations between discourse entities corresponding to the semantic interpretation of the four semantically interpretable subgraphs have been computed.

3 Evaluation Framework

In this section, we describe the framework for the evaluation of our approach to semantic interpretation. Since there are two major variants of SYNDIKATE, one for medicine and one for information technology (henceforth IT), two domains were covered by the empirical study. Although the comparison of the semantic interpretation in the medical vs. IT domain reveals interesting results, we will here focus on medicine.

The text collection was extracted from the hospital information system of the University Hospital in Freiburg (Germany) [5]. All finding reports in histopathology from the first quarter of 1999 were initially included, altogether 4,973 documents. However, for the time being MEDSYDIKATE covers especially the subdomain of gastro-intestinal diseases. Thus, 752 texts out of these 4,973 were extracted semi-automatically in order to guarantee a sufficient coverage of domain knowledge.[1] From this selection, a random sample of 90 texts was taken and divided into two sets. 60 texts served as the training set which was used for parameter tuning of the system. The remaining 30 texts were then used to measure the performance of the MEDSYNDIKATE system with unseen data. Therefore, the state of the system was frozen prior to analyzing the test set.

In the empirical study proper, three basic configurations of minimal interpretable subgraphs were evaluated, viz. ones containing genitives, constructions including modal verbs or auxiliaries and, finally, prepositional phrases. For each instance of these configurations a semantic interpretation was automatically computed the result of which was judged for accuracy by two skilled raters.

Still, the way how a (gold) standard for semantic interpretation can be set up is an issue of hot debates. In fact, conceptually annotated text corpora do not exist at all, at least for the German language. At this level, the ontology we have developed eases judgements since it is based on a fine-grained relation hierarchy with clear sortal restrictions for role fillers. In anatomy, e.g., we use relations such as ANATOMICAL-PART-OF, which is itself a subrelation of PHYSICAL-PART-OF and PART-OF, and specialize it in order to account for specific PART-OF relationships. A very special relation such as ANATOMICAL-PART-OF-MUCOSA refers to a precise subset of entities to be related by the interpretation process. Therefore, relating BRAIN to MUCOSA by ANATOMICAL-PART-OF-MUCOSA obviously would be con-

---

[1] The domain ontologies of SYNDIKATE consists of 2,500 concepts and relations in an upper ontology that is complemented by 1,500 concept and relations in the IT domain and another 2,000 in the medical domain.

sidered as incorrect, whereas relating LAMINA-PROPRIA-MUCOSAE is definitely an appropriate interpretation (cf. Figure 2).

4   Quantitative Analysis of Semantic Interpretation

The following tables contain the assessment data for the quality of the semantic interpretation as obtained for the different configurations for both the training set and the test set. Besides providing data for recall and precision, the tables are divided into two assessment layers: *"without interpretation"* means that the system was not able to produce an interpretation because of specification gaps, i.e., at least one of the two content words in a minimal dependency graph under consideration was not specified. Note that even for the training set which was intended to generate optimal results we were unable to formulate reasonable and generally valid concept definitions for some of the content words we encountered (e.g., for fuzzy expressions of locations: *"In der Tiefe der Schleimhaut"* (*"In the depth of the mucosa"*)). The second group *"with interpretation"* is divided into four categories. The label *correct (non-ambiguous)* qualifies, if just a single and correct conceptual relation was computed by the semantic interpretation process. However, if the result was correct but yielded more than one conceptual relation, the label *correct (ambiguous)* was assigned. An interpretation was considered *incorrect* when a conceptual relation was inappropriate. Finally, *NIL* was used to indicate that an interpretation was performed (both concepts for the content words were specified) but no conceptual relation could be computed.

Table 1. Evaluation of the Semantic Interpretation of Genitives

	Training Set	Test Set
Recall	92%	93%
Precision	93%	93%
# occurrences ...	168	91
... **with interpretation**	158 (94%)	86 (95%)
[confidence intervals]	[89%-97%]	[90%-98%]
......correct (non-ambiguous)	125.5 (75%)	48.5 (53%)
......correct (ambiguous)	22 (13%)	33 (36%)
......incorrect	6.5	3.5
......NIL	4	1
... **without interpretation**	10 (6%)	5 (5%)
# Nominalizations ...	42	23
...with interpretation	41	23
......correct (non-ambiguous)	41	23
......correct (ambiguous)	0	0

Genitives. In the medical domain, as indicated by Table 1 the recall and precision values for the interpretation of genitives are very encouraging both for the training set (92% and 93%) and the test set (93% and 93%), respectively.[2] However, since genitives, in general, provide no additional constraints how the conceptual correlates of the two content words involved can be related (for details, cf. [8]), the number of ambiguous interpretations amounts to 13% and 36%, respectively.

For genitives, nominalizations play an interesting role. Consider the phrase *"an inflammation of the stomach"*. An INFLAMMATION is a PROCESS that acts on some anatomical structure. The corresponding thematic role derived by the interpretation process is INFLAMMATION-PATIENT. The phrase *"a surface gastritis of the antrum"* is interpreted in the same spirit considering the ANTRUM as the anatomical structure on which the GASTRITIS acts. However, at the lexical level *"Gastritis"* is definitely not a nominalization, whereas at the ontological level it is a subconcept of PROCESS. This determines the interpretation as a kind of *genitivus objectivus* even if a derivation from a verb cannot be determined directly. This way, we gather indications from the source data to maintain and adapt the structure of the ontology in the light of empirical evidence.

Table 2. Evaluation of the Semantic Interpretation of Modal Verbs and Auxiliaries

	Training Set	Test Set
Recall	94%	80%
Precision	98%	84%
# occurrences ...	131	55
... **with interpretation**	125 (95%)	52 (95%)
[confidence intervals]	[92%-99%]	[84%-99%]
...... correct (non-ambiguous)	122 (93%)	43,5 (79%)
...... correct (ambiguous)	1	0
...... incorrect	0	0,5
...... NIL	2	8 (15%)
... **without interpretation**	6 (5%)	3 (5%)

Auxiliaries and Modals. Table 2 contains the results for minimal interpretable graphs with modal verbs or auxiliaries, a mediated linkage structure. Since modal verbs and auxiliaries can be combined in various ways, subgraphs of this type may consist of up to five nodes in German. In our data, however, just 2 out of 186 occurrences contained four nodes, the rest was composed of three nodes. A semantic interpretation of modal/auxiliary verb complexes relates a content-bearing verb with the conceptual correlate of the syntactic subject. In case of a passive construction the direct-object-to-subject normalization has to be carried out.

Recall and precision for the training set are very good (94% and 98%, respectively) and, therefore, indicate that semantic interpretation can cope with almost all occurrences given an optimal degree of specification. The values for recall and precision dropped to 80% and 84%, respectively, in the test set. The increase of

---

[2] Confidence intervals for .95 probability are given in square brackets.

NIL results reveals that the granularity of the underlying domain model is insufficient as far as conceptual relations are concerned. Although the corresponding concepts are modelled, no conceptual relation between them exists.

Table 3. Evaluation of the Semantic Interpretation of Prepositional Phrases

	Training Set	Test Set
Recall	85%	85%
Precision	79%	81%
# occurrences ...	562	278
...**with interpretation**	548 (98%)	253 (91%)
[confidence intervals]	[96%-99%]	[86%-93%]
......correct (non-ambiguous)	401,5 (71%)	167 (60%)
......correct (ambiguous)	32,5 (6%)	37,5 (13%)
......incorrect	43 (8%)	30,5 (11%)
......NIL	71 (13%)	18 (6%)
...**without interpretation**	14 (2%)	25 (9%)
interrater reliability (n = 2)	$\kappa = 0,591$	$\kappa = 0,774$
significance	$z = 5,72$	$z = 6,41$

Prepositional phrases (henceforth, PPs) are crucial for the semantic interpretation of a text, since they introduce a wide variety of conceptual relations, such as spatial, temporal, causal, or instrumental ones. The importance of PPs is reflected by their relative frequency. In the training set and the test set, we encountered 1,108 prepositions, which is a little bit less than 10% of the words in both sets (approximately 11,300).[3] Provided also that the preposition's syntactic head and its modifier participate in the interpretation, at the phrase level, more than 25% of the texts' contents is encoded by PPs (certainly, this data also reflects a considerable degree of genre dependency).

At the level of semantic interpretation, the values for recall and precision are almost the same for the training set and the test set. Recall reached 85% for both the training set and the test set, whereas precision amounted to 79% for the training set and 81% for the test set.[4] The lower numbers for recall and precision in the trainings set clearly indicate that even under optimal conditions there are PPs that are not interpretable with our approach to semantic interpretation. However, getting almost the same performance for the test set shows a stable level of semantic interpretation of PPs.[5]

---

[3] Only 940 of these 1,108 were included in the empirical analysis, since 168 did not form a minimal subgraph. Phrases like *"zum Teil"* (*"partly"*) map to a single meaning — as evidenced by the English translation correlate — and were therefore excluded.

[4] We are only able to provide a κ-statistics [9] for PPs, since for both genitives and modal verbs or auxiliaries the differences in the judgments of the two raters were too small. This means the expectation value was almost 1. For PPs the significance threshold of $z = 2.32$ for $\alpha = 0.01$ has been surpassed.

[5] The corresponding values for the IT domain are not as good as for the medical domain. For genitives, recall was 75% and 53% and precision was determined with

5 Qualitative Yield: Guiding Ontology Maintenance

We complemented the quantitative assessment of the results of semantic interpretation with qualitative considerations related to the structural organization of the underlying ontology. It turned out that certain interpretation patterns hint at hidden commonalities at the ontology layer.

In order to illustrate the effects from the qualitative analysis, we focus on one of the most frequent prepositions in our sample. About thirty different prepositions are present in the 940 PPs. Just twenty-one of them, however, occur more than ten times. On the other hand, the three German prepositions *"mit"*, *"in"* and *"von"* are responsible for 599 PPs. It is not surprising that these three prepositions are highly ambiguous in the way they have to be interpreted semantically. In the following, we will just consider the types of PPs containing *"von"* in the training set, which sum up to 103 occurrences.

Altogether 48 of 103 *"von"*–PPs showed the pattern of Sentence (2), where some type information (*"antrum type"*) is provided for an anatomical structure *"gastric mucosa"*. So nearly half of the sample fits this pattern.

(2)   *Erfaßt wurde eine Magenschleimhaut vom Antrumtyp. (48/103)*
       [A gastric mucosa of the antrum type was seized.]

Another 30 of the 103 occurrences linked a verb nominalization with its *subject* or *direct-object*, if transformed to a denominalized verb phrase (cf. Sentence (3)). *"Nachweis von Helicobacter-pylori"* (*"evidence for helicobacter-pyolori"*), where *"Helicobacter-pylori"* is interpreted in terms of the PATIENT of the underlying conceptual representation.

(3)   *Der Befund entspricht einer Gastritis mit Nachweis von Helicobacter-*
       pylori. (30/103)
       [The findings correspond to a gastritis with evidence for helicobacter-
       pylori.]

In German, the preposition *"von"* can also introduce an AGENT in a passive sentence as illustrated by Sentence (4). Therefore, the participle perfect passive *"gesäumt"* (*"bordered"*) is modified by the *"von"*–PP *"von Epithelien"* (*"by epithelia"*), a pattern that is mapped to an AGENT reading at the conceptual level.

(4)   *Die Foveolen sind von Epithelien gesäumt. (17/103)*
       [The foveolae are bodered by epithelia.]

The next pattern in Sentence (5) with 4 occurrences refers to a SOURCE reading: *"ein vom Magen ausgehender Tumor"* (*"a tumor emanating from the stomach"*). The metastasis originates from a primary tumor in the stomach.

97% and 83% in the training set and the test set, respectively. The values for modals and auxiliaries are: recall 85%/ 85% and precision 96%/ 98%, while those for PPs are: recall 70%/ 64% and precision 77%/ 66%. A reasonable argument why we achieved better results in the medical domain than in the IT world might be that in the medical texts a considerably lower degree of linguistic variation is encountered.

(5)   *Es handelt sich um einen vom Magen ausgehenden Tumor. (4/103)*
        [It is a matter of a tumor emanating from the stomach.]

Another example for introducing prepositional objects is illustrated by Sentence
(6) with 3 occurrences. The prepositional phrase *"von der Probe"* (*"of the sample"*) introduces an object that is affected by the action of producing something
(*"anfertigen"*).

(6)   *Von der Probe werden weitere Schnittstufen angefertigt. (3/103)*
        [Further "cut levels" will be made of the sample.]

Finally, in the phrase *"Tumor von 45 bis 55 cm"* (*"Tumor from 45 to 55 cm"*)
– occurring just once – information about the spatial location of a tumor in
the gastro-intestinal tract is given. However, such a dense utterance can hardly
be interpreted, unless in-depth knowledge is available such that, by convention,
there exists a longitudinal orientation of the gastro-intestinal tract. Obviously,
this kind of reasoning goes far beyond the semantic interpretation capabilities
we suggest in this paper.

As a result of investigating the regularities how concepts are combined by
different types of natural language expressions, we obtain important cues how
conceptual relations might be treated at the ontological level. We certainly do
not give up the idea that the core of a medical ontology be language-independent
(following Rector's idea of a general-purpose terminology server [7]). However,
the frequent combination of concepts in typical interpretation patterns gives us
hints how systematic natural language usage patterns might be reflected at the
level of ontology design. For example, in our ontology GASTRITIS is subsumed by
INFLAMMATION which is a BODY-PHENOMENON-PROCESS which is a PROCESS.
The concept PROCESS is a top-level node of the ontology for *verb* concepts and
provides thematic roles such as PATIENT. This kind of modeling decision might
not have been taken by *prima facie* inspection of plain language data.

6   Conclusions

In this paper, we presented an evaluation for an approach to the semantic interpretation of dependency structures. In order to assess the quality of our approach
three types of phrases were analyzed in depth, viz. genitives, constructions involving modal verbs or auxiliaries, as well as prepositional phrases. The data
reveals that the interpretation of genitives exhibits an real satisfactory level of
accuracy (93% recall and precision), while the remaining two patterns vary on
the order of 80% to 85% in terms of recall and precision — a result that obviously
reflects the text genre we use (medical finding reports).

Besides assessing the accuracy of semantic interpretation in metrical terms,
we also examined co-occurrences of conceptual patterns within a qualitative
analysis of semantic interpretation data. It seems that ontological regularities
are mirrored in actual language use. These observations can then be used, in
turn, to refine and, hopefully, improve medical ontologies without giving up

the basic claim that the core of any ontology should abstract from linguistic phenomena.

Acknowledgements. We would like to thank our colleagues in the CLIF group and the Department of Medical Informatics for fruitful discussions. M. Romacker was supported by a grant from DFG (Ha 2097/5-2).

References

1. C. Friedman and G. Hripcsak. Evaluating natural language processors in the clinical domain. *Methods of Information in Medicine*, 37(4/5):334–344, 1998.
2. C. Friedman, G. Hripcsak, W. DuMouchel, S. Johnson, and P. Clayton. Natural language processing in an operational clinical information system. *Natural Language Engineering*, 1(1):83–108, 1995.
3. U. Hahn, M. Romacker, and St. Schulz. MEDSYNDIKATE: Design considerations for an ontology-based medical text understanding system. In J. M. Overhage, editor, *AMIA 2000 – Proc. of the Annual Symposium of the American Medical Informatics Association*, pages 330–334. Los Angeles, CA, November 4-8, 2000. Philadelphia, PA: Hanley & Belfus, 2000.
4. G. Hripcsak, C. Friedman, P. Alderson, W. DuMouchel, S. Johnson, and PD. Clayton. Unlocking clinical data from narrative reports: a study of natural language processing. *Annals of Internal Medicine*, 122(9):681–688, 1995.
5. R. Klar, A. Zaiß, A. Timmermann, and U. Schrader. The information system of the Freiburger University Hospital. In K. Adlassnig et al., editor, *MIE'91 – Proceedings of the Medical Informatics Europe 1991*, pages 46–50. Berlin: Springer, 1991.
6. A. Nazarenko, P. Zweigenbaum, J. Bouaud, and B. Habert. Corpus-based identification and refinement of semantic classes. In R. Masys, editor, *AMIA'97 – Proc. of the 1997 AMIA Annual Fall Symposium (formerly SCAMC)*, pages 585–589. Philadelphia, PA: Hanley & Belfus, 1997.
7. A. Rector, D. Solomon, W. Nowlan, and T. Rush. A terminology server for medical language and medical information systems. *Methods of Information in Medicine*, 34(2):147–157, 1995.
8. M. Romacker, St. Schulz, and U. Hahn. Small *is* beautiful: Compact semantics for medical language processing. In W. Horn, Y. Shahar, G. Lindberg, S. Andreassen, and J. Wyatt, editors, *AIMDM'99 – Proc. of the Joint European Conference on Artificial Intelligence in Medicine and Medical Decision Making*, pages 400–410. Berlin: Springer, 1999.
9. S. Siegel and J. Castellan. *Nonparametric statistics for the behavioral sciences.* New York: McGraw-Hill, 2 edition, 1988.
10. W. Woods and J. Schmolze. The KL-ONE family. *Computers & Mathematics with Applications*, 23(2/5):133–177, 1992.
11. P. Zweigenbaum, J. Bouaud, B. Bachimont, J. Charlet, and J.-F. Boisvieux. Evaluating a normalized conceptual representation produced from natural language patient discharge summaries. In R. Masys, editor, *AMIA'97 – Proc. of the 1997 AMIA Annual Fall Symposium (formerly SCAMC)*, pages 590–594. Philadelphia, PA: Hanley & Belfus, 1997.

Medical Knowledge Acquisition from the Electronic Encyclopedia of China[1]

Cungen Cao

Intelligent Information Processing Laboratory, Institute of Computing Technology
Chinese Academy of Sciences, Beijing 100080, China

Abstract. The Encyclopedia of China contains considerably complete medical knowledge in unrestricted text. We have been developing a new method for extracting medical knowledge from the Electronic Encyclopedia of China. The method consists of two major parts: a high-level conceptual description language for use by knowledge engineers to formalize the text and a knowledge compiler for compiling the formalized text to a conceptual model.

1 Introduction

Knowledge acquisition from text is one of the current research areas [e.g. 1-9]. The challenge of extracting medical knowledge from text is that the texts are generally unrestricted and unstructured. In the literature on knowledge acquisition from text, two methodologies can, more or less, be identified. The first methodology relies on general-purpose algorithms to extract concepts and their relations from texts [3, 4, 5, 6, 7, 8]. As reported, this methodology can extract a considerable amount of knowledge from texts. However, because of the extreme complexity in a natural language, text knowledge acquisition may not be completely automated.

The second methodology is moderate in the sense that the process of text knowledge acquisition is aided by or interacted with knowledge engineers, or works with semantically tagged texts [1, 2, 8]. In this paper, we present a method of extracting medical concepts and their relations from the medicine volume of the Electronic Encyclopedia of China. The method falls into the second category of methods.

Our method consists of two major parts: a high-level conceptual language (or HLCL) for use by knowledge engineers to formalize medical text knowledge, and a HLCL compiler for compiling a HLCL text into knowledge code (IO-model). In addition, the compiler also locates common concepts and their relations in separate IO-models in order to connect the IO-models into larger ones through the common concepts. This connecting of IO-models is very important, because descriptions of a concept are usually scattered in different paragraphs and chapters. Since the model connection is automated, our text knowledge acquisition method is *superior* to any manual knowledge acquisition method from text.

---

[1] This work is supported by a grant from the Chinese Academy of Sciences (#2000-4010), and a grant from the Foundation of Chinese Natural Science (#20010010-A).

S. Quaglini, P. Barahona, and S. Andreassen (Eds.): AIME 2001, LNAI 2101, pp. 268–271, 2001.

2 The High-Level Conceptual Language

A HLCL text consists of a sequence of context-free statements, separated by a *semantically close* delimiter (i.e. ".##"). Here, the context-freeness of HLCL statements is actually a requirement to knowledge engineers in using HLCL to formalize texts: They must replace ambiguous terms with proper concepts. This is generally not difficult for knowledge engineers, but is very difficult (if not impossible) for automatic language understanding systems.

A HLCL statement is simple or compound. A *simple* statement is of the form <subject> <relation> [<object>], where <subject> consists of one or more concepts, <relation> is composed of one or more verbs, and <object> (if any) consists of one or more concepts. When using HLCL to formalize text assertions, we put one or more extra white spaces before <relation> and after <relation> to segment it from <subject> and <object>.

In the HLCL, concepts are classified into *atomic concepts, and-concepts, or-concepts*, and *and/or-concepts*. Atomic concepts represent inseparable and independent meanings in a domain of discourse. An and-concept consists of a number of atomic concepts, each of which is delimited by the constructor **and**. Or-concepts are a disjunction of a number of atomic concepts and and-concepts, delimited by the constructor **or**. For example, "diabetes, **or** Type I diabetes, **and** Type II diabetes" is an or-concept with one atomic concept (i.e. "diabetes"), and one and-concept (i.e. "Type I diabetes, **and** Type II diabetes").

In HLCL, we use the construct '<attribute> **of** <concept>' to indicate that <attribute> is an attribute of <concept>. For example, in "the former name **of** Type I diabetes", "the former name" is an attribute of the concept "Type I diabetes".

HLCL has some special conceptual relations induced from a considerable portion of the *entire* Electronic Encyclopedia of China, and we identified 27 categories of special conceptual relations, such as **be formally defined as, be formerly called, be classified into, be part of, no cases of, most cases of, imply**, and **to cause**.

A compound HLCL statement consists of simple HLCL statements, joined by a number of constructors, e.g. "**Because** <HLCL statement>, <HLCL statement>" and "**If** <HLCL statement>, <HLCL statement>".

For illustration, let us look at the following unstructured text:

Diabetes is classified into two types. In Type I, or insulin-dependent diabetes mellitus (IDDM), formerly called juvenile-onset diabetes, the onset usually occurs before or around puberty. In Type II, or non-insulin-dependent diabetes mellitus (NIDDM), formerly called adult-onset diabetes, the onset usually occurs after the age of 40.

This unstructured text is formalized in HLCL as follows:

Diabetes **is classified into** Type I diabetes, **and** Type II diabetes.## The formal name **of** Type I diabetes **is** insulin-dependent diabetes mellitus.## The acronym **of** insulin-dependent diabetes mellitus **is** IDDM.## Type I diabetes **is formerly called** juvenile-onset diabetes.## The onset **of** Type I diabetes **is usually before or around** puberty. The formal name **of** Type II diabetes **is** non-insulin-dependent diabetes mellitus.## The acronym **of** insulin-dependent diabetes mellitus **is** NIDDM. ## Type II diabetes **is formerly called** adult-onset diabetes.## The onset **of** Type II diabetes **is usually after** the age **of** 40.##

3 The HLCL Knowledge Compiler

The HLCL compiler first parses the formalized medical text and, if no grammatical error is found, generates the knowledge code from the text.

The knowledge code language is based on the notion of *IO-model*, a special directed hyper-graph. These graphs facilitate the retrieval of concepts, attributes and relations in IO-model connection.

In an IO-model, each node represents a concept, attribute or relation, and has an IO-queue to represent the connections between concepts/attributes and relations. The content of an IO-queue of a node is of the form (<source >, <target >, <node role>), where <node rule> indicates the role of the node in the context (<source >, <target >, <node role>), which assumes one of *concept, attribute*, and *relation* as value. The notion of node role is important, and it distinguishes concepts from attributes – in some assertions, concepts are attributes, but in some others attributes are concepts.

As illustration, the left part of Fig.1 shows two IO-models for the two statements "Type I diabetes **is formerly called** juvenile-onset diabetes" and "Type I diabetes **is formerly called** juvenile-onset diabetes", respectively. Nodes for **and, or, and/or,** and **of** are labeled with M*x*, and other nodes are labeled with N*x*. N*x*.io (M*x*.io) indicates the content(s) of the IO-queue of N*x* (M*x*).

```
{
    M01=and
    N02=diabetes
    N03=is classified into
    N04=Type I diabetes                          {
    N05=Type II diabetes                             M01=and
                                                     N02=diabetes
    N02.io=* N03 concept                             N03=is classified into
    N03.io=N02 M01 relation                          N04=Type I diabetes
    M01.io=N03 N04 * relation:N03 N05 relation       N05=Type II diabetes
    N04.io=M01 * concept                             N06=is formerly called
    N05.io=M02 *concept                              N07=juvenile-onset diabetes
}
{                                                    N02.io=* N03 concept
                                                     N03.io=N02 M01 relation
    N01=type I diabtes                               M01.io=N03 N04 * relation:N03 N05 relation
    N02=is former called                             N04.io=M01 * concept:* N06 concept
    N03=juvenile-onset diabetes                      N05.io=M02 * concept
                                                     N06.io=N04 N07 concept
    N01.io=* N02 concept                             N07.io=N06 * concept
    N02.io=N01 N03 relation                      }
    N03.io=N02 * concept
}
```

connect

Fig. 1. Connecting two IO-models

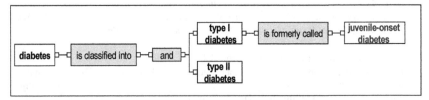

Fig. 2. Graphical View of the Connected IO-model

To connect the second IO-model with the first one, the compiler retrieves the first IO-model to locate the concepts "Type I diabetes" and "juvenile-onset diabetes". The retrieval is successful, because the concept "Type I diabetes" is found in the first IO-model. Then, the compiler connects the two models through the common concept (i.e. Type I diabetes). The connected IO-model is depicted in Fig. 2.

4 Conclusion

We believe that some sort of human aid or intervention is necessary for knowledge acquisition from unrestricted and unstructured texts. In our work, we designed a high-level conceptual language (HLCL) for use by knowledge engineers to formalize medical texts from the Electronic Encyclopedia of China. HLCL statements are generally natural and readable, making the proofreading and error-checking of HLCL texts considerably easy.

We have implemented a HLCL parser in Microsoft VJ 6.0. The compiler parses and analyzes HLCL texts into IO-models. It also connects different IO-models to generate bigger, more complete IO-models. So far, we have extracted more than 150,000 concepts from the Electronic Encyclopedia of China.

References

1. Bowden, P.R., Halstead, P., Rose, T.G.: Extracting Conceptual Knowledge from Text Using Explicit Relation Markers. In: Shadbolt, N., Ohara, K, Schreiber, G. (eds.): Advances in Knowledge Acquisition. Lecture Notes In Artificial Intelligence, Vol. 1076. Springer-Verlag, Berlin Heidelberg New York (1996) 147-162.
2. Delisle, S., Barker, K., Copek, T., Szpakowicz, S.: Interactive Semantic Analysis of Technical Texts. Int. J.Comp. Intell., 12 (1996), 273-306.
3. Hahn, U., Romacker, M.: Content Management in the SYNDIKATE System - How Technical Documents Are Automatically Transformed to Text Knowledge Bases. IEEE Transactions on Data & Knowledge Engineering 35 (2000) 137-159.
4. Hearst, M.A.: Untangling Text Data Mining. In: Proceedings of the 37th Annual Meeting of the Association for Computational Linguistics (invited paper).
5. Hull, R., Gomez, F.: Automatic Acquisition of Biographic Knowledge from Encyclopedic Texts. Int. J. Exp. Sys. with Appl. 16 (1999) 261-270.
6. Kazawa, K. Fujimoto, K., Matsuzawa, K.: Attribute Dependency Acquisition from Formatted Text. In: Proceedings of the 3rd International Conference on Knowledge-Based Intelligent Information Engineering Systems (1999) 464-468.
7. Plant, R.T.: Techniques for Knowledge Acquisition from Text. Int. J. Comp. Info. Sys. 35 (1994) 64-70.
8. Lu, R., Cao, C.: Towards Knowledge Acquisition from Domain Books. In: Wielinga, B, Gaines, B., Schreiber, G., Vansomeren, M. (eds.): Current Trends in Knowledge Acquisition. Amsterdam: IOS Press (1990), 289-301.
9. Sato, H., Fujimoto, K.: A New Approach to Semantic Word-matching for Knowledge Acquisition from Text Containing Daily-used Words. In Mohammadian, M. (ed.): Advances in Intelligent Systems: Theory and Applications. Frontiers in Artificial Intelligence and Applications, Vol. 59 (2000), 135-140.

Quantitative and Qualitative Approaches to Reasoning under Uncertainty in Medical Decision Making

John Fox, David Glasspool, and Jonathan Bury

Imperial Cancer Research Fund Labs
Lincoln's Inn Fields
London WC2A 3PX
United Kingdom
jf@acl.icnet.uk; dg@acl.icnet.uk; jb@acl.icnet.uk

Abstract. Medical decision making frequently requires the effective management and communication of uncertainty and risk. However a tension exists between classical probability theory, which is precise and rigorous but which people find non-intuitive and difficult to use, and qualitative approaches which are *ad hoc* but can be more versatile and easily comprehensible. In this paper we review a range of approaches to uncertainty management, then describe a logical approach, argumentation, which subsumes qualitative as well as quantitative representations and has a clear formal semantics. The approach is illustrated and evaluated in five decision support applications.

1 Introduction

Representing and managing uncertainty is central to understanding and supporting much clinical decision-making and is extensively studied in AI, computer science and psychology. Implementing effective decision models for practical clinical applications presents a dilemma. On the one hand, informal and qualitative representations of uncertainty may be natural for people to understand but they often lack formal rigour. On the other hand formal approaches based on probability theory are precise but can be awkward and non-intuitive to use. While in many cases probability theory is an ideal for optimal decision-making it is often impractical.

In this paper we review a range of approaches to uncertainty representation, then describe a logical approach, argumentation, which can subsume both qualitative and quantitative approaches within the same formal framework. We believe that this may enable improvements in both the scope and comprehensibility of decision support systems and illustrate the approach with five decision support applications developed by our group.

2 Decision Theory and Decision Support

It is generally accepted that human reasoning and decision-making can exhibit various shortcomings when compared with accepted prescriptive theories derived from mathematical logic and statistical decision-making, and there are systematic patterns of distortion and error in people's use of uncertain information [1,2,3,4]. In the 1970s and 1980s cognitive scientists generally came to the view that these characteristic failures come about because people revise their beliefs by processes that bear little resemblance to formal mathematical calculation. Kahneman and Tversky developed a

S. Quaglini, P. Barahona, and S. Andreassen (Eds.): AIME 2001, LNAI 2101, pp. 272–282, 2001.

celebrated account of human decision-making and its weaknesses in terms of what they called heuristics and biases [5]. They argued that people judge things to be highly likely when, for example, they come *easily to mind* or are *typical* of a class rather than by means of a proper calculation of the relative probabilities. Such heuristic methods are often reasonable approximations for practical decision making but they can also lead to systematic errors.

If people demonstrate imperfect reasoning or decision-making then it would presumably be desirable to support them with techniques that avoid errors and comply with rational rules. *Mathematical logic* (notably "classical" propositional logic and the predicate calculus) is traditionally taken as the gold standard for logical reasoning and deduction, while *expected utility theory* (EUT) plays the equivalent role for decision-making. A standard view on the "correct" way to take decisions is summarised by Lindley as follows:

> "... there is essentially only one way to reach a decision sensibly. First, the uncertainties present in the situation must be quantified in terms of values called probabilities. Second, the consequences of the courses of actions must be similarly described in terms of utilities. Third, that decision must be taken which is expected on the basis of the calculated probabilities to give the greatest utility. The force of 'must' used in three places there is simply that any deviation from the precepts is liable to lead the decision maker in procedures which are demonstrably absurd" [6], p.vii.

However, many people think that this overstates the value of mathematical methods and understates the capabilities of human decision makers. There are a number of problems with EUT as a practical method for decision making, and there are indications that, far from being "irrational", human decision processes depart from EUT because they are optimised to make various tradeoffs to address these problems in practical situations.

An expected-utility decision procedure requires that we know, or can estimate reasonably accurately, all the required probability and utility parameters. This is frequently difficult in real-world situations since a decision may still be urgently required even if precise quantitative data are not available. Even when it is possible to establish the necessary parameters, the cost of obtaining good estimates may outweigh the expected benefits. Furthermore, in many situations a decision is needed before the decision options, or the relevant information sources, are fully known. The complete set of options may only emerge as the decision making process evolves. The potential value of mathematical decision theory is frequently limited by the lack of objective quantitative data on which to base the calculations, the limited range of functions that it can be used to support, and the problem that the underlying numerical representation of the decision is very different from the intuitive understanding of human decision makers.

Human decision-making may also not be as "absurd" as the normative theories appear to suggest. One school of thought argues that many apparent biases and shortcomings are actually artefacts of the highly artificial situations that researchers create in order to study reasoning and judgement in controlled laboratory conditions. When we look at real-world decision-making we see that human reasoning and decision-making is more impressive than the research implies.

Shanteau [7] studied *expert* decision-making, "investigating factors that lead to competence in experts, as opposed to the usual emphasis on incompetence". He identified a number of important positive characteristics of expert decision-makers: First, they know what is relevant to specific decisions, what to attend to in a busy environment, and they know when to make exceptions to general rules[1]. Secondly, experts know a lot about what they know, and can make decisions about their own decision processes: they know which decisions to make and when, and which to skip, for example. They often have good communication skills and the ability to articulate their decisions and how they arrived at them. They can adapt to changing task conditions, and are frequently able to find novel solutions to problems. Classical deduction and probabilistic reasoning do not deal with these meta-cognitive skills.

It has also been strongly argued that people are well adapted for making decisions under adverse conditions: time pressure, lack of detailed information and knowledge etc. Gigerenzer, for instance, has suggested that people make decisions in a "fast and frugal" way, which is to say human cognition is rational in the sense that it is optimised for speed at the cost of occasional and usually inconsequential errors [4].

2.1   Tradeoffs in Effective Decision-Making

The strong view expressed by Lindley and others is that the only rational or "coherent" way to reason with uncertainty is to require that we comply with certain mathematical axioms - the axioms of EUT. In practice compliance with these axioms is often difficult because there is insufficient data to permit a valid calculation of the expected utility of the decision options, or a valid calculation may require too much time. An alternative perspective is that human decision-making is rational in that it incorporates practical tradeoffs that, for example, trade a lower cost (e.g. errors in decision-making) against a higher one (e.g. the amount of input data required or the time taken to calculate expected utility).

Tradeoffs of this kind not only simplify decision-making but in practice may entail only modest costs in the accuracy or effectiveness of decision-making. Consequently the claim that we should not model decision-support systems on human cognitive processes is less compelling than it may at first appear.

This possibility has been studied extensively in the field of medical decision-making.

In the prediction of sudden infant death, for example, Carpenter et al. [8] attempted to predict death from a simple linear combination of eight variables. They found that weights can be varied across a broad range without decreasing predictive accuracy.

In diagnosing patients suffering from dyspepsia, Fox et al. [9] found that giving all pieces of evidence equal weights produced the same accuracy as a more precise statistical method (and also much the same pattern of errors). In another study [10] we developed a system for the interpretation of blood data in leukaemia diagnosis, using the EMYCIN expert system shell. EMYCIN provided facilities to attach numerical "certainty factors" to inference rules. Initially a system was developed

---

[1]   "Good surgeons, the saying goes, know how to operate, better surgeons know when to operate and the best surgeons know when not to operate. That's true for all of medicine" Richard Smith, Editor of the *British Medical Journal*.

using the full range of available values (-1 to +1). These values were then replaced with just two: if the rule made a purely categorical inference the certainty factor was set to be 1.0 while if there was any uncertainty associated with the rule the certainty factor was set to 0.5. The effect was to *increase* diagnostic accuracy by 5%!

In a study of whether or not to admit patients with suspected heart attacks to hospital by O'Neil and Glowinski [11] no advantage was found of a precise decision procedure over simply "adding up the pros and cons". A similar comparison by Pradhan *et al* in a diagnosis task [12] showed a slight increase in accuracy of diagnosis with precise statistical reasoning, but the effect was so small it would have no practical clinical value.

While the available evidence is not conclusive, a provisional hypothesis is that for some decisions strict use of quantitatively precise decision-making methods may not add much practical value to the design of decision support systems over simpler, more "ad hoc" methods.

3   Qualitative Methods for Decision Making

Work in artificial intelligence raises an even more radical option for the designers of decision support systems. The desire to develop versatile automata has stimulated a great deal of research in new methods of decision making under uncertainty, ranging from sophisticated refinements of probabilistic methods such as Bayesian networks and Dempster-Shafer belief functions to non-probabilistic methods such as fuzzy logic and possibility theory. Good overviews of the different approaches and their applications are [13, 14].

These "non-standard" approaches are similar to probability methods in that they treat uncertainty as a matter of *degree*. However, even this apparently innocuous assumption has also been widely questioned on the practical grounds that they also demand a great deal of quantitative input data and also that decision-makers often find them difficult to understand because they do not capture intuitions about uncertainty - the nature of "belief", "doubt" and the form of natural justifications for decision-making.

Consequently, interest has grown in AI in the use of non-numerical methods that seem to have some "common-sense" validity for reasoning under uncertainty but are not *ad hoc* from a formal point of view. These include *non-classical logics* including non-monotonic logics, default logic and defeasible reasoning. Cognitive approaches, sometimes called *reason-based* decision making, are also gaining ground, including the idea of using informal endorsements for alternative decision options [15] and formalisations of everyday strategies of reasoning about competing beliefs and actions based on logical arguments [16, 17, 18]

Argumentation is a formalisation of the idea that decisions are made on the basis of arguments for or against a claim. Fox and Das [19] propose that argumentation may be the basis of a generalised decision theory, embracing standard probability theory as a special case, as well as other qualitative and semi-quantitative approaches. To take an example, suppose we wished to make the following informal argument:

If three or more first degree relatives of a patient have contracted breast cancer, then this is one reason to believe that the patient carries a gene predisposing to breast cancer.

In the scheme of [19] arguments are defined as logical structures having three terms:

(Claim, Grounds, Qualifier)

In the example the *Claim* term would be the proposition "this patient carries a gene predisposing to breast cancer" and the *Grounds* "three or more first degree relatives of this patient have contracted breast cancer" is the justification for the argument. The final term, *Qualifier*, specifies the nature and strength of the argument which can be drawn from the grounds to the claim. In the example the qualifier is informal "this is one reason to believe", but it could be more conventional, as in "given the *Grounds* are true the *Claim* is true with a conditional probability of 0.43".

Qualifiers are specified with reference to a particular *dictionary* of terms, along with an *aggregation function* that specifies how qualifiers in multiple arguments are to be combined. One possible dictionary is the set of real numbers from 0.0 to 1.0, which would allow qualifiers to be specified as precise numerical probability values and, with an appropriate aggregation function based on the theorems of classical probability, would allow the scheme to reduce to standard probability theory.

In many situations little can be known of the strength of arguments, other than that they indicate an increase or decrease in the overall confidence in the claim. In this case the dictionary and aggregation function might be simpler. In [20] for example we describe a system which assesses carcinogenicity of novel compounds using a dictionary comprising the symbols + (argument in favour), - (argument against). The aggregation function in this case simply sums the number of arguments in favour of a proposition minus those against. Other dictionaries can include additional qualifiers, such as ++ (the argument confirms the claim) and -- (the argument refutes the claim).

Another possible dictionary adopts *linguistic* confidence terms (e.g. *probable, improbable, possible, plausible* etc.) and requires a logical aggregation function that provides a formalised semantics for combining such terms according to common usage. Such terms have been formally categorised by their logical structure for example [21, 22].

A feature of argumentation theory is that it subsumes these apparently diverse approaches within a single formalism which has a clear consistent formal semantics [19]. Additionally, argumentation gives a different perspective on the decision making process which we believe to be more in line with the way people naturally think about probability and possibility than standard probability theory. Given the evidence reviewed above that people do not naturally use EUT in their everyday decision making, our tentative position is that expressing a preference or confidence in terms of arguments for and against each option will be more accessible and comprehensible than providing a single number representing its aggregate probability.

We have developed a number of decision support systems to explore this idea. In the next sections we describe a technology which supports an argument-based decision procedure, then outline several applications which have been built using it, and finally consider quantitative evaluations of the applications.

4   Practical Applications of the Argumentation Method

We have used the argumentation framework in designing five decision support systems to date.

4.1   CAPSULE

The CAPSULE (Computer Aided Prescribing Using Logic Engineering) system was developed to assist GPs with prescribing decisions [19,23]. CAPSULE analyses patient notes and constructs a list of relevant candidate medications, together with arguments for and against each option (based on nine different criteria, including efficacy, contra-indications, drug interactions, side effects, costs etc).

4.2   CADMIUM

The CADMIUM radiology workstation is an experimental package for combining image processing with logic-based decision support. The main use that CADMIUM has been applied to is in screening for breast cancer, in which an argument based decision procedure has the dual function of controlling image processing functions which extract and describe micro-calcifications in breast x-rays and interprets the descriptions in terms of whether they are likely to indicate benign or malignant abnormalities. The decision procedure assesses the arguments and presents them to the user in a structured report.

4.3   RAGs

The RAGs (Risk Assessment in Genetics) system allows the user to describe a patient's family tree incorporating information on the known incidence of cancers within the family. This information is evaluated to assess the likelihood that a genetic predisposition to a particular cancer is present. The software makes recommendations for patient managementin language which is comprehensible to both clinician and patient.

A family tree graphic is used for incremental data entry (Figure 1). Data about relatives are added by clicking on each relative's icon, and completing a simple form. RAGs analyses the data and provides detailed assessments of genetic risk by weighing simple arguments like the example above rather than using numerical probabilities. Based on the aggregate genetic risk level the patient is classified as at high, moderate or low risk of carrying a BrCa1 genetic mutation, which implies an 80% lifetime risk of developing breast cancer. Appropriate referral advice can be given for the patient based on this classification. The software can provide a comprehensible explanation for its decisions based on the arguments it has applied (Figure 1).

RAGs uses a set of 23 risk arguments (e.g. if the client has more than two first-degree relatives with breast cancer under the age of 50 then this is a risk factor) and a simple dictionary of qualifiers which allows small positive and negative integer values as well as plus and minus infinity (equivalent to confirming or refuting the claim). This scheme thus preserves relative rather than absolute weighting of different factors in the analysis.

4.4   ERA

Patients with symptoms or signs which may indicate cancer should be investigated quickly so that treatment may commence as soon as possible. The ERA (Early Referrals Application) system has been designed in the context of the UK Department of Health's (DoH) "2 week" guideline which states that patients with suspected cancer should be seen and assessed by an appropriate specialist within 2 week of their presentation. Referral criteria are given for each of 12 main cancer groups (e.g. Breast, Lung, Colorectal).

The practical decision as to whether or not to refer a particular patient is treated in ERA as based on a set of patient-specific arguments (see figure 2). The published referral criteria have been specifically designed to be unambiguous and easy to apply. Should any of the arguments apply to a particular patient, an early referral is warranted. Qualifiers as to the weight of each argument are thus unnecessary, with arguments generally acting categorically in an *all or nothing* fashion. An additional feature of this domain is that there are essentially no counter-arguments. The value of argumentation in this example lies largely in the ability to give meaningful explanations in the form of reasons for referral expressed in English.

4.5   REACT

The applications described so far involve making a single decision - what drug to prescribe, or whether to refer a patient. Most decisions are made in the context of plans of action, however, where they may interact or conflict with other planned actions or anticipated events. REACT (Risk, Events, Actions and their Consequences over Time) is being developed to provide decision support for extended plans. In effect REACT is a logical spreadsheet that allows a user to manipulate graphical widgets representing possible clinical events and interventions on a timeline interface and propagates their implications (both qualitative and quantitative) to numerical displays of risk (or other parameters) and displays of arguments and counter-arguments.

While the REACT user creates a plan, a knowledge-based DSS analyses it according to a set of definable rules and provides feedback on interactions between events. Rules may specify, for example, that certain events are mutually exclusive, that certain combinations of events are impossible, or that events have different consequences depending on prior or simultaneous events). Global measures (for example the predicted degree of risk or predicted cost or benefit of combinations of events) can be displayed graphically alongside the planning timeline. Qualitative arguments for and against each individual action proposed in the plan can be reviewed, and can be used to generate recommended actions when specified combinations of plan elements occur.

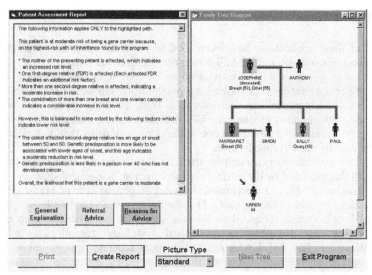

Fig. 1. The RAGs software application. A family tree has been input for the patient Karen, who has had three relatives affected by relevant cancers. The risk assessment system has determined a pattern of inheritance that may indicate a genetic factor, and provides an explanation in the left-hand panel. Referral advice for the patient is also available.

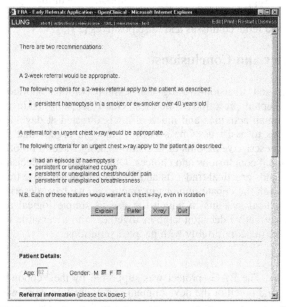

Fig. 2. The ERA early referral application. After completing patient details on a form, the program provides referral recommendations with advice, and can contact the hospital to automatically make an appointment.

5   Evaluations

A number of these applications have been used to carry out controlled evaluations (with the exception of ERA and REACT which are still in development).

In the case of the CAPSULE prescribing system a controlled study with Oxfordshire general practitioners showed the potential for substantial improvements in the quality of their prescribing decisions [23]. With decision support there was a 70% increase in the number of times the GPs decisions agreed with those of experts considering the cases, and a 50% reduction in the number of times that they missed a cheaper but equally effective medication.

The risk classifications generated by the RAGS software was compared for 50 families with that provided by the leading probabilistic risk assessment software. This uses the Claus model [27], a mathematical model of genetic risk of breast cancer based on a large dataset of cancer cases. Despite the use of a very simple weighting scheme the RAGs system produced exactly the same risk classification (into high, medium or low risk, according to established guidelines) for all cases as the probabilistic system [24, 25]. RAGs resulted in more accurate pedigree taking and more appropriate management decisions than either pencil and paper or standard probabilistic software [26].

In the CADMIUM image-processing system users are provided with assistance in interpreting mammograms using an argument-based decision making component. Radiographers who were trained to interpret mammograms were asked to make decisions as to whether observed abnormalities were benign or malignant, with and without decision support. The decision support condition produced clear improvements in the radiographers' performance, in terms of increased hits and correct rejections and reduced misses and false positives [27].

6   Summary and Conclusions

Human reasoning and decision-making can exhibit various shortcomings when compared with accepted prescriptive theories. Good decision-making is central to many important human activities and much effort is directed at developing decision support technologies to assist us. One school of thought argues that these systems must be based on prescriptive axioms of decision-making since to do otherwise leads inevitably to irrational conclusions and choices. Others argue that decision-making in the real world demands practical tradeoffs and a failure to make those tradeoffs would be irrational. Although the debate remains inconclusive, we have described a number of examples of medical systems in which the use of simple logical argumentation appears to provide effective decision support together with a versatile representation of uncertainty which fits comfortably with people's intuitions.

Acknowledgements. The RAGs project was supported by the Economic and Social Research Council, and much of the development and evaluation work was carried out by Andrew Coulson and Jon Emery. Michael Humber carried out much of the implementation of the ERA system.

References

1. Kahneman D., Slovic P. and Tversky A. (eds): Heuristics and Biases. Cambridge University Press, Cambridge (1982)
2. Evans J. st B. and Over D.E.: Rationality and reasoning. Psychology press, London (1996)
3. Wright G. and Ayton P. (eds): Subjective Probability. Wiley, Chichester, UK (1994)
4. Gigerenzer G. and Todd P.M.: Simple heuristics that make us smart. Oxford University Press, Oxford (1999)
5. Kahneman, D. and Tversky, A.: Judgement under Uncertainty: Heuristics and Biases. Science, Vol. 185, 27 (1974) pp. 1124-1131.
6. Lindley DV.: Making Decisions (2nd Edition). Wiley, Chichester, UK (1985)
7. Shanteau, J.: Psychological characteristics of expert decision makers. In , J Mumpower (ed) Expert judgement and expert systems. NATO ASI Series, volume F35 (1987)
8. Carpenter R G, Garnder A, McWeeny P M. and Emery J L.: Multistage scoring system for identifying infants at risk of unexpected death. Archives of disease in childhood, 53(8), (1977) pp.600-612
9. Fox J. Barber DC. and Bardhan KD.: Alternatives to Bayes? A quantitative comparison with rule-based diagnosis. Methods of Information in Medicine, 10 (4) (1980) pp.210-215
10. Fox, J. Myers CD., Greaves MF. and Pegram S.: Knowledge acquisition for expert systems: experience in leukaemia diagnosis. Methods of Information in Medicine, 24 (1) (1985) pp.65-72
11. O'Neil MJ. and Glowinski AJ.: Evaluating and validating very large knowledge-based systems. Medical Informatics, 15 (3) (1990) pp.237-251
12. Pradhan M.: The sensitivity of belief networks to imprecise probabilities: an experimental investigation. Artificial Intelligence Journal, 84 (1-2) (1996) pp.365-397
13. Krause P. and Clark C.:   Uncertainty and Subjective Probability in AI Systems In Wright G & Ayton P (Eds) Subjective Probability, Wiley J & Sons (1994) pp.501-527
14. Hunter, A. and Parsons, S. (Editors) Applications of uncertainty formalisms, Springer Verlag, LNAI 1455, (1998)
15. Cohen P.R.: Heuristic Reasoning: An Artificial Intelligence Approach. Pitman Advanced Publishing Program, Boston (1985)
16. Fox J.: On the necessity of probability: Reasons to believe and grounds for doubt. In Wright G, Ayton, P, eds., Subjective Probability. John Wiley, Chichester (1994)
17. Fox J, Krause P. and Ambler S.: Arguments, contradictions and practical reasoning. In Neumann B, ed. Proceedings of the 10th European Conference on AI (ECAI92), Vienna, Austria (1992) pp.623-627
18. Curley SP. and Benson PG.: Applying a cognitive perspective to probability construction. In G Wright & P Ayton (eds.), Subjective Probability. John Wiley & Sons. Chichester, England (1994) pp. 185-209
19. Fox J. and Das S K.: Safe and Sound: Artificial Intelligence in Hazardous Applications, American Association of Artificial Intelligence and MIT Press (2000)
20. Tonnelier CAG., Fox J., Judson P., Krause P., Pappas N. and Patel M.: Representation of Chemical Structures in Knowledge-Based Systems. J. Chem. Inf. Sci. 37 (1997) pp.117-123.
21. Elvang-Goransson M, Krause P.J and Fox J.: Acceptability of Arguments as Logical Uncertainty. In: Clarke M, Kruse R and Moral S, eds. Symbolic and Quantitative Approaches to Reasoning and Uncertainty. Proceedings of European Conference ECSQARU93. Lecture Notes in Computer Science 747. Springer-Verlag (1993) pp.85-90.
22. Glasspool DW. and Fox J.: Understanding probability words by constructing concrete mental models. In Hahn M, Stoness, SC, eds, Proceedings of the 21st Annual Conference of the Cognitive Science Society (1999) pp.185-190.

23. Walton RT, Gierl C, Yudkin P, Mistry H, Vessey MP & Fox J.: Evaluation of computer support for prescribing (CAPSULE) using simulated cases. *British Medical Journal* 315 (1997) pp.791-795.
24. Emery J, Watson E, Rose P and Andermann, A. A systematic review of the literature exploring the role of primary care in genetic services. Fam. Prac. 16 (1999) pp.426-45.
25. Coulson AS, Glasspool DW, Fox J and Emery J. Computerized Genetic Risk Assessment from Family Pedigrees. MD computing, in press.
26. Emery J., Walton, R., Murphy, M., Austoker, J., Yudkin, P., Chapman, C., Coulson, A., Glasspool, D. and Fox, J.: Computer support for interpreting family histories of breast and ovarian cancer in primary care: comparative study with simulated cases. British Medical Journal, 321 (2000) pp.28-32.
27. Claus E, Schildkraut J, Thompson WD and Risch, N. The genetic attributable risk of breast and ovarian cancer. *Cancer* 1996; 77, pp. 2318-24.
28. Taylor, P, Fox J and Todd-Pokropek, A "The development and evaluation of CADMIUM: a prototype system to assist in the interpretation of mammograms" *Medical Image Analysis,* 1999, 3 (4), 321-337.

Comparison of Rule-Based and Bayesian Network Approaches in Medical Diagnostic Systems*

Agnieszka Onisko[1], Peter Lucas[2], and Marek J. Druzdzel[3]

[1] Białystok University of Technology, Institute of Computer Science, Białystok,
15–351, Poland, aonisko@ii.pb.bialystok.pl
[2] Department of Computing Science, University of Aberdeen, Aberdeen AB24 3UE,
Scotland, UK, plucas@csd.abdn.ac.uk
[3] Decision Systems Laboratory, School of Information Sciences, Intelligent Systems
Program, and Center for Biomedical Informatics, University of Pittsburgh,
Pittsburgh, PA 15260, U.S.A., marek@sis.pitt.edu

Abstract. Almost two decades after the introduction of probabilistic expert systems, their theoretical status, practical use, and experiences are matching those of rule-based expert systems. Since both types of systems are in wide use, it is more than ever important to understand their advantages and drawbacks. We describe a study in which we compare rule-based systems to systems based on Bayesian networks. We present two expert systems for diagnosis of liver disorders that served as the inspiration and vehicle of our study and discuss problems related to knowledge engineering using the two approaches. We finally present the results of a simple experiment comparing the diagnostic performance of each of the systems on a subset of their domain.

1 Introduction

Two major classes of expert systems are those based on rules, known as *rule-based expert systems*, and those based on probabilistic graphical models, often referred to as *probabilistic expert systems* or *normative systems*. Rule-based expert systems, originating from the pioneering work of Buchanan and Shortliffe on the Mycin system [1], aim at capturing human expertise in terms of rules of the form **if** *condition* **then** *action*. There is overwhelming psychological evidence (e.g., [9]) that such rules are capable of modelling the human thought process. A set of rules can capture a human expert's relevant knowledge of a domain and can be subsequently used to reproduce the expert's problem solving in that domain. Probabilistic expert systems originate from research at the intersection of statistics and artificial intelligence. This research focuses on the concepts of relevance and probabilistic independence and has led to the development of intuitive and efficient graphical tools for knowledge representation. A prominent tool for

---

* The following grants supported our work: KBN 8T11E02917, W/II/1/00, AFOSR F49620–00–1–0112, NSF IRI–9624629, NATO PST.CLG.976167.

S. Quaglini, P. Barahona, and S. Andreassen (Eds.): AIME 2001, LNAI 2101, pp. 283–292, 2001.

capturing expert knowledge in this approach are *Bayesian networks* [11], often referred to, somewhat imprecisely, as *causal networks*, because of their ability to capture causal relations. Bayesian networks, while also aim at capturing expert knowledge, are based on the mathematical foundations of probability theory. When used in reasoning, they apply mathematical formalism and make no claim about reproducing the expert's thought process.

Several authors have studied theoretical differences between rule-based expert systems and normative systems (e.g., [2,6,13]), in particular with respect to handling uncertainty. Much less work, however, has been done on studying the implications that choosing one approach over the other has on the knowledge engineering effort and overall system performance. Today, theoretical developments and practical experiences with the probabilistic systems are matching those of rule-based expert systems. Both rule-based and probabilistic systems are in wide use and it is more than ever important to understand the advantages and drawbacks of each of the approaches.

Our paper focuses on comparing the two approaches in the context of a challenging practical problem that we worked on independently, using both rule-based and probabilistic approaches: diagnosis of liver disorders. Expert systems that we have developed are of considerable size and have taken several years to build. Hepatology, the study of diseases of the liver and biliary tract, is an excellent domain for such comparison, as it is complex, contains both rare and frequently occurring disorders, disorders for which both much biomedical knowledge is available and which are described only in terms of symptoms and signs.

The remainder of this paper is structured as follows. Section 2 summarises the main principles of the rule-based and probabilistic expert systems, and introduces the systems on which our comparison is based. Section 3 focuses on the qualitative comparison of the two systems and, in particular, on the knowledge engineering aspects of the two approaches. Section 4 describes the results of a study that aimed at evaluating the diagnostic performance of the two systems. Finally, Section 5 summarises our most important findings.

2   The Basics

The systems, HEPAR and HEPAR II (a successor of another HEPAR project!), focus on the diagnosis of liver disorders. *Hepar* is Greek for *liver* and this explains similarity in names of the systems, which have been conceived independently. We realize that these names may lead to confusion on the part of the reader and, therefore, we will refer to them in this paper by HEPAR-RB and HEPAR-BN respectively. HEPAR-RB is a rule-based system which was developed from 1984 to 1990 [8]. Its development was a joint work of Roelof Janssens (hepatologist, St Elisabeth Hospital, Leidschendam, The Netherlands) and Peter Lucas; the latter has since then also done work on probabilistic and decision-theoretic systems. HEPAR-BN, still under development, is a probabilistic system and it is a collaborative effort of Agnieszka Oniśko, Marek Druzdzel and Hanna Wasyluk (hepatologist, Medical Centre for Postgraduate Education, Warsaw, Poland) [10].

2.1   Rule-Based Expert Systems and the HEPAR-RB Project

A rule-based expert system $\mathcal{S}$ can be defined as a triple $\mathcal{S} = (\Delta, \Phi, \mathcal{R})$, with a set of possible conclusions Δ, a set of observable findings Φ, and a set of generalised Horn clauses, or *rules*, $\mathcal{R}$ taking the form:

$$(e_1 \wedge \cdots \wedge e_p \wedge \sim f_1 \wedge \cdots \wedge \sim f_q) \to d_x \tag{1}$$

where $d \in \Delta$ and $e_i, f_j \in (\Delta \cup \Phi)$ (the subscript x of d is discussed below). The negation sign $\sim$ in a rule denotes a special type of closed-world assumption, called *negation by absence* [7]. Negation by absence was especially designed to accommodate the way medical doctors handle patient findings: usually only positive (present) findings are recorded, whereas only a small proportion of negative (absent) findings are written down. A finding may only be assumed to be absent when the corresponding test has been performed. For example, $\sim(jaundice \in$ Signs) is true when an attempt has been made to observe signs in the patient, and no jaundice was observed; formally: $((\text{Signs} \neq unknown) \wedge (jaundice \notin \text{Signs}))$.

If $H \subseteq \Delta$ is a set of possible diagnostic conclusions, called the *hypothesis set*, and $E \subseteq \Phi$ is the set of observed patient findings, then a *diagnosis* D is defined as follows [5]:

$$D = \{d \in H \mid \mathcal{R} \cup E \vdash_{\text{NA}} d\}$$

where $\vdash_{\text{NA}}$ denotes logical deduction using negation by absence. Note that this definition implies that rule-based systems of the Mycin type are deductively incomplete. However, this incompleteness has no significant drawback. On the contrary, it even has an advantage: it reduces the amount of information requested from the user [5].

A traditionally popular way to deal with uncertainty in rule-based expert systems has been the certainty-factor calculus as originally developed for the (E)Mycin system by Shortliffe and Buchanan [1]. The subscript x in rule (1) expresses uncertainty with respect to d given absolute certainty of the rule's conditions. Although the certainty-factor calculus has attracted a fair amount of criticism, the model is in fact related to encoding and processing uncertainty in Bayesian networks, as was only recently shown [6].

HEPAR-RB [7] is a rule-base expert system which is structured along the lines briefly discussed above. The system is able to differentiate among nearly 80 disorders of the liver and biliary tract. It uses a hierarchical reasoning strategy, as illustrated in Fig. 1. The system includes 118 different variables, some of which are multivalued. Only non-invasive tests are included; liver biopsy, for example, is not included, as one of the aims of the development of the system was to assist clinicians in the appropriate selection of patients who need to be submitted to such invasive tests.

A performance evaluation has been carried out twice, using data from the Rotterdam University Hospital (Dijkzigt Hospital) [8]. The second of these datasets, which includes 181 patient cases after removal of patients of whom the diagnosis was unclear, will be used in this paper as one of the datasets for a comparative quantitative analysis of HEPAR-RB and HEPAR-BN. This dataset will be referred to in the sequel as the *DH dataset*.

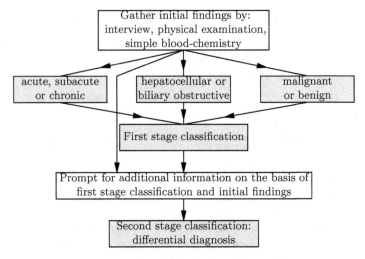

Fig. 1. Diagnostic strategy in HEPAR-RB.

2.2   Probabilistic Expert Systems and the HEPAR-BN Project

A probabilistic expert system consists of a Bayesian network with a set of algorithms to manipulate its incorporated probabilistic information. More formally, a Bayesian network is defined as a pair $\mathcal{B} = (G, \mathrm{Pr})$, where G is an acyclic directed graph, modelling probabilistic (in)dependencies among variables, and Pr is a set of local conditional probability distributions, which together define a joint probability distribution on the variables. The graphical part of a Bayesian network normally reflects the causal structure of a problem. Fig. 2 shows a simplified fragment of the HEPAR-BN Bayesian network model. The network models 18 variables related to diagnosis of a small set of hepatic disorders: three risk factors, 12 symptoms and test results, and three disorder nodes.

Given a patient's case E, i.e., values of some of the modelled variables, such as risk factors, symptoms, and test results, a probabilistic system derives the posterior probability distribution over the possible disorders D: $\mathrm{Pr}(d \mid E)$, for each $d \in D$. This probability distribution can be directly used in diagnostic decision support.

To give the reader an idea of the number of numerical parameters needed to quantify a Bayesian network, let us assume for simplicity that each variable in the model in Fig. 2 is binary. The complete joint probability distribution for 18 binary variables would contain $2^{17} = 131{,}072$ independent parameters (we take here into account that for every propositional variable x, $\mathrm{Pr}(\overline{x}) = 1 - \mathrm{Pr}(x)$). Explicit information about independencies included in the model allows for specifying the joint probability distribution by means of a series of conditional probability distribution tables (CPTs) of individual nodes conditional on their direct predecessors. A CPT for a binary variable with n binary predecessors requires specification of 2^n independent parameters. A popular approximation of the in-

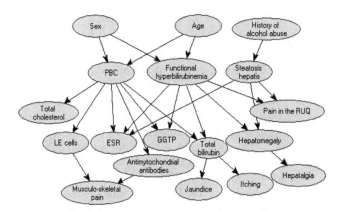

Fig. 2. A Bayesian network (a simplified fragment of the HEPAR-BN model).

teraction between a node and its direct predecessors in a Bayesian network is the Noisy–OR gate [11]. In Noisy–OR gates, each of the arcs is described by a single number expressing the causal strength of the interaction between the parent and the child. If there are other, unmodelled causes of a, we need one additional number, known as the *leak probability* [3], denoting the cumulative causal strength of all unmodelled causes of a. If each of the interactions in our model is approximated by a leaky Noisy–OR gate, only 43 numbers suffice to specify the entire joint probability distribution. It is apparent from the above example that Bayesian networks offer a compact representation of joint probability distributions and are capable of practical representation of large models.

The HEPAR-BN model [10] is a causal Bayesian network involving a subset of the domain of hepatology: 11 liver diseases (described by 9 disorder nodes), 18 risk factors, and 44 symptoms and laboratory tests results. It was designed for gathering and processing clinical data of patients with liver disorders and, through its diagnostic capabilities, reducing the need for liver biopsy. An integral part of the HEPAR system is its dataset, created in 1990 and thoroughly maintained since then at the Gastroentorogical Clinic of the Institute of Food and Feeding in Warsaw (we will refer to this dataset as the *IFF dataset*). The current IFF dataset contains over 800 patient records and its size is still growing. Each hepatological case is described by over 200 different medical findings.

3 Qualitative Comparison

There are numerous structural, qualitative differences between rule-based and Bayesian network systems which determine the way these systems diagnose disorders in patients. These differences also give rise to different methodologies for the development of such systems. Due to space constraints, we will compare HEPAR-RB and HEPAR-BN only with regard to multiple-disorder diagnosis and knowledge modelling.

3.1 Single versus Multiple Disorder Diagnosis

The *single disorder assumption* takes that a patient only suffers from one disorder at the same time, i.e., disorders are assumed to be *mutually exclusive*. This is often unnecessarily restrictive, as it happens fairly often that a patient suffers from *multiple disorders* and a single disorder may not account for all observed findings. This is certainly the case for liver diseases, where an initial disease process may give rise to multiple disorders.

As diagnostic problem solving in rule-based systems is taken as logical deduction, the capability of producing multiple, alternative diagnostic solutions is dependent on the freedom allowed in the syntax of rules. Multiple disorder diagnosis is only possible when disjunctions are allowed in the rules, i.e., when rules are non-Horn clauses. As many rule-based systems, including HEPAR-RB, restrict rules to the (generalised) Horn-clause format, multiple disorder diagnoses such as $d_1 \vee (d_2 \wedge d_3)$, the patient has either d_1 or both d_2 and d_3, is not possible. Instead, diagnostic conclusions have the form $D = \{d_{x_1}^1, \ldots, d_{x_k}^k\}$, to be interpreted as: $d_{x_1}^1 \wedge \cdots \wedge d_{x_k}^k$. This conjunction consists of diagnostic conclusions $d_{x_j}^j$ with a measure of uncertainty x_j. HEPAR-RB includes a multi-valued variable 'diagnosis' which can take on disorders as values. A simple type of multiple disorder diagnosis is therefore obtained in HEPAR-RB, as values are not assumed to be mutually exclusive.

In the case of a Bayesian network, the single disorder diagnosis assumption is modelled by using a single diagnostic variable D, which takes disorders as its possible values. Due to the axiom $\sum_{d \in \rho(D)} \Pr(D = d) = 1$, where $\rho(D)$ is the domain of the variable D, the disorders are *mutually exclusive*. This was one of the underlying assumptions of an initial version of HEPAR-BN, influenced by the IFF dataset that was available to us that had every patient case ultimately diagnosed with only one liver disorder.

Instead of representing all disorders by a single variable, every disorder can also be represented by a separate variable. This allows for exploiting the multiple disorder assumption in Bayesian networks. Normally, a Bayesian network algorithm is used to compute the posterior probability:

$$\Pr(d \mid E) \tag{2}$$

for each $d \in \Delta$, where Δ is the set of disorder variable, and E is the set of patient findings. However, the probability of this co-occurrence is actually:

$$\Pr(D \mid E) \tag{3}$$

where $D \subseteq \Delta$; for example $D = \{d_1, d_2\}$. Bayesian networks incorporate the necessary probabilistic information to compute probability (3). Computing the probability distribution over all possible combinations of diseases is for a sufficiently large set of diseases infeasible. Many Bayesian-network systems including HEPAR-BN, therefore, compute the probability distributions (2), and do not attempt to do full multiple disorder diagnosis.

We may conclude that although the foundations of HEPAR-RB and HEPAR-BN are quite different, the systems implement essentially the same restricted type of multiple disorder diagnosis. This facilitates the comparison of the systems' diagnostic performances.

3.2   Knowledge Modelling

Development of a rule-based expert system amounts to eliciting heuristic knowledge of the type Features $\Rightarrow$ Class, where 'Features' is a Boolean expression involving features relevant with respect to the class, and $\Rightarrow$ a classification relation. For example, one of classification relations underlying one of the logical rules in HEPAR-RB is the following:

(Chronic_disorder $\wedge$ Female_gender $\wedge$ $(age > 40)$ $\wedge$ (Raynaud's_phenomenon $\vee$
  $\{burning\_eyes, dry\_mouth\} \subseteq$ Signs) $\wedge$ Biliary-obstructive_type) $\Rightarrow$ PBC

Development of a Bayesian network usually involves causal modelling, where one attempts to acquire knowledge of the form $Cause_1, \ldots, Cause_n \to$ Effect. For example, in HEPAR-BN one of the underlying causal relations is:

Cirrhosis, Total_proteins_low $\to$ Ascites

For rule-based systems, the essential modelling problem is to decide which features to include in the classification relation, and which to leave out, as this will have a significant bearing on the quality of the system. The decision which variables to include in a causal relation when developing a Bayesian network is less hard, as experts are usually confident about the factors influencing another factor. Moreover, acquiring information about the actual interaction among the factors involved in a causal relation is dealt with separately, when acquiring probabilistic information. This seems to suggest that the development of a Bayesian network may require less time than the development of a corresponding rule-based system. On the other hand, the developer of a rule-based system has a more direct control over the diagnostic behaviour of the system, whereas in the case of a Bayesian network, insight into possible changes in behaviour is mainly obtained by examining the model's result for test cases.

   HEPAR-RB was developed over a period of four years, during regular meetings with Dr. Roelof Janssens, taking a total of approximately 150 hours. Certainty-factors were gathered by using the direct scaling method, i.e., a scale from -100 to 100 was used, and the hepatologist was asked to indicate his belief concerning certain statements on this scale. Subsequently, considerable time has been invested in refining the rule base using patient data [4].

   In case of the HEPAR-BN system, we elicited the structure of the model based on medical literature and conversations with our domain expert, Dr. Hanna Wasyluk. We estimate that elicitation of the structure took approximately 50 hours with the experts (in addition to Dr. Wasyluk, we verified the parts of the model with Drs. Daniel Schwartz and John Dowling of the University of Pittsburgh). Access to the IFF dataset allowed us to learn all the numerical parameters of the model from data rather than eliciting them from experts.

4 Quantitative Comparison

In this section, we compare the two systems HEPAR-RB and HEPAR-BN in quantitative terms, using data from two different datasets mentioned earlier: the DH dataset from Rotterdam and the IFF dataset from Warsaw.

4.1 Patient Data

As the diagnostic categories distinguished in the systems HEPAR-RB and HEPAR-BN are different, so are the patient findings used in order to diagnose disorders. Both the IFF and DH datasets had to be converted to make comparison between the systems possible, which is not a straightforward process. First, we focused on identifying those medical findings that are common for them. Those attributes whose values were not mutually exclusive were broken down into several attributes. This is a simple consequence of the probabilistic constraint that the outcomes of a random variable must be mutually exclusive. We also assumed that missing values of attributes correspond to values *absent*, which is a popular assumption in case of medical datasets [12].

We identified 46 findings that were common for both systems. Due to different disorder mapping in both data sets, we found only two common disorders: *primary biliary cirrhosis* and *steatosis hepatis*. Of these two, primary biliary cirrhosis (PBC) was the only one with a reasonable number of patient cases in both data sets and, therefore, we focused on PBC in our experiment.

4.2 Results

The results of our experiment are presented in Tables 1(a) through 1(f). Our first observation was that in a significant portion of the cases HEPAR-RB was not able to reach a conclusion. If the most likely disease is the one that the system recommends, HEPAR-BN will always make a diagnosis. To make the comparison fair, we assumed that there is a probability threshold that has to be crossed in order for the system to make a diagnosis with a reasonable confidence. We would like to point out that in practice this threshold depends on the utility of correct diagnosis and misdiagnosis (which are disease-dependent). The threshold can be naturally introduced into a probabilistic system using decision-theoretic methods. In our experiments, we chose a fixed threshold of 50%, which is rather conservative towards HEPAR-BN. HEPAR-BN was not able to cross this threshold in a number of cases that is comparable to HEPAR-RB.

Tables 1(a) and 1(b) summarise the results of both systems when tested with the 699 IFF patients. Similarly, Tables 1(c) and 1(d) present the results for HEPAR-RB and HEPAR-BN, respectively, for the 181 DH patients. In both cases, the performance of HEPAR-BN was determined by cross-validation using the leave-one-out method. Table 1(e) gives the results for HEPAR-BN trained on the DH dataset and tested with the IFF dataset, whereas the results of Table 1(f) were obtained the other way around. Note that the results of Table 1(e) are inferior to those given in Table 1(f).

Table 1. Comparison of diagnostic accuracy of HEPAR-RB (**H-RB**) and HEPAR-BN (**H-BN**); PBC+ and PBC− stand for PBC present and absent, respectively; UC: unclassified.

Results (a) and (b) for 699 IFF patients.

H-RB	**Patients** PBC+	(%)	PBC−	(%)	Total
PBC+	174	(62)	15	(4)	189
PBC−	11	(4)	85	(20)	96
UC	95	(34)	319	(76)	414
Total	280	(100)	419	(100)	699

(a)

H-BN	**Patients** PBC+	(%)	PBC−	(%)	Total
PBC+	263	(94)	61	(15)	324
PBC−	13	(5)	190	(45)	203
UC	4	(1)	168	(40)	172
Total	280	(100)	419	(100)	699

(b)

Results (c) and (d) for 181 DH patients.

H-RB	**Patients** PBC+	(%)	PBC−	(%)	Total
PBC+	11	(73.3)	1	(1)	12
PBC−	2	(13.3)	143	(86)	145
UC	2	(13.3)	22	(13)	24
Total	15	(100)	166	(100)	181

(c)

H-BN	**Patients** PBC+	(%)	PBC−	(%)	Total
PBC+	12	(80)	1	(1)	13
PBC−	3	(20)	65	(39)	68
UC	0	(0)	100	(60)	100
Total	15	(100)	166	(100)	181

(d)

Results of HEPAR-BN for (e) 699 IFF and (f) 181 DH patients.

H-BN	**Patients** PBC+	(%)	PBC−	(%)	Total
PBC+	170	(60.7)	12	(2.9)	182
PBC−	9	(3.2)	76	(18.1)	85
UC	101	(36.1)	331	(79)	432
Total	280	(100)	419	(100)	699

(e)

H-BN	**Patients** PBC+	(%)	PBC−	(%)	Total
PBC+	14	(93)	57	(34.3)	71
PBC−	1	(7)	71	(42.8)	72
UC	0	(0)	38	(22.9)	38
Total	15	(100)	166	(100)	181

(f)

5 Discussion

It seems that building the models in each of the two approaches has its advantages and disadvantages. One feature of the rule-based approach that we found particularly useful is that it allows testing models by following the trace of the system's reasoning. A valuable property of Bayesian network-based systems is that models can be trained on existing data sets. Exploiting available statistics and patient data in a Bayesian network is fairly straightforward. Fine-tuning a rule-based system to a given dataset is much more elaborate.

Rule-based systems capture heuristic knowledge from the experts and allow for a direct construction of a classification relation, while probabilistic systems capture causal dependencies, based on knowledge of pathophysiology, and enhance them with statistical relations. Hence, the modelling is more indirect, although in domains where capturing causal knowledge is easy, the resulting diagnostic performance may be good. Rule-based systems may be expected to perform well for problems that cannot be modelled using causality as a guiding principle, or when a problem is too complicated to be modelled as a causal graph.

Our experiments have confirmed that a rule-based system can have difficulty with dealing with missing values: around 35% of the IFF patients remained unclassified by HEPAR-RB, while in HEPAR-BN only 2% of IFF patients remained unclassified. Note that this behaviour is due to the semantics of negation by absence, and in fact a deliberate design choice in rule-based systems. Refraining from classifying is better than classifying incorrectly, although it will be at the cost of leaving certain cases unclassified. In all cases, the true positive rate for HEPAR-BN was higher than for HEPAR-RB, although sometimes combined with a lower true negative rate.

Both systems were in general more accurate when dealing with their original datasets. The reason is that the systems were using then all available data, not only the common variables. We have noticed some indications of overfitting in case of HEPAR-BN, visible especially in those results, where the system was trained and tested on different data sets.

References

1. B.G. Buchanan and E.H. Shortliffe (Eds.). *Rule-Based Expert Systems: The MYCIN Experiments of the Stanford Heuristic Programming Project.* Addison-Wesley, Reading, MA, 1984.
2. D. Heckerman. Probabilistic interpretations for Mycin's certainty factors. In: L.N. Kanal and J.F. Lemmer (Eds.). *UAI 1* (Elsevier, NY, 1986) 167–196.
3. M. Henrion. Some practical issues in constructing belief networks. In: L.N. Kanal, T.S. Levitt, and J.F. Lemmer (Eds.). *UAI 3* (Elsevier, NY, 1989) 161–173.
4. P.J.F. Lucas. Refinement of the HEPAR expert system: tools and techniques. *Artificial Intelligence in Medicine* 6(2) (1994) 175–188.
5. P.J.F. Lucas. Symbolic diagnosis and its formalisation. *The Knowledge Engineering Review* 12(2) (1997) 109–146.
6. P.J.F. Lucas. Certainty-like structures in Bayesian belief networks. *Knowledge-based Systems* (2001).
7. P.J.F. Lucas and A.R. Janssens. Development and validation of HEPAR. *Medical Informatics* 16(3) (1991) 259–270.
8. P.J.F. Lucas, R.W. Segaar, and A.R. Janssens. HEPAR: an expert system for diagnosis of disorders of the liver and biliary tract. *Liver* 9 (1989) 266–275.
9. A. Newell and H.A. Simon. *Human Problem Solving.* Prentice-Hall, Englewood Cliffs, NJ, 1972.
10. A. Oniśko, M.J. Druzdzel, and H. Wasyluk. Extension of the Hepar II model to multiple-disorder diagnosis. In: S.T. Wierzchoń M. Kłopotek, M. Michalewicz (Eds.). *Intelligent Information Systems.* Advances in Soft Computing *Series* (Physica-Verlag Heidelberg, 2000) 303–313.
11. J. Pearl. *Probabilistic Reasoning in Intelligent Systems: Networks of Plausible Inference.* Morgan Kaufmann, San Mateo, CA, 1988.
12. M. Peot and R. Shachter. Learning from what you don't observe. In: *UAI–98* (Morgan Kaufmann, San Francisco, CA, 1998) 439–446.
13. L.C. van der Gaag. *Probability-Based Models for Plausible Reasoning.* PhD thesis, University of Amsterdam, Amsterdam, The Netherlands, 1990.

Parts, Locations, and Holes — Formal Reasoning about Anatomical Structures

Stefan Schulz[1] and Udo Hahn[2]

[1] Abteilung Medizinische Informatik
Universitätsklinikum Freiburg, Stefan-Meier-Str. 26, D-79104 Freiburg
[2] Linguistische Informatik / Computerlinguistik
Universität Freiburg, Werthmannplatz 1, D-79085 Freiburg

Abstract. We propose an ontology engineering framework for the anatomy domain, focusing on mereotopological properties of parts, locations and empty spaces (holes). We develop and formally describe a basic ontology consisting of the mutually disjoint primitives solid object, hole and boundary. We embed the relations *part-of* and *location-of* into a parsimonious description logic (ALC) and emulate advanced reasoning across these relations - such as transitivity at the T-Box level - by taxonomic subsumption. Unlike common conceptualizations we do not distinguish between solids and the regions they occupy, as well as we allow solids to have holes as proper parts. Concrete examples from human anatomy are used to support our claims.

1 Introduction

Physical entities, such as body parts, organs, cells etc. constitute the location of physiological and pathological processes, as well as the targets of diagnostic procedures and therapeutic measures. Hence, they play a crucial role in the design of the basic ontologies covering these domains [11,1,14]. Such foundational models should also be portable across subdomains and applications, and simultaneously be usable for formal reasoning devices.

In our previous work on anatomical knowledge representation, we already developed a formal solution for the seamless integration of partonomic and taxonomic reasoning [7] in the context of $\mathcal{ALC}$-style description logics [21]. This approach has already proved useful for the construction of a large terminological knowledge base [16]. Recently, we proposed an extension of this approach covering aspects of spatial reasoning as related to anatomical topology [17]. In the present paper, we intend to enhance the notion of strict mereology, i.e. the study of *parts*, by including spatial *location*, as well. As a consequence, we also have to provide an adequate representation of empty spaces, i.e., *holes* in a very general sense. Based on a careful design of the underlying ontology and the provision of a composite data structure for the encoding of physical concepts, we are able to render complex mereotopological reasoning feasible without computationally expensive extensions of the underlying description logics.

S. Quaglini, P. Barahona, and S. Andreassen (Eds.): AIME 2001, LNAI 2101, pp. 293–303, 2001.

2   Basic Mereological Categories Revisited

Parts. A concise semantic characterization of the parthood relation has to incorporate observations from a cognitive/linguistic perspective. Numerous examples have been brought forward which challenge the general validity of the assumption that mereological relations, in common-sense reasoning, at least, be transitive and propagate roles across partitive hierarchies. Cruse [4] cited the following examples from anatomy: *a head has ears, ears have lobes*: *? a head has lobes?*; or *an arm has a hand, a hand has fingers*: *? an arm has fingers?*. Winston, Chaffin and Herrmann [20] argued in a similar vein noting that subrelations of part-of can be considered transitive as long as "a single sense of part" is kept. This view contrasts with the formal/philosophic understanding of parthood in classical mereology (e.g., Lesniewski's *General Extensional Mereology*, GEM, referred to in [19]). Here, the part-of relation is axiomatized as being reflexive, antisymmetric and transitive. Varzi [19] claims, however, that both approaches can coexist when a single general part-of relation is assumed which subsumes all specialized part-of relations and fulfills the axioms of classic mereology, as well.

We consider Varzi's proposal apt for describing spatial entities in our domain. Whereas *transitivity* can be plausibly assumed with regard to the broadest possible notion of parthood, p, *reflexivity* is only partially compatible with shared intuitions about parthood in anatomy. A part of a brain , e.g., must not be classified as brain, nor a part of hand, stomach, etc. Here, parthood has to be understood as *proper* parthood pp which excludes equality. However, parthood in the broadest sense holds with respect to mass concepts and collections of elements, according to the typology of Gerstl and Pribbenow [6]. The *lymphocytes* of the spleen can be considered both a *subset of* all lymphocytes and a *kind of* lymphocytes. Similar considerations apply to mass concepts, such as *blood*. If we take a part of a blood sample, we obtain just another blood sample.

Location. Spatial location refers to a defined space in which (i) some event takes place or (ii) some object can be placed. The relevance of the first meaning for the medical domain is evident: Physiological or pathological changes take place at a certain location, e.g., hematopoesis in the bone marrow, nephritis in the kidney and the extraction of a tooth takes place in the mouth.[1]

The second meaning of location can be illustrated as follows: If an object is part of another one, it is also *located* in it. Given that the brain is *part of* the head, we may infer that it is also located in the head. Considering solid objects, the inversion of this implication leads hardly to counterexamples, e.g., the bone marrow is located in the bone, it is also part of the bone. This assumption does no longer hold when *holes*[2] come into the play. A gall stone is *not* part of a gallbladder, although it is located within the

---

[1] The inferences on events and locations, however, are not so straightforward: An appendicitis is an inflammatory process located at the appendix, a colitis is an inflammatory process located at the colon. Yet colitis does not subsume appendicitis though the appendix is a part of the colon. By way of contrast, nephritis (an inflammatory process located at the kidney) does subsume glomerulonephritis (an inflammatory process located at the glomerula), glomerula being part of the kidney (for a formal solution to cope with these pheneomena of role propagation across part-whole hierarchies, cf. [7]).

[2] We use the term *'hole'* in a very general way, following the typology of Casati and Varzi [2], according to which a *'hole'* includes also surface depressions, hollows, tunnels and cavities.

gallbladder. An embryo is located within an uterus, but is is, of course, not part of an uterus. Whether a liver tumor can be considered a part of a liver or not, is a matter of debate, but without any doubt, it is located within the liver.[3] Following a suggestion of Casati and Varzi [3], we here introduce the relation *whole location* (wl): A wl B means that A is entirely (but not necessarily exactly) located within the boundaries of B.

Holes. In our ontology, locative relations boil down to mereological relations when restricted to 3-D solid objects, i.e., objects which coincide with the region they occupy. As we have seen, this restriction becomes obsolete when *holes* are introduced. Accordingly, we have to define the ontological status of holes in our domain. Nearly all macroscopic anatomical objects exhibit holes, at least contain spaces within the blood vessels, and it is consensual in our domain that not all objects contained by these spaces are necessarily parts of the macroscopic object, as already discussed. Hence, we will axiomatically define the status of holes in mereological terms.

In standard mereotopological theories holes or empty spaces are not parts of their "hosts". Moreover, they constitute a part of their exterior space [2]. This view is hardly tenable for anatomical entities due to its cognitive inadequacy. The particular epistemological status attributed to holes in anatomical structure is evident in existing ontologies, such as the *Digital Anatomist*, where, e.g., the spaces in the thorax such as the mediastinum are classified as parts of the thorax [9]. Consequently, we include holes in the region a spatial object occupies. More specifically, we state that solid objects ontologically coincide with the spatial region given by their convex hull. An example is the mastoid bone. Any bony material and airy cells in its interior is part of it, and the region given by its geometrical outline is the same as the object itself. This axiomatic assumption is admittedly unorthodox, but is dictated by our domain.[4] It may, however, lead to possibly unwarranted consequences: In our understanding of spatial overlap — the overlap of regions equivalent to the mereological overlap (cf. [17]) — a portion of the optic nerve would belong to the sphenoid bone because the optic channel is part of this bone. Unfortunately, this is entirely implausible. Thus, an axiomatization of holes is required which allows distinctions at a finer granularity level. Summarizing our considerations, we then make the following assumptions:

- No ontological distinction is made between a solid physical entity and its convex hull (see the above characterization of spongiform objects).
- Holes are always part of at least one solid entity (e.g., the cranial cavity is part of the skull).
- Solid objects can never be *parts* of holes, while they still can be *located* inside holes (e.g., the brain is located in the cranial cavity).
- Solid objects wholly located in a hole can also be parts of solid objects which host that hole (e.g., the brain is located within the cranial cavity which is part of the head, but it is also part of the head).[5]

---

[3] We only mention here the distinction between partitive and locative relations in linguistic terms (genitive attributes vs. prepositional phrases). E.g., a metastasis of_{part} a prostatic carcinoma $in_{location}$ the liver is not a tumor of_{part} the liver.

[4] This is certainly in contrast to geographic entities often referred to in the spatial reasoning community. Here, the ontological distinction, e.g., between 'Switzerland' as political entity and the 2-D region it occupies is obvious.

[5] This supposition will also solve the spatial overlap puzzle, as mentioned above.

 – Given a solid object C (e.g., a brain metastasis of a carcinoma) which is located in another solid object D (e.g., the brain) without being part of it, this implies the existence of a hole H which it fills out completely.

These claims are supported by looking at the, up to now, most comprehensive approach to ontology engineering for anatomy, *viz.* the Digital Anatomist (UWDA) [14]. In its 2001 release (included in the UMLS metathesaurus [10]), from a total of 38,811 anatomy concepts 1,145 are associated with the concept *Body Space NOS*, and 132 are associated with the concept *Orifice or Ostium*. Most of them are found to be part of a non-space entity, e.g., the UWDA concept *esophageal lumen* is related to *esophagus* by a *part-of* relation; the same applies to *vertebral foramen* and *vertebra*, etc.

3   A Terminological Knowledge Representation Language

The formal framework we provide for deductive reasoning over parts and locations is based on $\mathcal{ALC}$, a parsimonious variant of descriptions logics (DL, for a survey, cf. [21]). [6] The syntax and semantics of $\mathcal{ALC}$ are summarized in Table 1. $\mathcal{ALC}$ has several constructors combining *atomic* concepts, roles and individuals to define the terminological theory of a domain. *Concepts* are unary predicates, *roles* are binary predicates over a domain Δ, with *individuals* being the elements of Δ. We assume a common set-theoretical semantics for this language – an interpretation $\mathcal{I}$ is a function that assigns to each concept symbol (from the set **A**) a subset of the domain Δ, $\mathcal{I} : \mathbf{A} \to 2^{\Delta}$, to each role symbol (from the set **P**) a binary relation of Δ, $\mathcal{I} : \mathbf{P} \to 2^{\Delta \times \Delta}$, and to each individual symbol (from the set **I**) an element of Δ, $\mathcal{I} : \mathbf{I} \to \Delta$.

Table 1. Syntax and Semantics for the Description Logic Language $\mathcal{ALC}$

Syntax	Semantics
C	$\{d \in \Delta^{\mathcal{I}} \mid \mathcal{I}(C) = d\}$
$C \sqcap D$	$C^{\mathcal{I}} \cap D^{\mathcal{I}}$
$C \sqcup D$	$C^{\mathcal{I}} \cup D^{\mathcal{I}}$
$\neg C$	$\Delta^{\mathcal{I}} \setminus C^{\mathcal{I}}$
R	$\{(d,e) \in \Delta^{\mathcal{I}} \times \Delta^{\mathcal{I}} \mid \mathcal{I}(R) = (d,e)\}$
$\forall R.C$	$\{d \in \Delta^{\mathcal{I}} \mid R^{\mathcal{I}}(d) \subseteq C^{\mathcal{I}}\}$
$\exists R.C$	$\{d \in \Delta^{\mathcal{I}} \mid R^{\mathcal{I}}(d) \cap C^{\mathcal{I}} \neq \emptyset\}$

Concept terms and *role terms* are defined inductively. Table 1 states corresponding constructors for concepts and roles, together with their semantics. C and D denote concept terms, while R and Q denotes role terms. $R^{\mathcal{I}}(d)$ represents the set of *role fillers* of the individual d, i.e., the set of individuals e with $(d, e) \in R^{\mathcal{I}}$.

---

[6] The DL knowledge representation paradigm is already well-known in the medical informatics community, too (cf. [11,18]).

Table 2. Terminological Axioms

Axiom	Semantics	Axiom	Semantics
$A \doteq C$	$A^{\mathcal{I}} = C^{\mathcal{I}}$	$Q \doteq R$	$Q^{\mathcal{I}} = R^{\mathcal{I}}$
$A \sqsubseteq C$	$A^{\mathcal{I}} \subseteq C^{\mathcal{I}}$	$Q \sqsubseteq R$	$Q^{\mathcal{I}} \subseteq R^{\mathcal{I}}$

By means of *terminological axioms* (cf. Table 2) a symbolic name can be defined for each concept and role term. We may supply necessary and sufficient constraints (using "$\doteq$") or only necessary constraints (using "$\sqsubseteq$") for concepts and roles. A finite set of such axioms, $\mathcal{T}$, is called the *terminology* or *TBox*.

In the following, we will sketch a complex, though computationally neutral data structure encoding of concepts which supports the emulation of part-whole reasoning by taxonomic subsumption. This approach will then be extended to the notion of spatial location in Section 5. In Section 6 stipulations on upper-level categories as given in Section 2 are refined and translated into the data structure approach previously introduced which leads us to a reconstruction of *holes* in DL terms.

4   The Part-of Relation in DL

In our approach, partonomic reasoning is based on the notion of SEP triplets, which are used to emulate the transitivity property of the *part-of* relation p. An SEP triplet (cf. Figure 1) consists, first of all, of a composite 'structure' concept, the so-called **S-node** (cf. C_S in Figure 1, e.g., *Hand-Structure*), a representational artifact required for the formal reconstruction of systematic patterns of transitive part-whole reasoning. The two direct subsumees of an S-node are the corresponding **E-node** ('entity') and **P-node** ('part'), e.g., *Hand* and *Hand-Part*, respectively (cf. C_E and C_P in Figure 1). Unlike an **S-node**, these nodes refer to concrete ontological objects. The E-node denotes the whole entity to be modeled, whereas the P-node is the common subsumer of any of the parts of the E-node. Hence, for every P-node there exists a corresponding E-node as filler of the role p. Transitivity is emulated at the TBox level because any subsumee of a P-node has p filled by the corresponding E-node. The E-node, S-node and P-node must always be of a physical nature, though no restrictions apply with regard to being a 3-D-region, hole or boundary.

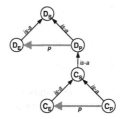

Fig. 1. SEP Triplet Encoding of the Relation *Part-Of*

For a formal reconstruction of these considerations, let us consider the following TBox. We assume C_E and D_E to denote E-nodes, C_S and D_S to denote S-nodes that subsume C_E and D_E, respectively, and C_P and D_P to denote P-nodes related to C_E and D_E, respectively, via the role p. Also, since C is modeled as being one of the parts associated with D, D_P subsumes C_S (cf. Figure 1):

$$C_E \sqsubseteq C_S \sqsubseteq D_P \sqsubseteq D_S \sqsubseteq PhysicalEntity \qquad (1)$$

$$D_E \sqsubseteq D_S \qquad (2)$$

$$D_P \doteq D_S \sqcap \exists p.D_E \qquad (3)$$

Since C_E is subsumed by D_P (condition 1), we infer that the relation p holds also between C_E and D_E. It is obvious that, using this pattern across various physical concepts linked with each other via the p relation, the deductions are the same — as if p were really transitive at the T-box level. 'Chains' of concepts, one having the other as filler of the role p, are modeled as P-node/S-node links between the corresponding SEP triplets. To obviate reflexivity (cf. Section 2) we add a disjointness criterion to condition (3) where necessary:

$$D_P \doteq D_S \sqcap \neg D_E \sqcap \exists p.D_E \qquad (4)$$

In the following, we will substantiate the claim that this framework can be enlarged to meet the requirements for an adequate representation of location, using a construction pattern that complies with the restrictions entailed by $\mathcal{ALC}$.

5 DL Reconstruction of Spatial Location

We reconstruct spatial location on the basis of SEP triplets by adding a second artifact, the so-called L-node (cf. C_L in Figure 2), yielding a so-called LSEP compound. L-nodes subsume S-nodes and are, furthermore, linked to the corresponding E-nodes by the relation wl (whole location), a reflexive, antisymmetric and transitive relation, such as introduced by Casati & Varzi [3].

The TBox specifications from Section 4 — expressions (1) to (3) — are modified as follows. Let us assume that C is wholly located inside D, but C is not a part of D.

$$D_L \doteq PhysicalEntity \sqcap \exists wl.D_E \qquad (5)$$

$$C_L \doteq D_L \sqcap \exists wl.C_E \qquad (6)$$

$$C_E \sqsubseteq C_S \sqsubseteq C_L \qquad (7)$$

$$D_E \sqsubseteq D_S \sqsubseteq D_L \qquad (8)$$

$$D_P \doteq D_S \sqcap \exists p.D_E \qquad (9)$$

The L-node subsumes exactly all those concepts which are physically located at the corresponding E-node. Since all E-nodes are subsumees of $PhysicalEntity$, L does not capture other types such as events (physiological processes, diseases, procedures, etc.). Physical location has to be understood as *whole* location: Objects located within an

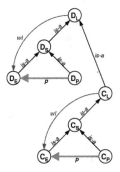

Fig. 2. LSEP Encoding of the Relation *Whole Location* (wl)

instance of D must not exceed the boundaries of D but they need not fill D completely. In a similar way as sketched with the *part-of* relation, transitivity (at the TBox level) of wl is emulated by the L-node construct, because any subsumee of an L-node has wl filled by the corresponding E-node. If a *part-of* relation holds between C and D an additional S-P link is added by substituting formula (7) by (10):

$$C_E \sqsubseteq C_S \sqsubseteq D_P \tag{10}$$

A hierarchical *part-of* link – realized as an *is-a* link between an S-node and a P-node – must therefore be accompanied by the subsumption of the corresponding L-nodes.

6 A Basic Ontology for Anatomy

In Section 2, we introduced two major categories of domain concepts, *viz. holes* and *solids*. We now add *boundary* (cf. [17]) as a third major category and introduce *3-D region* as the disjunction of solids and holes.

Figure 3 depicts this basic ontology, a TBox consisting of four SEP triplets. The topmost triplet is RE (*3-D region*). Its S-node RE_S (which stands for 3-D regions or parts of 3-D regions) subsumes the whole domain. It is equal to $PhysicalEntity$ in expression (1). The E- and S-nodes are designed as usual. No disjointness between E and S node is assumed.

$$RE_E \sqsubseteq RE_S \tag{11}$$
$$RE_P \doteq RE_S \sqcap \exists p.RE_E \tag{12}$$

Any boundary is part of a 3-D region, while no boundary or boundary part is a 3-D region. In addition, boundaries cannot exist autonomously. A more thorough analysis of boundaries lies beyond the scope of this paper (cf. [17]).

$$BD_S \sqsubseteq RE_P \sqcap \neg RE_E \tag{13}$$

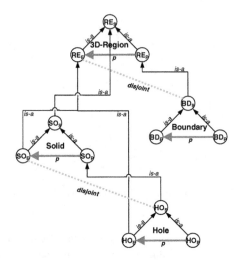

Fig. 3. Basic Ontology for Anatomy

3-D regions are either solids or holes. Any hole is part of a solid. Holes cannot have solids as parts.

$$SO_S \sqsubseteq RE_S \tag{14}$$

$$SO_E \sqsubseteq SO_S \sqcap RE_E \tag{15}$$

$$SO_P \doteq SO_S \sqcap \exists p.SO_E \tag{16}$$

$$HO_S \sqsubseteq SO_P \sqcap \neg SO_E \tag{17}$$

$$HO_E \sqsubseteq HO_S \sqcap RE_E \tag{18}$$

$$HO_P \sqsubseteq HO_S \sqcap \exists p.HO_E \tag{19}$$

We now combine this basic ontology with the LSEP construct for location.

With the technical conventions just introduced we are able to deal with holes as *parts* of solid physical entities (the hosts of the holes), as well as with objects which are located in these holes without being part of their hosts. Figure 4 depicts a TBox for the example mentioned in Section 2 including the upper level categories *hole HO* and *solid SO*. The four concepts *head, skull, brain* (solids) and *cranial cavity* (hole) are modeled as LSEP compounds. From this model, we are able to derive:

1. The skull is part of the head and located in the head.
2. The cranial cavity and all parts of it are parts of the skull and located within the skull. The model allows to infer (by transitivity) that the cranial cavity is located in the head and is part of it, too. No solid must be part of the cranial cavity (HO_S and SO_E are disjoint, cf. Fig. 3)
3. The brain, as well as any part of it, is located within the cranial cavity. However, the brain, as well as any part of it, is not part of the cranial cavity. Nor is it part of the skull.
4. The brain, as well as any part of it, is part of the head and is located within the head.

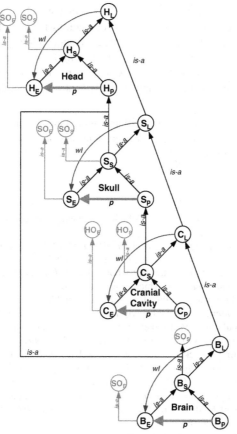

Fig. 4. Example for Parts and Locations using LSEP compounds (shaded concepts refer to the basic ontology depicted in Figure 3)

7   Related Work and Conclusions

Most basic ontologies related to anatomy are merely descriptive in the sense of a generalized anatomical typology (e.g., organs, tissues, cells etc.), known as *nomina generalia* from the *Terminologia Anatomica* [5]. A more precise typology is provided in the *Digital Anatomist* project [14]. In its upper ontology anatomical empty spaces are clearly distinguished from anatomical structure and body substance. Formal reasoning, however, – beyond a vague notion of part-whole transitivity – is not supported. The ontological engineering efforts of Schubert *et al.* [15] aim at the support of a terminological 3-D atlas of anatomy. They propose a fine-grained "mereological classification" and add a set of constraints on allowed associations between classes. Yet a formal semantics, the backbone of DL systems (cf. Table 1), is not given. Neither is a clear distinction between parts and locations proposed in any of these approaches, nor is the special epistemological status of holes accounted for in any of these frameworks. This criticism applies also to the GALEN ontology [12,13], one of the few formal models of anatomical reasoning. Proper ontological distinctions and formal foundations for knowledge representation, however, are indispensable for inference-intensive applications [8]. Our approach tries to fill this gap by proposing an ontology engineering framework based on a parsimonious terminological language. The price we have to pay is the proliferation of a constant number of artificial and, hence, computationally neutral concept definitions.

Acknowledgements. We would like to thank our colleagues in the CLIF group and the Department of Medical Informatics for fruitful discussions. S. Schulz was supported by a grant from DFG (Ha 2097/5-2).

References

1. K. Campbell, A. Das, and Musen M. A logical foundation for representation of clinical data. *JAMIA*, 1(3):218–232, 1994.
2. R. Casati and A. Varzi. *Holes and other Superficialities*. MIT Press, 1994.
3. R. Casati and A. Varzi. *Parts and Places*. MIT Press, 1999.
4. D. Cruse. On the transitivity of the part-whole relation. *J. of Linguistics*, 15:29–38, 1979.
5. FCAT. *Terminologia Anatomica*. Thieme-Verlag, 1998.
6. P. Gerstl and S. Pribbenow. Midwinters, end games and body parts: a classification of part-whole relations. *International Journal of Human-Computer Studies*, 43:865–889, 1995.
7. U. Hahn, S. Schulz, and M. Romacker. Partonomic reasoning as taxonomic reasoning in medicine. In *Proceedings of the AAAI'99*, pages 271–276, 1999.
8. Udo Hahn, Martin Romacker, and Stefan Schulz. Discourse structures in medical reports – watch out! *International Journal of Medical Informatics*, 53(1):1–28, 1999.
9. J. Mejino and C. Rosse. Conceptualization of anatomical spatial entities in the Digital Anatomist foundational model. In *Proceedings of the AMIA'99*, pages 112–116, 1999.
10. National Library of Medicine. *Unified Medical Language System*. Bethesda, MD: National Library of Medicine, 2001.
11. A. Rector, S. Bechhofer, C. Goble, I. Horrocks, W. Nowlan, and W. Solomon. The GRAIL concept modelling language for medical terminology. *Artificial Intelligence in Medicine*, 9:139–171, 1997.
12. A. Rector, A. Gangemi, Galeazzi E., A. Glowinski, and Rossi-Mori A. The GALEN model schemata for anatomy. In *Proceedings of the MIE'94*, pages 229–233, 1994.
13. J. Rogers and A. Rector. GALEN's model of parts and wholes: Experience and comparisons. In *Proceedings of the AMIA 2000*, pages 714–718, 2000.
14. C. Rosse, J. Mejino, B. Modayur, R. Jakobovits, K. Hinshaw, and J. Brinkley. Motivation and organizational principles for anatomical knowledge representation: The Digital Anatomist symbolic knowledge base. *JAMIA*, 5(1):17–40, 1998.
15. R. Schubert, K. Priesmeyer, H. Wulf, and K. Höhne. VOXEL-MAN (WEB) – Basistechnologie zur modellbasierten multimedialen Repräsentation von komplexen räumlichen Strukturen. *Künstliche Intelligenz*, 14(1):44–47, 2000.
16. S. Schulz and U. Hahn. Knowledge engineering by large-scale knowledge reuse: experience from the medical domain. In *Proceedings of the KR 2000*, pages 601–610, 2000.
17. S. Schulz, U. Hahn, and M. Romacker. Modeling anatomical spatial relations with description logics. In *Proceedings of the AMIA 2000*, pages 779–783, 2000.
18. K. Spackman and K. Campbell. Compositional concept representation using SNOMED: towards further convergence of clinical terminologies. In *Proceedings of the AMIA 1998*, pages 740–744, 1998.

19. A. Varzi. Parts, wholes, and part-whole relations: The prospects of mereotopology. *Data & Knowledge Engineering,* 20(3):259–268, 1996.

20. Morton Winston, Roger Chaffin, and Douglas J. Herrmann. A taxonomy of part-whole relationships. *Cognitive Science,* 11:417–444, 1987.

21. W. Woods and J. Schmolze. The KL-ONE family. *Computers & Mathematics with Applications,* 23(2/5):133–177, 1992.

Abductive Inference of Genetic Networks

Blaž Zupan[1,3], Ivan Bratko[1,2], Janez Demšar[1], J. Robert Beck[3], Adam Kuspa[4,5], and Gad Shaulsky[5]

[1] Faculty of Computer and Information Science, University of Ljubljana Slovenia
[2] Jožef Stefan Institute, Ljubljana, Slovenia
[3] Office of Information Technology and Dep. of Family and Community Medicine
[4] Department of Biochemistry and Molecular Biology
[5] Department of Molecular and Human Genetics
Baylor College of Medicine, Houston, TX, USA

Abstract. GenePath is an automated system for reasoning on genetic networks, wherein a set of genes have various influences on one another and on a biological outcome. It acts on a set of experiments in which genes are knocked out or overexpressed, and the outcome of interest is evaluated. Implemented in Prolog, GenePath uses abductive inference to elucidate network constraints based on prior knowledge and experimental results. Two uses of the system are demonstrated: synthesis of a consistent network from abduced constraints, and qualitative reasoning-based approach that generates a set of networks consistent with the data. In practice, illustrated by an example using Dictyostelium aggregation, a combination of constraint satisfaction and qualitative reasoning produces a small set of plausible networks.

1 Introduction

Genetic analysis often defines a framework for the elucidation of biological mechanisms. Mutations are the main tool used by geneticists to investigate biological phenomena. Initially, mutations help define and catalogue genes that participate in a biological mechanism. Relationships between the genes are then determined using combinations of mutations in two or more genes.

Genetic networks that outline the molecular details of a biological mechanism are generated by integration of the relationships between pairs of genes. The method used for ordering gene function is fairly straightforward and requires only a short time relative to the time required to obtain the experimental data. However, accounting for all the data becomes complicated when the amount of data increases as the number of possible genetic networks grows combinatorially with the number of genes. We therefore sought to develop an automated tool that will assist the geneticist in considering all the available data in a consistent manner.

The program we developed, GenePath, receives genetic information in a variety of forms, including prior knowledge, and provides an output in the form of a genetic network. Its primary source of data is a set of genetic experiments,

S. Quaglini, P. Barahona, and S. Andreassen (Eds.): AIME 2001, LNAI 2101, pp. 304–313, 2001.

where genes are either knocked out or activated, and specific functions (phenotype, *i.e.*, outcome of experiment and its magnitude) are analyzed. To relate genes and outcomes, GenePath uses a set of expert defined patterns, which, when applied to the data, identify constraints on the genetic network. GenePath constructs the genetic network either from such constraints directly, or combines constraints with a qualitative reasoning-based algorithm to identify a number of possible networks.

GenePath allows the user to examine the experimental evidence and the logic that were used to determine each relationship between genes. This feature allows a geneticist to interact with the data without becoming an expert in the specific problem under investigation. Furthermore, GenePath can generate several models that are consistent with the data and propose experimental tests that may help determine the most likely model. As such, GenePath is not intended to replace the researcher, but rather supports the process of cataloging and explorating genetic experiments and the derivation of genetic networks.

Notice that GenePath performs abductive inference. Given a *Theory* and *Observation*, the goal of abduction [3] is to find an explanation such that

$$Theory \cup Explanation \models Observation$$

That is, *Observation* follows logically from *Theory* and *Explanation*. In GenePath, *Observation* is a set of genetic experiments, *Theory* a background knowledge, and *Explanation* a set of constraints over the genetic network which are (in their form) limited with expert-defined inference patterns.

GenePath is implemented in the Prolog computer language [1]. Since it is a declarative language based on logic, Prolog is an excellent environment for this purpose: Prolog makes it easy to consistently encode the data, background knowledge and expert-defined patterns, and allows for a relatively straightforward integration of different GenePath's components.

The current paper begins with a general description of GenePath's architecture. An example of genetic data is given next, and in further sections the example is used to illustrate techniques developed within GenePath. Finally, we mention a few other successful cases of GenePath's use, briefly discuss the utility of GenePath, and conclude with a list of ideas for further work.

2   GenePath's Architecture

GenePath was designed to solve the following problem: given a set of genetic experiments and an optional background knowledge in the form of already known relations among genes and outcomes, derive the genetic network that is consistent with the data and background knowledge.

GenePath implements a framework for reasoning about genetic experiments and hypothesizing genetic networks. It consists of the following entities:

– *genetic data*, *i.e.*, experiments with mutations and corresponding outcomes,

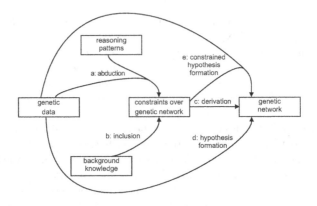

Fig. 1. GenePath's architecture

- *prior knowledge* in the form of known gene-to-gene and gene-to-outcome relations,
- *expert-defined patterns*, which are used by GenePath to abduce gene relations from genetic experiments,
- *abductive inference engine*, which is implemented in Prolog by matching encoded patterns with genetic data to obtain constraints over genetic network,
- *network synthesis methods*, that form networks (hypotheses) that are consistent with genetic data, abduced constraints and prior knowledge. A genetic network is a graph whose nodes correspond to genes and phenotypes, and arcs correspond to direct influences of genes on other genes and phenotypes.

The architecture of GenePath is shown in Figure 1. GenePath starts with abduction of relations between genes and outcomes (Figure 1.a). Additional relations directly obtained from prior knowledge are also added to the collection of abduced relations (b). They can be used directly to obtain a single genetic network (c). A set of possible genetic networks can also be derived through qualitative modeling directly from the data (d). In practice, a combined approach (e) may work best, where the abduced relations are used as constraints to filter out inconsistent networks generated by the qualitative approach.

3 Data and Background Knowledge

Experiments GenePath can consider are tuples of mutations and outcomes. Mutations are specified as a set of one or more genes with information on the type of mutation. A gene can be either knocked out (loss of function) or overexpressed (constitutive function). The outcome of an experiment is assessed through the description of a specific phenotype (e.g., cells grow, or cells do not grow, etc).

A data set that will be used to illustrate some of GenePath's functions is given in Table 1. The data comes from the studies of *Dictyostelium discoideum*, an organism that has a particularly interesting developmental cycle from single independent cells to a multicellular sluglike form (Figure 2). The transition from ordinary single cells to a multicellular structure is of great interest for biologists interested in the evolution and development of multicellular organisms [8,6,5].

Table 1. Genetic data set: aggregation of *Dictyostelium*

#	Genotype	Aggregation
1	wild-type	+
2	yakA-	-
3	pufA-	++
4	gdtB-	+
5	pkaR-	++
6	pkaC-	-
7	acaA-	-
8	regA-	++
9	acaA+	++
10	pkaC+	++
11	pkaC-, regA-	-
12	yakA-, pufA-	++
13	yakA-, pkaR-	+
14	yakA-, pkaC-	-
15	pkaC-, yakA+	-
16	yakA-, pkaC+	++
17	yakA-, gdtB-	±

The example data set focuses on cell aggregation. It includes seven genes: yakA, pufA, gdtB, pkaR, pkaC, acaA, and regA. Seventeen experiments were performed: in each (except for wild type) selected genes were either knocked out or overexpressed (denoted with "-" or "+", respectively). Observed aggregation was either normal ("+"), excessive ("++"), reduced ("±") or absent ("-"). Note that the aggregation level is an ordinal variable, with the order being -, ±, +, ++.

Background (prior) knowledge may be given to GenePath in the form of known parts of networks. For our example, GenePath was informed that it is already known that acaA inhibits pkaR, pkaR inhibits pkaC, which in turn excites aggregation. This can be formally denoted with a single path of acaA ⊣ pkaR ⊣ pkaC → aggregation, where → denotes excitation and ⊣ inhibition (for qualitative definition of these relations, see Section 5.2). The ultimate network is expected to include the partial networks given as prior knowledge.

4   Expert-Defined Patterns

GenePath's patterns determine the type of constraints that are abduced from data. They are implemented as Prolog clauses, and for a specific **Phenotype**, are used to determine the relation between two genes or the relation between

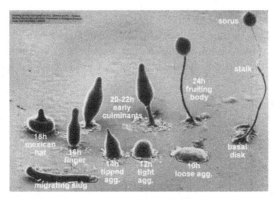

Fig. 2. Development of *Dictyostelium* (R. Blanton, M. Grimson, Texas Tech. Univ.)

a gene and an outcome. Every relation found is supported by the evidence in the form of the name of the pattern that was used to find the relation and experiments that support it. Where the pattern includes an `Influence`, this can be either "excites" or "inhibits" and is determined directly from the data. GenePath currently implements twelve patterns of four types:

1. *parallel*: both `GeneA` and `GeneB` influence `Phenotype`, but are on separate (parallel) paths;
2. *precedes*: `GeneA` precedes `GeneB` in a path for `Phenotype` (both genes are therefore on the same path);
3. *influences*: `GeneA` either excites or inhibits (`Influence`) the `Phenotype` or a downstream gene;
4. *not_influences*: `GeneA` does not influence the `Phenotype`.

One or more patterns exist for each type. For instance, there are three `precedes` and two `influences` patterns. To illustrate how the patterns are composed and matched with the data, we will discuss two patterns in detail.

4.1 A Pattern for Parallel Relation

There is currently a sole pattern for parallel relation called `parDiff`. It is implemented through the following predicate:

`parallel(GeneA,GeneB,parDiff:Exp1/Exp2/Exp3,Phenotype)`: *Let us have three experiments: single mutation of* `GeneA` *and outcome* `OA` *(Exp1), single mutation of* `GeneB` *and outcome* `OB`, *and double mutation of both* `GeneA` *and* `GeneB` *and outcome* `OAB`. *If* `OA` ≠ `OB`, `OA` ≠ `OAB`, *and* `OB` ≠ `OAB` *then* `GeneA` *and* `GeneB` *are on parallel paths to* `Phenotype`.   □

Two pairs of genes were matched by the above pattern:

```
parallel(yakA, pkaR, parDiff:2/5/13, aggregation)
parallel(yakA, gdtB, parDiff:2/4/17, aggregation)
```

GenePath has thus found that yakA should be on a different path to aggregation than pkaR, and on a different path to aggregation than gdtB. Notice also that the evidence for above is stated in terms of corresponding trio of experiments (Table 1) that matched the `parDiff` pattern. In this way, the geneticist can trace GenePath's findings back to the experiments.

4.2   A Pattern for Precedes Relation

One of the most important patterns for the construction of genetic networks in GenePath is pRev:

precedes(GeneA,GeneB,Influence,pRev:Exp1/Exp2/Exp3,Phenotype): *Let us have three experiments,* Exp1, Exp2, *and* Exp3. Exp1 *with mutations of* GeneA *and of some other, possibly empty set of genes* GeneSet, *has outcome* OA. Exp2 *with mutations of* GeneA, GeneB *and* GeneSet *has outcome* OAB. Exp3 *with mutations of* GeneB *and* GeneSet *has outcome* OB. *If* OAB = OB, *and the outcomes are ordered such that* WildType > OAB > OA *or* WildType < OAB < OA, *then* GeneB *is in the same path but after* GeneA.   □

Three sets of experiments matching `pRev` were found, identifying three important gene-to-gene relations:

```
precedes(regA,pkaC,inhibits,pRev:11/8/6, aggregation)
precedes(yakA,pkaC,excites, pRev:16/2/10,aggregation)
precedes(yakA,pufA,inhibits,pRev:12/2/3, aggregation)
```

5   Synthesis of Genetic Networks

GenePath can derive genetic networks either by satisfaction of abduced network constraints, by semi-arbitrary construction of genetic networks that are then tested on consistency with data through qualitative reasoning, and by a combined approach.

5.1   Derivation through Constraint Satisfaction

The mutual consistency of abduced network constraints is tested first. If conflicts are found – such as, for instance, a gene reported to not influence the phenotype and at the same type involved in corresponding precede relation – they are shown to the domain expert and resolved either by removal of one of the constraints in conflict, or through proper revision of data (if the error has been found there). For the paper's example, no conflicts in abduced constraints were detected. Upon examination by the domain expert (GS), we found that the constraints were also consistent with his knowledge. An exception was gene gdtB, which was found by GenePath to inhibit aggregation. Relying on the expert's comment, this constraint and gdtB were removed from further analysis. To the biologically oriented reader: the effect of mutating gdtB alone is not manifested in the aggregation step of development, but is revealed when aggregation is severely reduced by the absence of yakA. This is a common finding in genetics. We expect that biochemical studies will be required to decipher the function of gdtB and its relationship to yakA.

The construction of the genetic network is based on identification of *directly* related genes. GeneA and GeneB are assumed to be in direct relation if they are not on parallel paths and if no other gene is found that precedes GeneA and is at the same time preceded by GeneB. GenePath considers all the genes that influence the outcome and removes the genes that influence any other gene in the group. The remaining genes influence the outcome directly.

From our data set, three genes in direct relation were found: yakA → pkaC, regA ⊣ pkaC, and yakA ⊣ pufA. Together with prior knowledge, and GenePath's finding that all the genes from the experiments influence the aggregation, the resulting genetic network is as shown in Figure 3.a.

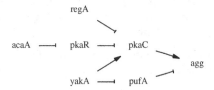

Fig. 3. Constraint satisfaction-derived genetic network

The constructed genetic network was examined by the domain expert (GS). He immediately realized that, while the network was in general consistent with his domain knowledge, the direct influence of pufA to aggregation was not expected. He commented that it is immediately evident (from the network and the set of neighboring genes) that relations between regA and most of the other genes, and between pufA and pkaC were not determined. Tracing this back to data, it is evident that experiments that would include any of these pairs are missing.

5.2   Derivation through Qualitative Reasoning

Alternatively to the approach described above, GenePath can in effect search through all potential networks and expose those that are consistent with the data. The method starts by determining how genes influence the outcome (Influences), constructs a candidate Network that accounts for these influences and checks if the Network is consistent with the data.

Influences are determined directly from single mutation experiments. To construct a Network that accounts for all the Influences, the following procedure is executed: For each influence path(Node1,Sign,Node2) it is ensured that there is a path in Network from Node1 to Node2 with cumulative influence Sign. Network is constructed gradually, starting from the initial network that contains no arcs. Then for each influence path(N1,Sign,N2) do:

if there is a path in the current network from N1 to N2 with
the cumulative influence Sign then do nothing,
else either add to the current network arc(N1,N2,Sign),
or add arc(N1,N,Sign1) for some node N in the current network, and
call the construct predicate recursively so that it also takes care
of another influence path(N,Sign2,N2) where Sign1*Sign2=Sign

Obviously, explaining the observed influences by constructing corresponding network models is a combinatorial process that involves search. This search is controlled by the following mechanisms that were elicited from the geneticists and reflect their preferential bias: (1) Among the models consistent with the data, look for models that minimize the total number of arcs. (2) Among the models with equal total number of arcs, first look for models with the smallest number of nodes' inputs.

The constructed models are checked for consistency with all the experiments by carrying out a qualitative simulation [7]. This simulation uses a qualitative semantics of the genetic networks. For instance, A→ B means: If A increases and all other things in the network stay equal, B also increases. For multiple direct influences (e.g., when the state of gene C directly depends on genes A and B), the meaning of the combined influence of A and B on C was chosen to be the qualitative summation.

The qualitative simulation-based approach was applied to our sample data set. Several thousands of networks comprising six to eight edges and consistent with the data set were derived – an obviously too large a number to be searched and analyzed by the expert.

5.3   Combined Approach

The combined approach derives genetic networks through qualitative reasoning, except that only those candidate networks that are consistent with the abduced constraints are considered. This substantially narrows the search space, and results in only four networks of low complexity (six edges in the network) that are consistent with abduced constraints and with experimental data (Figure 4).

The networks from Figure 4.c and d were discarded because they are inconsistent with our biochemical knowledge of the system. Although we preferred the network from Figure 4.a which is completely consistent with our knowledge and experience in the domain, we did not have experimental evidence in our sample data set (Table 1) to discard the network from Figure 4.b. Without that knowledge, additional experiments with appropriate Dictyostelium mutants would be required to decide in favor of one or the other.

6   Discussion

Besides a *Dictyostelium* aggregation genetic network, in its year-long existence GenePath has been tried on a number of other problems. Using 28 experiments,

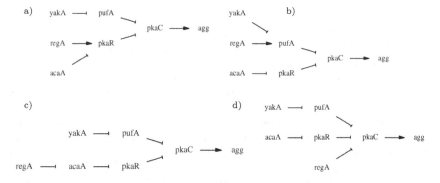

Fig. 4. Genetic networks proposed by combined approach

GenePath found a correct genetic network for growth and development of *Dictyostelium* that includes 5 genes [6,5]. From the data on 20 experiments, it successfully reconstructed the programmed cell death genetic network of *C. elegans* that involves four genes [4]. In its most severe test, 79 experiments involving 16 genes were presented to GenePath. Data was encoded: genes where not named but rather given an ID number, origin of data was unknown. At the start, GenePath pointed out the inconsistencies in the data and suggested a single gene that was a source of them. After that gene was excluded, GenePath developed a single solution in the form of a (linear) path that, when presented to the owner of the data, was confirmed to be correct and consistent with the one published [2].

What the case with aggregation of Dictyostelium and other cases tested by GenePath indicate, is that the constraints obtained through abduction are very useful. Since they are based on expert-defined patterns, they speak their language and are found easy to interpret. While the constraint satisfaction approach does not (formally) guarantee a solution consistent with the data (it only guarantees consistency with constraints abduced from data), it was often found that where there were enough experiments, it was this approach that found a sole (and correct) solution. However, especially when used in the domains where genetic networks are yet unknown, the combined approach should be the one of choice. In such setups, GenePath should be used as an intelligent assistant to support reasoning on network constraints, hypothesize a number of plausible networks, and (further work!) suggest experiments that would narrow down the choice of networks leading to a most probable and hopefully correct one.

With respect to scalability, the abductive part of GenePath should scale well: most GenePath's patterns are defined over a couple of genes and although the corresponding search space grows exponentially with number of genes considered, geneticists would usually investigate on regulatory networks that include at most a few dozen of genes. On the other hand, the complete hypothesis generator that involves qualitative reasoning may have problems. However, the types of experiments GenePath interprets are not in abundance: it often takes weeks of laboratory work for a single experiment in Table 1. GenePath performance is already sufficient for problems that involve up to 20 genes: this is also a current upper bound on the number of genes most usually considered in a geneticist's quest.

7 Conclusion

GenePath has been a subject of experimental verification for over a year, and is now approaching the point where it can assist geneticists, scholars and students in discovering and reasoning on genetic networks. There are a few improvements under development: a web-based interface to GenePath, and an enhancement that allows GenePath to propose experiments. These developments should enable GenePath to mature into a seamless intelligent assistant for reasoning on genetic networks.

References

[1] I. Bratko. *Prolog Programming for Artificial Intelligence*. Pearson Education / Addison-Wesley, Reading, MA, third edition, 2001.

[2] d. L. Riddle, M. M. Swanson, and P. S. Albert. Interacting genes in nematode dauer larva formation. *Nature*, (290):668–671, 1981.

[3] P. Flach. *Simply Logical: Intelligent Reasoning by Example*. John Wiley & Sons, 1994.

[4] M. M. Metzstein, G. M. Stanfield, and H. R. Horvitz. Genetics of programmed cell death in *C. elegans*: past, present and future. *Trends in Genetics*, 14(10):410–416, 1998.

[5] G. M. Souza, A. M. da Silva, and A. Kuspa. Starvation promotes dictyostelium development by relieving PufA inhibition of PKA translation through the YakA kinase pathway. *Development*, 126(14):3263–3274, 1999.

[6] G. M. Souza, S. Lu, and A. Kuspa. Yaka, a protein kinase, required for the transition from growth to development in *Dictyostelium*. *Development*, 125(12):2291–2302, 1998.

[7] D. S. Weld and J. de Kleer. *Readings in Qualitative Reasoning about Physical Systems*. Morgan Kaufmann, Los Altos, CA, 1990.

[8] C. Zimmer. The slime alternative. *Discover*, pages 86–93, May 1998.

Interface of Inference Models with Concept and Medical Record Models

Alan L. Rector[1], Peter D. Johnson[2], Samson Tu[3], Chris Wroe[1], and Jeremy Rogers[1]

[1]Medical Informatics Group, Dept of Computer Science, University of Manchester, UK
(arector jrogers wroec)@cs.man.ac.uk
[2]Sowerby Centre for Health Informatics in Newcastle, University of Newcastle upon Tyne, UK
pete@mimir.demon.co.uk
[3]Stanford Medical Informatics, Stanford University, USA
tu@SMI.Stanford.EDU

Abstract. Medical information systems and standards are increasingly based on principled models of at least three distinct sorts of information – patient data, concepts (terminology), and guidelines (decision support). Well defined interfaces are required between the three types of model to allow development to proceed independently. Two of the major issues to be dealt with in the defining of such interfaces are the interaction between ontological and inferential abstractions – how general notions such as 'abnormal cardiovascular finding' are abstracted from concrete data – and the management of the meaning of information in guidelines in different contexts. This paper explores these two issues and their ramifications.

1. Introduction

Medical Information systems and standards are increasingly based on principled models. Recent papers by two of the authors [1] [2] discussed the interface between three different types of models used by different groups to represent different aspects of clinical information:

1. *'Information' or 'patient-data' models* – the structure of the information to be stored, e.g. HL7's Reference Information Model (RIM) [3], CEN's Electronic Healthcare Record Architecture [4] or the models underlying GEHR's architecture [5, 6] typically expressed in UML object models. Also referred to as the 'Patient Data Model' [2]

2. *'Concept models' or 'ontologies'* – the meaning of what is stored (referred to in [2] as the 'medical specialty model'). In this framework, a 'terminology' consists of the combination of a 'concept model' plus one or more 'lexicons' supplying natural language words to signify the concepts. For example, SNOMED-RT's compositional representation [7] or GALEN's Common Reference Model [8, 9] are concept models in this sense. Concept models are typically expressed in hierarchies, frame systems, or their more modern successors, description logics.

3. *'Inference' models* – models that encapsulate knowledge needed to derive the conclusions, decisions, and actions that follow from what is stored. In this paper,

S. Quaglini, P. Barahona, and S. Andreassen (Eds.): AIME 2001, LNAI 2101, pp. 314–323, 2001.

4. we will use models of clinical guidelines and protocols as examples of such inference models, although the issues discussed here apply to medical decision-support systems more generally *e.g.* Medical Logic Modules (MLMs) [10] EON [11], Prodigy [12], *PROF*orma [13] or GLIF [14].

This tripartite functional division mirrors an analysis of the operational information requirements of guideline-based decision-support systems in which those information needs are divided into two broad categories and the second category divided again into two further categories as follows:

1. *Information about specific patients and clinical situations* – information gathered from healthcare workers about clinical observations and results and also, potentially, inferences made by guidelines or other software agents based on the human input.

2. *General patient-independent information about medicine and medical practice (also known as 'domain knowledge')* This information can be subdivided further:

2a. *Guideline independent static knowledge* – definitions and intensions of concepts and closely associated facts such as indications and contraindications of drugs, causes and symptoms of diseases, and mechanisms of tests and procedures which are both relatively independent of individual guidelines and directly linked to particular concepts without complex inference.

2b. *Guideline dependent dynamic knowledge* – the model of how to infer conclusions and decisions from the patient specific information and guideline independent facts.

Our assumption is that the goal is to express protocols or guidelines for care in an executable form that interacts with an electronic patient record (and broader clinical information systems). We assume that the key elements in inference models are 'criteria' – logical expressions which trigger inferences or actions. In order to execute a guideline for a specific patient, criteria from the inference model must be transformed into queries against the corresponding electronic patient record. We assume that in principle each model specifies a corresponding repository of information - patient records, dynamic executable guidelines, and static domain information respectively. We assume, however, that electronic patient records and clinical information systems will continue to be designed largely independently from any reusable guideline-based decision-support systems. Therefore it is essential to design a clean and well defined interface between them.

This architecture is shown graphically in Figure 1. The three models are shown as boxes shadowed by their respective repositories. For clarity, the number referring to the type the classification above is shown in brackets with each repository. The interfaces are shown as 'lenses'. Each interface is bi-directional. In each direction, each interface filters and transforms information so that the receiving model sees only that portion of the originating model and associated repository that is relevant for its own purposes – as symbolised by the arrows emerging from each model as multiple broad lines and continuing on from the interface as single thin lines. As well as carrying information, the arrows carry obligations. Each interface places mutual obligations on the two models it connects, and all these obligations must be coherent – as symbolised by the overlap of the interfaces at the centre of the drawing.

The architecture in figure 1 raises many questions. This paper examines two important issues –

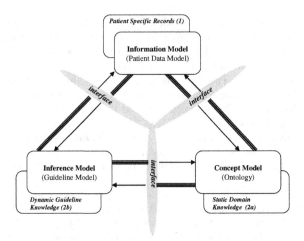

Fig. 1. Interfaces, Models and corresponding repositories

1. Expressing the abstractions in guideline criteria operationally in terms of the patient-specific information in the medical record
2. Relating patient independent information to individual patients in the clinical context and how to partition this information between the concept and inference models.

The ideas will be illustrated by examples drawn from the UK Department of Health sponsored PRODIGY project developing guidelines for chronic disease prescribing in primary care [12].

2. Abstraction and Operationalisation

The main barriers to successfully expressing guideline criteria in a form compatible with an electronic patient record (EPR) system are closely related:

1. *Differences in granularity and axes of classification:* The information in the criteria may not be expressed at the same granularity as in the medical record or the relevant abstraction may be missing in the terminology used in the record, e.g. there is no single code for "steroid" in most standard drug classifications, although there are codes for all of the individual drugs in question and abstractions for covering various subclasses of steroids (e.g. "topically applied steroids").
2. *Need for inferential abstractions:* Some information may be recorded as raw measurements which need to be interpreted before use - *e.g.* "elevated white cell count" may never be explicitly recorded by the user but must instead be inferred from a range of values. .
3. *Ambiguity of operational meaning:* The criteria in a written guideline may not correspond to any obvious information likely to be ever recorded in the medical record, *e.g.* "tendency to prolonged ST interval".
4. *Differences in encapsulation and form of expression:* There are almost always many different ways in which the same information can be packaged or 'encapsulated' (see [1]). Information expected as a code-value pair in one

('melanoma' + 'metastatic'), may be represented as a single code ('metastatic melanoma'), or as a code plus a series of modifiers in the other ('neoplasm' + 'melanocyte' + 'malignant' + 'metastatic').

Each of the above issues will be discussed in turn.

2.1 Ontological and Inferential Abstractions

The information recorded in medical records is usually fine grained and specific – concrete findings, diagnoses, drugs, procedures, etc. The criteria in guidelines are usually expressed as abstractions of such findings. Ontological abstraction bridges the difference in granularity between the information in the record and that being looked for by the guidelines. Roughly, the requirement is that the concept model be capable of classifying the information in the medical record under the abstractions used in the guideline.

Unfortunately, many standard terminologies cannot make this link reliably. For example, the example of the absent category "Steroid" in the current drug classifications used by the British National Formulary (BNF) is typical: although the classification provides for various types of steroids, e.g. "topical steroids," it does not provide all needed generalisations at the correct granularity.

There are at least two reasons for these failures or omissions:

1. The axis of classification required may not exist in the concept system or may not exist consistently throughout the system – e.g. 'indication' may not be used consistently as an axis and 'contraindication' may not exist as an axis of classification at all.
2. The concept system may be structured primarily for navigation using mixed axes, i.e. they are structured as 'thesauri' rather than as formal classifications [9]. Abstraction works reliably only along strict subsumption ("is-a") hierarchies in formal classifications. ICD, the Read Codes v1 and v2 and most drug classifications are examples of thesauri in this sense.

Inferential abstraction, by contrast, is required when a criterion used in a protocol cannot be determined by simple logical operations directly from the meaning of individual terms in the medical record. This occurs in several situations:

1. When a single quantitative item of data or very specific observation needs to be converted to a qualitative abstraction using mathematical or logical inferences beyond the restricted set provided by the concept model – e.g. to convert a blood pressure of 190/110 to "elevated blood pressure".
2. When a quantitative summary value must be calculated from several other values in the medical record – e.g. body mass index, predicted peak expiratory flow rate, or cardiovascular risk probability.
3. When a temporal abstraction must infer a state or trend from several items of information in the record – e.g. to obtain an abstraction such as "rising blood pressure" or "on steroids for more than three months". Such inferences often depend on the clinical context and locality as well as the raw data (see [15]).
4. When the required abstraction cannot reliably be found in the medical record and must be inferred from proxies.

It is a common feature of inferential abstraction that it is defeasible, i.e. that subsequently acquired information may invalidate an earlier inference. This is particularly common in dealing with temporal abstraction or proxies in the medical record.

The details of inferential abstraction depend on three sets of issues:

1. *Operational issues* – what information is likely, in practice, to be in the patient record. Presented with a paper guideline, human readers will make the necessary inferential leaps. Computer assisted guidelines must specify them explicitly, which involves formalising the intuitions by which by which much medical data is actively reconstructed as part of the decision making process rather than predefined [16]. This is made more difficult by the fact that the medical record is rarely either complete or consistent - *e.g.*a recent British study found that "Ischaemic Heart Disease" was recorded in less than half the relevant cases in general practice [17].

2. *Issues of clinical context* – what are the criteria for a given inference and in what contexts is it permissible, safe, and/or necessary to make it. These often involve subtle distinctions in usage – the entry criteria for an asthma treatment guideline may be different from the criteria used to trigger warnings concerning drugs contraindicated in asthma – or local conventions – *e.g.* Two different guidelines may have different entry criteria, or two different authorities may have different criteria for when the risk of bronchospasm is sufficient to trigger a warning

3. *Formal issues* – how should the criteria be expressed formally internally and with respect to the information and terminology models.

As a practical example, in the PRODIGY guidelines it has been determined *operationally* by experience that a diagnosis of "asthma" is not always recorded in patients who should be recognised as matching the criterion "contraindicated in asthma". *Clinically* it has been decided that more than one episode of "wheezing" in the past year is but one of the proxy criteria sufficient to count as "asthma" for these purposes. *Formally* the criteria are represented as logical expressions in which the terms ultimately map to sets of Clinical Terms (Read Codes).

2.2   Ambiguity of Operational Meaning

Written guidelines are written for human interpretation. It is not sufficient to represent a notion found in a text guideline or warning 'literally'; it must also be operationally and clinically useful and effective to do so.

For example the British National Formulary contains references to drugs being contraindicated in the presence of a "tendency to prolonged ST intervals". Even an experienced physician might have to think twice as to what this meant in terms of the concepts represented in an electronic patient record. However, since it is a recurring phrase, it is worth attempting to capture it in a general way, *e.g.* as any suggestion of heart block. This in turn suggests defining an inferential abstraction for "suggestion of heart block".

2.3   Differences in Encapsulation and Structure amongst Models

The structure of encapsulation used in various inference and information models differs widely. Encapsulation is a key issue for the interface between the information and concept models [1], and analogous issues exist with the inference model.

For example, the Arden Syntax assumes that patient data can be represented as lists of time-stamped values [18]. It defines a criteria language that includes operators to manipulate such lists (e.g., *latest* or *merge*) and make comparisons of values and of timestamps (e.g., *greater than* or *is before*). Prodigy, by contrast, assumes that information about patients can be expressed as instances of structured objects, such as *Investigation_Result* and *Note_Entry,* having time stamps or time intervals denoting periods of validity. A *Note_Entry*, for example, specifies a domain concept and a time interval during which the condition represented by the concept is present. Eon, meanwhile, represents information as part of a temporal database that permits complex temporal queries and abstractions. None of these three inference models correspond directly to any commonly used medical record model.

There are three approaches to this problem:

1. *Ad hoc* mapping
2. *Use a standards-based information model* such the HL7 RIM, CEN's EHRC or GEHR.
3. *Creating a virtual medical record* within the inference model and define a mapping from that model to each individual information model

In the *ad hoc* approach, exemplified by Arden Syntax for Medical Logic Modules, differences in encapsulation are dealt with by *ad hoc* programmes. The alternative is to base the mapping on a standard information model and associated interchange format such as the HL7 RIM or CEN's EHRC.

There are two difficulties with this approach: a) Achieving a standard view to meet the requirements of both the interface and information models may be difficult. b) No currently existing medical record systems are based firmly on the RIM or any similar standard, although several are in construction. To circumvent these problems both the PRODIGY and EON systems have defined 'virtual medical record systems' – in effect medical record models tailored to the needs of the guideline system.

3. Static Domain Information and Context

One of the major benefits of using modern ontological methods is that they are an effective means of organising complex sets of special cases along multiple axes. For example systematically creating notions such as "normal range for haemoglobin for a patient in renal failure". In principle, this can even be extended to capture local policies   "maximum dose of inhaled steroid for a patient on local research on research protocols".

This approach provides two important benefits:

1. *Safety and consistency* – General policies can be implemented that can only be overridden explicitly – *e.g.* to express a generalisation that "beta blockers are contraindicated by the risk of bronchospasm" but include specific exceptions for certain beta blockers in specific clinical situations. In this way any new beta blocker will 'inherit' the contraindication unless it is explicitly overridden.
2. *Scalability* – The total number of such special cases is potentially combinatorially explosive. As the number of guidelines and variants increases, managing the underlying information consistently becomes increasingly difficult. This is most obvious currently in fields such as drug information, but as guideline libraries grow in size, it can be expected to become an increasingly important issue.

Given such a broader ontological knowledge base, there may be tight integration between ontological and inferential abstraction and between the concept and inference models. For inferential abstraction, the inference itself must be represented in the inference model, but the information used by the inference and further abstractions from that initial inference may be represented in the ontology – *e.g.* both the concept of the lower bound for a normal white-blood cell count (WBC) and the concept represented by the qualitative abstraction – *e.g.* "leukopoenia" – might be represented in the ontology. The inference from a specific measured value to the corresponding qualitative abstraction – *i.e.*, the criteria that relates the lower bound to the abstraction – resides in the inference model.

4. Example

Consider the criteria in the example below of a condition action rule from a decision support system:

IF
CRITERIA:
    a patient has a diagnosis of *confirmed hypertension* recorded AND the patient has either
        diabetes mellitus OR
        persistent highly elevated cholesterol OR
        a *family history of heart disease*
    AND the patient has *no renal disease*
    AND the patient is on no *drug* with a *serious interaction* to *chronic therapy* with *ACE inhibitors*
THEN
INFERENCE: an *ACE inhibitor* is a candidate treatment for the *hypertension*"

Taking the concepts in turn, the construct "a diagnosis of … recorded" must be mapped to a corresponding encapsulation in the information model.

"Confirmed hypertension" may be specific to this protocol *"confirmed hypertension as per guideline_h_23"*. Alternatively, it may be a locally tailorable notion in the ontology used by several different guidelines, or a widely agreed concept within a clinical community. Whichever, the implication is that it is a predefined notion either entered directly by a clinician or, alternatively, was inferred earlier from a machine analysis of a series of documented blood pressure readings. It may be that the ontology allows for specialisations of such concepts, so that it includes, for example, "confirmed surgical hypertension", "confirmed essential hypertension", "confirmed renin dependent hypertension", etc. An ontology might provide a range of such notions, possibly with criteria for each. Alternatively, a post-co-ordinated concept system might provide a general notion of 'confirmed' which could be either entered or inferred.

The concept *"diabetes mellitus"* may be found literally or, more likely, will require simple ontological abstraction from either "insulin dependent diabetes mellitus" or "non-insulin dependent diabetes mellitus", being those terms at the minimum level of disambiguation that is clinically useful or necessary and, therefore, what is likely to be in the record. Additionally, it might be inferred by proxy for patients taking injectable insulin even in the absence of any diabetes-related diagnosis term.

"Persistent highly elevated cholesterol" by contrast will usually require two steps of inferential abstraction. Step one is to abstract from each numerical measurement of cholesterol, to determine whether or not it meets the definition of "highly elevated cholesterol". The second, to abstract from a temporal series of such abstractions, determining whether the elevation is persistent. Alternatively, a more sophisticated temporal abstraction mechanism might perform the two operations together.

"Family history of heart disease" and *"no renal disease"* present superficially analogous problems. Firstly the encapsulation and representation of "family history of ..." and "no ..." must be determined from the interface to the information model. Secondly, there is the question of what constitutes "Heart disease" and "Renal disease". In principle, the second step ought to be a matter of ontological abstraction. In the case of "family history of heart disease" this is probably sufficient or at least all that is possible. However, in context, this may not be sufficient for "no renal disease". Since this is in the context of a contraindication, it should be reformulated as a more sensitive criterion such as "no evidence suggesting renal disease" and inferred from the medical record.

"No serious contraindication to *chronic therapy* with *ACE inhibitors"* requires coping with the issues of negation and the interface to the information model for drugs, and a rich ontological knowledge base able to perform the ontological abstractions indicated by *"...serious contraindication* to *chronic therapy* with..."

5. Consequences for the Interface

The above analysis suggests a number of requirements for the interface from the inference model to the information and concept models and amongst the three models.
1. Amongst the three models:
   - *Consistency of meaning:* The meaning of all concepts used, wherever they appear, must be the same. In principle, all should be derived from the definitions in the concept model.
   - *Unambiguous encapsulation of information between information and concept models:* In order for "family history of heart disease" and "no renal disease" to be represented unambiguously, the interface between the concept model and the information model must specify responsibility and structures for status concepts such as "family history of ..."
2. From the inference model to the patient information model
   - *Adequacy of structure:* The information model must hold the patient information necessary to determine if criteria are satisfied, in the example above this implies at least "observation", "diagnosis", "laboratory test result", "drug sensitivity" and "medication", but a more complete analysis would extend this list.
3. From the inference model to the concept model
   - *Axes of the concept model and ontological knowledge base:* The interaction check requires that interactions be held in the ontological KB, in the example that it include an appropriate notion of the seriousness, and that the use of the

drug and whether it is acute or chronic be axes along which interactions are classified.

- *Level of abstraction in the concept model:* The inference model requires abstractions at the level of "diabetes mellitus", "renal disease" and "heart disease" to be provided by the concept model.
- *Content of the ontological knowledge base:* The inferential abstraction from laboratory values to "persistently highly elevated cholesterol" will require relevant thresholds to be stored in the ontological knowledge base. If "no renal disease" is to be obtained by inferential abstraction, it too will require relevant thresholds in the ontological knowledge base.

6. Discussion

Parts of the architecture in Figure 1 have been implemented in by various groups, but a complete implementation in which the interfaces are well enough specified to allow easy integration and scaling has yet to be achieved.

For example, the 'virtual medical record' in PRODIGY and EON can be regarded as a 'thick' version of the interface between the inference and information models. The inference model side of the interface is well defined, but the information model and its mapping to site-specific electronic medical-record system consists still of *ad hoc* programming[2]. HL7's Message Development Framework (MDF) [19] with its progression from a Reference Information Model (RIM) through a Message Information Model (MIM) to a Refined Message Information Model (R-MIM) represents one part of an interface from the Information Model to the Inference Model, which potentially deals with many issues of encapsulation and transformation, but within a framework in which each message must be worked out (almost) individually. GALEN's perspective mechanism [20] and the proposed SNOMED-CT subset mechanism [21], each provide parts of the interface between the ontological knowledge base and the inference and information models, but neither is fully formalised and neither deals adequately with the mutual obligations required to represent unambiguously negation and notions such as "family history of" ('status concepts'). A more systematic approach to these issues is sketched in a previous paper [1] but is far from being implemented.

Standard frame systems such as those derived from PROTÉGÉ used in EON provide a knowledge base linked to a relatively simple ontology. The UK Drug Ontology is moving towards representation of context within the ontological knowledge base as did the PEN&PAD user interface [22], but the mechanisms used need to be generalised and formalised.

There remains a question as to whether 'abstraction' in the sense used in this paper should remain an emergent property of cooperation between the three models or requires a separate mechanism such as the Tzolkin module used in the EON architecture [2].

Putting all of the pieces together remains a challenge. New technical frameworks such as those provided by Franconi [23] for schema evolution and the development of standards for computable ontologies – the Ontology Inference Layer (OIL) [24] may provide further tools. However, what is urgently needed are practical tools for defining each interface.

References

1. Rector, A.L. The Interface between Information, Terminology, and Inference Models. in Medinfo-2001 (2001) (in press).
2. Tu, S.W. and M.A. Musen. Modeling data and knowledge in the EON guideline architecture. in Medinfo 2001 (2001) (in press).
3. HL7, HL7 Data Model Development, (2000), http://www.hl7.org/library/data-model/
4. CEN/WG1, ENV13606: Electronic Healthcare Record Architecture, . 1999, CEN.
5. Ingram, D., GEHR: The Good European Health Record, in Health in the New Communications Age, M. Laires, M. Ladeira, and J. Christensen, Editors. IOS Press: Amsterdam. (1995) 66-74.
6. Education, C.f.H.I.a.M., The GEHR Homepage, (1997), http://www.cww.chime.ucl.ac.uk/HealthI/GEHR/
7. Spackman, K.A., K.E. Campbell, and R.A. Côté, SNOMED-RT: A reference Terminology for Health Care. Journal of the American Medical Informatics Association (JAMIA), ((Symposium special issue)): .(1997) 640-644.
8. OpenGALEN, *Open*GALEN Home Page, www.opengalen.org
9. Rector, A., Thesauri and formal classifications: Terminologies for people and machines. Methods of Information in Medicine, . 37(4-5): .(1998) 501-509.
10. Pryor, T. and G. Hripscsak, The Arden syntax for medical logic modules. Int J Clin Monit Comput, . 10(4): .(1993) 214-224.
11. Tu, S.W. and M.A. Musen. A flexible approach to guideline modelling. in AMIA Fall Symposium. Hanley and Belfus (1999) 420-424.
12. Johnson, P.D., *et al.*, Using scenarios in chronic disease management guidelines for primary care. JAMIA, (Symposium Special Issue): .(2000) 389-393.
13. Fox, J. and S. Das, Safe and Sound. , Cambridge MA: MIT Press. (2000) .
14. Peleg, M., *et al.* GLIF3: The evolution of a guideline representation format. in AMIA Fall Symposium (2000) 645-649.
15. Shahr, Y. Timing is everything: temporal reasoning and temporal data maintenance in medicine. in Seventh Joint European Conference on Artificial Intelligence in Medicine and Medical Decision Making. Springer Verlag (1999)
16. Berg, M., Medical work and the computer-based patient record: A sociological perspective. Methods of Information in Medicine, . 37: .(1998) 294-301.
17. Bray, J., *et al.*, Identifying patients with ischaemic heart disease in general practice: cross sectional study of paper and computerised medical records. British Medical Journal, . 321: .(2000) 548-050.
18. Hripscak, G., *et al.* The Arden Syntax for Medical Logic Modules. in Fourteenth Annual Symposium on Computer Applications in Medical Care (SCAMC-90). McGraw Hill (1990)
19. HL7, HL7 Home Page, www.hl7.org
20. Solomon, W., *et al.*, Having our cake and eating it too: How the GALEN Intermediate Repre-sentation reconciles internal complexity with users' requirements for appropriateness and simplicity. Journal of the American Medical Informatics Association, (Fall Symposium Special Issue): .(2000) 819-823.
21. College of American Pathologists, SNOMED Home Page, www.snomed.org
22. Nowlan, W.A., Clinical workstation: Identifying clinical requirements and understanding clinical information. International Journal of Bio-Medical Computing, . 34: .(1994) 85-94.
23. Franconi, E. A Semantic approach for schema evolution and versioning in object-oriented databases. in 6th International Conference on Rules and Objects in Databases (DOOD'2000) (2000)
24. The OIL Home Page, (2000), www.ontoknowledge.org/oil/

Integrating Ripple Down Rules with Ontologies in an Oncology domain

Rodrigo Martínez-Béjar[1][*], Francisca Ibañez-Cruz[1], Paul Compton[3],

Jesualdo Tomás Fernández-Breis[1] and Manuel De las Heras-González[2]

[1]Departamento de Ingeniería de la Información y de las Comunicaciones, Universidad de Murcia, 30071 Espinardo (Murcia), Spain. Phone: + 34 968 364634, Fax: + 34 968 364151, E-mail: rodrigo@dif.um.es; jfernand@perseo.dif.um.es

[2]Oncology Service, Virgen de la Arrixaca Hospital, Murcia, Spain

[2]Department of Artificial Intelligence, School of Computer Science and Engineering, University of New South Wales, Sydney, Australia. Phone:+61(0)293853980, Fax:+61(0)293851814, E-mail:compton@cse.unsw.edu.au

Abstract: An ontology can be seen as an specification of a domain knowledge conceptualisation. Nowadays, ontological engineering is a widespread manner to achieve knowledge reuse and sharing that has been applied to clinical domains. Ripple Down Rules is a user-centred approach that allows users to perform knowledge acquisition as well as system maintenance. In this work, we show an approach through which users can specify conceptualisations and perform knowledge acquisition and system maintenance. The approach has been applied in oncology.

1 Introduction

The motivation for this work is an ongoing project whose goal is that the users connected to a system be able to incrementally both fill knowledge bases and update them without any human support from their workplaces. In other words, there is a need for a user-centred approach. Nowadays, ontology engineering is an effective manner to ensure knowledge reuse and sharing [3]. Ontologies, which have been used for representing knowledge in clinical domains [4], are viewed as specifications of a domain knowledge conceptualisation [5] and are represented by means of *multiple hierarchical restricted domains* (MHRD), which are sets of concepts defined each through a set of attributes. Taxonomic and partonomic relations among concepts are admissible.

---

[*] Correspondence author

S. Quaglini, P. Barahona, and S. Andreassen (Eds.): AIME 2001, LNAI 2101, pp. 324–327, 2001.
Springer-Verlag Berlin Heidelberg 2001

On the other hand, Ripple-Down Rules (RDR) [1] is both an incremental Knowledge Acquisition (KA) technique and a knowledge-based system (KBS) construction methodology based on a user-centred philosophy.

The aim of this work was to develop an integrated knowledge-based solution that allowed users both to specify a conceptualisation (through ontological technology) and acquire as well as maintaining the KBS for which that conceptualisation had be done (through RDR technology). For it, Multiple Classification Ripple-Down Rules (MCRDR), now the most widely used RDR technology, is integrated with an ontological framework through which they can form cases and establish/maintain KBs. We illustrate the usefulness of the new approach with the application to an oncology domain, where a medical doctor built and maintained a KBS prototype.

2 About Ripple-Down Rules (RDR)

RDR [1, 2] provides both a methodology and specific technology. The key features of the methodology are the following. A task is identified which has the following characteristics: (1) there is an information system, which outputs case data; (2) there is a need for expert interpretation of this case data; (3) it is normal or convenient for experts to monitor the output case data, and in doing so can monitor the output of the KBS as a part of this activity. Sufficient data modelling and software engineering is carried out to enable case data to be passed to the KBS from the information system, processed by the KBS, and to be presented to experts in a suitable way for them to identify features and add rules. An RDR system embodying standard RDR technology, and the further developments required to deal with cases in the domain is then put into routine use. If during monitoring a case is identified where the KBS output is incorrect in some way, the expert enters the correct conclusion for that part of the output and the case is flagged for rule updating. The KBS is then updated. However, only a single component of the system is output – a single rule conclusion is corrected at a time.

When rules are updated, the expert is shown a display of the case, perhaps also a previously stored case (a cornerstone case) and perhaps also a list of the differences between the two cases which perhaps also highlights possibly important features. However, it should be noted that this assistance is not critical as the expert has already identified features in the case in deciding that the initial conclusion was incorrect. The expert selects sufficient features to construct a rule to eliminate relevant cornerstone cases, (the expert also has the option of assigning the conclusion to cornerstone cases, if appropriate. This can occur when a system is developed piecemeal, and it has become appropriate to make a more complete response to a case.). The system adds the rule to the KB, so that it will be evaluated in a fixed sequence, namely, the input case is added into the cornerstone case database and linked to the new rule, or either the case is rerun and more components of the conclusion may be changed by a repetition of the knowledge acquisition process. The major KA-related motivation of the present work is to provide an explicit ontological framework for Multiple Classification RDR (MCRDR) systems dealing with domains for which manual input and human judgement are required.

3 The Reusable, Shareable Framework

We have designed and implemented a software tool in Java with two modules supporting MCRDR inference and ontology construction respectively. The ontology is used for conceptualizing the domain so that, a consistent domain conceptualization can be obtained. On the other hand, the RDR part makes use of the ontological entities defined in the ontology. Therefore, the RDR and the ontological part are complementary each other. The ontology can be specified through a text file with the following format for each concept of the ontology: name of the concept; number and list of alternative names for the concept.; number and list of the specific attributes (name and values); number and list of mereological parent concepts; number and list of taxonomic parent concepts; number and list of specializations (pairs <name of attribute, name of taxonomic parent> standing that the current concept is a classification of this taxonomic parent through the attribute of the specialisation).

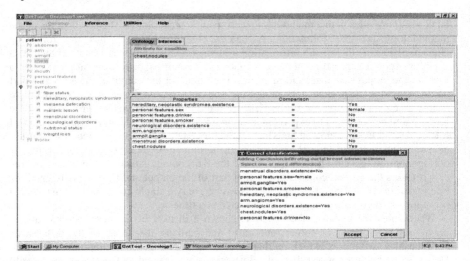

Fig. 1. A maintenance session with the tool.

Figure 1 shows an example of a maintenance session in an oncology domain. In this figure, by clicking on the ontology, the expert has formed an input case. Moreover, the differences between the input case and a cornerstone case associated with the ultimate true rule in the rule trace assist the medical doctor to select the features for the new rule, its location being supplied by the rule trace. Note also that the medical doctor decided to correct the previous conclusion with a new one and a condition list is shown to her/him from where conditions can be selected. With MCRDR there may be multiple cornerstone cases associated with a rule. For example at the top level all the cases in the system will reach a new rule. However, normally no more than two or three cases have to be seen it before all the cornerstone cases are excluded. In this context, our main evaluation of the tool has consisted of applying it to breast cancer diagnosis.

4 Conclusion

Ripple-down rules (RDR) can be viewed as a methodology for incrementally building knowledge-based systems where both the knowledge acquisition process and maintenance are performed by the domain experts. Despite the fact that RDR has been successful as a problem-solving method, this methodology fails to explicitly provide end-users with both the structure and the vocabulary associated to the domain knowledge they are dealing with for a particular task. This makes the approach of doubtful benefit when dealing with domains where the user manually constructs the case based on human judgement and more generally is an impediment for re-using and sharing domain knowledge.

Reusable, shareable domain knowledge ontologies constitute an important research area in the development of knowledge-based systems. Their purpose is to supply mechanisms for constructing domain knowledge from reusable components. In this work, we have utilised a formal framework that allows for the structured extraction and verification of domain knowledge ontologies while experts enter knowledge (through conceptual hierarchies) to an RDR system.

By integrating the ontology philosophy with the RDR one, we have described the main characteristics of a tool that enables experts to construct and verify domain knowledge ontologies for Multiple Classification (MC) RDR systems. As a first application of the tool, medical doctors succeeded in constructing a Knowledge Base containing knowledge to make cancer diagnoses from the symptoms and data contained in cases.

Acknowledgements: The last author is supported by the Fundación Séneca, Centro de Coordinación para la Investigación through the Programa Séneca.

References

[1] Compton, P., Horn, R., Quinlan, R. and Lazarus, L.: Maintaining an expert system, In J. R. Quinlan (Eds.), Applications of Expert Systems (1989), 366-385, London, Addison Wesley.
[2] Compton, P., and Jansen, R.: A philosophical basis for knowledge acquisition, Knowledge Acquisition, 2 (1990):241-257.
[3] Fridman-Noy, N. and Hafner, C. D.: Ontological foundations for experimental science knowledge bases, Applied Artificial Intelligence, 14 (2000):565-618.
[4] Shahar, Y., and Musen, M.A.: Knowledge-based Temporal Abstraction in Clinical Domains. Artificial Intelligence in Medicine 8(3) (1996) 267-298.
[5] Van Heijst, G., Schreiber, A. T., and Wielinga, B. J.: Using explicit ontologies in KBS development, International Journal of Human-Computer Studies (1997), 45: 183-292.

Towards a Simple Ontology Definition Language (SOntoDL) for a Semantic Web of Evidence-Based Medical Information

Rolf Grütter and Claus Eikemeier

Institute for Media and Communications Management, University of St. Gallen,
Müller-Friedberg-Strasse 8, CH-9000 St. Gallen, Switzerland
{rolf.gruetter, claus.eikemeier}@unisg.ch

Abstract. This paper documents the development of a Simple Ontology Definition Language (SOntoDL). The development is part of a project aimed at the implementation of an ontology-based semantic navigation through the glossary of an evidence-based medical information service on the WWW. The latest version of SOntoDL is integrated with the RDF/RDFS framework thereby providing for the foundation of a Semantic Web of evidence-based medical information.

1 Introduction

It is the vision of the protagonists of the Semantic Web to achieve „a set of connected applications for data on the WWW in such a way as to form a consistent logical web of data" ([1], p. 1). Therefore, the Semantic Web approach develops languages for expressing information in a machine-processable form. Particularly, the Resource Description Framework, RDF and RDF Schema, RDFS are considered as the logical foundations for the implementation of the Semantic Web.

This paper documents the development of a Simple Ontology Definition Language (SOntoDL). The development is part of a project aimed at the implementation of an ontology-based semantic navigation through the glossary of an evidence-based medical information service on the WWW. The latest version of SOntoDL is integrated with the RDF/RDFS framework thereby providing for the foundation of a Semantic Web of evidence-based medical information.

2 Methods: The Concept of the Ontology

The applied conceptual framework refers to the ontology as defined by Gruber [2]. According to Gruber, an ontology is a specification of a conceptualization, i.e., a formal description of the concepts and their relations for a „universe of discourse". The universe of discourse refers to the set of objects which can be represented in order to represent the (propositional) knowledge of a domain. This set of objects and the

S. Quaglini, P. Barahona, and S. Andreassen (Eds.): AIME 2001, LNAI 2101, pp. 328–331, 2001.
© Springer-Verlag Berlin Heidelberg 2001

describable relations among them are reflected in a representational vocabulary. In an ontology, definitions associate the names of objects in the universe of discourse with human-readable text, describing what the names mean, and formal axioms constrain the interpretation and well-formed use of the ontology. In short, an ontology consists of the triple (vocabulary, definitions, axioms). Formally, an ontology is the statement of a logical theory.

3 Results: Towards a Simple Ontology Definition Language

The development process of SOntoDL was guided by the following requirements (since the language should be kept as simple as possible, not all were specified in advance, instead, the list was completed during the development process):

(1) The language format must allow for an easy integration with the WWW.

(2) Since the knowledge base of the given domain evolves with time, the language must allow for an easy extension of the ontology without requiring the modification of the program, i.e., inference engine, that processes the ontology.

(3) The language should be applicable not only to the given application domain but also to additional domains.

(4) The language should support the physically dissociated (i.e., distributed) maintenance of representational vocabulary and human-readable definitions, as the two do not require the same frequency of updates and the respective editors may not be the same.

(5) The language should allow for the representation of complex, non-hierarchical knowledge structures.

(6) The language should allow to distinguish between generic (IS-A) and partitive (PART-OF) relations thereby providing enough conceptual expressiveness to support an easy handling of the representational vocabulary from a formal-logical point of view.

(7) The language should be integrated into a common logical framework for connected applications on the WWW thereby taking advantage of a range of tools (hopefully) being developed.

```
<!ELEMENT ontology (item*)>
<!ATTLIST ontology version CDATA  #FIXED "1.1">
<!ELEMENT item (identifier+,description, item*)>
<!ATTLIST item myID NMTOKEN #IMPLIED>
<!ELEMENT identifier (#PCDATA)>
<!ATTLIST identifier language (english | german | french)
#REQUIRED>
<!ATTLIST identifier format (short | long) #REQUIRED>
<!ELEMENT description (#PCDATA)>
<!ATTLIST description language (english | german | french)
#REQUIRED>
<!ATTLIST description implementation (html|url) #REQUIRED>
```

Fig. 1. Basic approach towards a simple ontology definition language

The basic approach defines an ontology definition language by an XML Document Type Definition (DTD) (Fig. 1). Most of the element types denote generic concepts such as item, identifier, and description. „Generic" means in this context that the concepts do not refer to a particular application domain (e.g., Evidence-Based Medicine, EBM). In addition, since the element type ontology includes zero, one or more item(s) (denoted by the symbol *) and each item, in turn, includes zero, one or more item(s), the ontology can be arbitrarily extended. To sum up, the requirements (1) - (3) are met by the basic approach.

```
<?xml version='1.0' encoding='ISO-8859-1'?>
<rdf:RDF
  xmlns:rdf="http://www.w3.org/1999/02/22-rdf-syntax-ns#"
  xmlns:rdfs="http://www.w3.org/2000/01/rdf-schema#"
  xmlns:o="http://ontoserver.aifb.uni-karlsruhe.de/schema/rdf">
  <rdf:Description ID="Item">
    <rdf:type resource="http://www.w3.org/2000/01/rdf-
schema#Class"/>
    <rdfs:subClassOf resource="http://www.w3.org/2000/01/rdf-
schema#Resource"/>
  </rdf:Description>
  <rdf:Description ID="childOf">
    <rdf:type resource="http://ontoserver.aifb.uni-
karlsruhe.de/schema/rdf#Irreflexive"/>
    <rdf:type resource="http://ontoserver.aifb.uni-
karlsruhe.de/schema/rdf#Asymmetric"/>
    <rdfs:domain rdf:resource="#Item"/>
    <rdfs:range rdf:resource="#Item"/>
    <o:isInverseRelationOf rdf:resource="#parentOf"/>
  </rdf:Description>
  <rdf:Description ID="siblingOf">
    <rdf:type resource="http://ontoserver.aifb.uni-
karlsruhe.de/schema/rdf#Irreflexive"/>
    <rdf:type resource="http://ontoserver.aifb.uni-
karlsruhe.de/schema/rdf#Symmetric"/>
    <rdf:type resource="http://ontoserver.aifb.uni-
karlsruhe.de/schema/rdf#Transitive"/>
    <rdfs:domain rdf:resource="#Item"/>
    <rdfs:range rdf:resource="#Item"/>
  </rdf:Description>
  <rdf:Description ID="parentOf">
    <rdf:type resource="http://ontoserver.aifb.uni-
karlsruhe.de/schema/rdf#Irreflexive"/>
<rdf:type resource="http://ontoserver.aifb.uni-
karlsruhe.de/schema/rdf#Asymmetric"/>
    <rdfs:domain rdf:resource="#Item"/>
    <rdfs:range rdf:resource="#Item"/>
  </rdf:Description>
</rdf:RDF>
```

Fig. 2. Integration of SOntoDL into RDF/RDFS

The basic version of SOntoDL has been applied in order to implement an ontology-based semantic navigation through the glossary of an evidence-based medical information service on the WWW [3]. Since the ontology is implemented as a single

XML file, the document is very large and hard to handle. Worse, all updates, be it of the representational vocabulary (element type identifier) or of the human-readable definitions (element type description), must be made in this central document. In order to anticipate these disadvantages (and to meet requirement 4), the option to implement the description as an URI reference instead of a CDATA section was added to the language (attribute implementation). Even though this extension of SOntoDL is marginal, it has a major impact on its applicability. Particularly, it is now possible to integrate external resources into the domain ontology.

The basic version of SOntoDL takes advantage of the intrinsic structuring capabilities of XML documents, i.e., the representational vocabulary is implemented as a hierarchy of items together with their identifiers and descriptions, whereby each item corresponds to a node of the document tree. The disadvantage of this approach is its limitation to a (mono-) hierarchical representation and the inability to represent more complex knowledge structures. In order to overcome this limitation, SOntoDL is integrated into the RDF/RDFS framework, i.e., the potential de facto standard for connected applications on the WWW. Thus, along with this development step, the requirements (5) - (7) are met in addition to (1) - (4)

In view of its conception, the basic approach is closely related to RDF/RDFS, and a re-definition mainly required the effort to become familiar with RDF/RDFS. The concept corresponding to the XML DTD is the RDF *Schema*. Therefore, SOntoDL is re-defined as an application-specific extension to RDFS (Fig. 2). In addition to the generic namespaces rdf and rdfs (referring to the RDF Schema), the namespace o [4] is used. The latter refers to a schema that provides an ontology meta-layer for the representation of axioms. These can be used to type relations (i.e., properties in terms of RDF/RDFS) thereby providing the basis for the implementation of integrity constraints for the ontology. While the re-definition of the so far latest version of SOntoDL has been completed, it has only been partially applied to the EBM domain in order to test its applicability (not shown).

References

1. Berners-Lee, T.: Semantic Web Road map. (1998) Retrieved December 28, 2000 from the World Wide Web: http://www.w3.org/DesignIssues/Semantic.html
2. Gruber, T.:. What is an Ontology? Retrieved October 13, 2000 from the World Wide Web: http://www-ksl.stanford.edu/kst/what-is-an-ontology.html
3. Grütter, R., Eikemeier, C., & Steurer, J. (2001). Up-scaling a Semantic Navigation of an Evidence-based Medical Information Service on the Internet to Data Intensive Extranets. In Proceedings of the 2nd International Workshop on User Interfaces to Data Intensive Systems (UIDIS 2001). Los Alamitos, California, USA: IEEE Computer Society Press.
4. Staab, S., Erdmann, M., Maedche, A., Decker, S.: An Extensible Approach for Modeling Ontologies in RDF(S). Institut für Angewandte Informatik und Formale Beschrei-bungsverfahren (AIFB), Universität Karlsruhe (2000). Retrieved July 21, 2000 from the World Wide Web:
http://www.aifb.uni-karlsruhe.de/~sst/Research/Publications/onto-rdfs.pdf

Knowledge Acquisition System to Support Low Vision Consultation

Cláudia Antunes [1] and J.P. Martins [2]

[1] Instituto Superior Técnico, Portugal
Claudia.Antunes@rnl.ist.utl.pt
[2] Instituto Superior Técnico, Portugal
jpm@gia.ist.utl.pt

Abstract. This paper describes an integrated system to support medical consultations, in particular low vision consultation. Low vision requires patient monitoring after the patient has lost some abilities due some functional changes at the organ level, caused by a lesion in the eye. In emerging domains where the population is reduced (such as low vision), traditional studies are difficult to conduct and not statistically representative.

This work contributes with the creation of an information system, which supports the entire consultation, and is based on three components: a transactional system, a rehabilitation system and a knowledge acquisition system. The transactional system records and manages patient data. It is done in a distributed way, making it possible to expand the system's utilization to similar consultations in different hospitals. The rehabilitation system provides a set of exercises to train eye movements. The knowledge acquisition system helps the discovery of relations between changes at the organ level and changes at the individual abilities level. This system is based on knowledge discovery from databases techniques.

1 Introduction

This work defines and describes an information system, able to support medical domains, where patient's situation is determined based on the combination of their impairment measure and the assessment of their disabilities. Low vision is a particular example of such a medical domain.

The approach presented allows the system, besides recording and managing patients data, to analyse data, in order to discover relations between impairments and disabilities. The system can be used in other medical domains, since transactional system and knowledge acquisition system are independent of the database design. To extend this system to other domains, it needs a new database, since system uses its meta-information to work. The system is composed of three modules: the transactional, the rehabilitation and the knowledge acquisition system. The first one records and manages the patient data, the second one presents a set of rehabilitation exercises and the last one to provides the means to discover relations in the recorded data.

In this paper, in the following section, it is presented a brief description of low vision. Section 3 describes the information system and explains its functionalities and architecture. Section 4 presents the knowledge acquisition system. The results are in Section 5 followed by the conclusions and future work.

S. Quaglini, P. Barahona, and S. Andreassen (Eds.): AIME 2001, LNAI 2101, pp. 332–338, 2001.

2   Low Vision

Low vision is a recent therapeutic domain, and is expressed as a partial vision loss that can't be resolved by traditional treatments. Like other medical domains, low vision requires patient monitoring when the patient has lost some abilities due some functional changes at the organ level, caused by a lesion in that organ. In low vision the affected organ is the eye, and lost abilities and functional changes are at the visual level. Again, like in many other medical domains, there is two distinct steps in the patient monitoring: assessment and rehabilitation. There are two important aspects in visual assessment: visual functions and functional vision. The term "visual functions" is used to refer to functional changes, also called impairments, and refers to the organ. Most of visual functions can be assessed quantitatively and expressed in units relative to a standard measurement (the most relevant are visual acuity and visual field). On the other side, functional vision refers to visual abilities, like reading or mobility, and could only be described qualitatively. It is interesting to see that "eye care professional typically describe the severity of a case in terms of impairment of visual function ('visual acuity has dropped by two lines'), and the patient, on the other hand, will usually couch the complaint in terms of loss of an ability ('Doctor, I am not able to read anymore')" [1]

The assessment issue here is to combine both aspects to establish the patient diagnosis, and therefore determine his rehabilitation plan. How to combine these different aspects is the great problem. Beside the evolution in this domain, the assessment stills usually be done exclusively based on the doctor's experience. There aren't standard measures for most of the visual functions (contrast and glare sensitivity, colour vision, binocularity and others) and functional vision stills be appreciated but not recorded. Due to the few number of patients with low vision, studying the impact of visual functions on functional vision is very difficult, and most of the time, these studies aren't statistically representative.

In visual rehabilitation, nothing can be done to improve the patient physical condition: low vision rehabilitation means the adoption of a set of visual strategies to surpass visual difficulties. At this level everything is to be done: rehabilitation plans aren't formalized and are exclusively based on the eye care professional experience.

3   Information System

The main goal of this project is to support the entire low vision consultation, including assessment and rehabilitation steps. Beside that, it aims to support low vision investigation.

To achieve these goals, the first step is creating an information system to record patient data. These data are typically composed by personal data, clinical history and results of anatomical examinations, which represent vision function assessment. Moreover it is necessary to record the functional vision performance, which is done by recording the patient's answers to questionnaires, where his abilities are assessed.

To be able to support all steps of low vision consultation, the information system must allow: to electronically record and access to patient data (in the maximum number of hospitals that would be possible), to support a set of rehabilitation exercises and plans, and finally allow performing studies on the collected data, so that relations between visual functions and functional vision, or between assessment and rehabilitation may be discovered.

The system is divided in three main modules: a transactional system, a rehabilitation system and a knowledge acquisition system. Both transactional and knowledge acquisition system have a client/server architecture and manipulate the data recorded in the database.

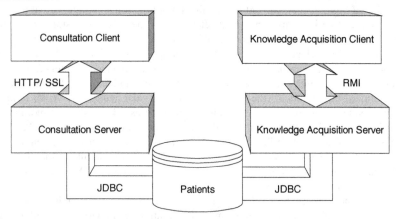

Fig. 1. System architecture

The database is the physical support to the patient data gathered during assessment. It has to have a flexible design, in order to be able to record either quantitative visual function values, either qualitative function visual assessment. Another important feature is to allow different records to different patients (like children versus adults or readers versus non readers). These different records refers mainly to the questionnaires posted to patients to assess his functional vision, and must be determined accordingly the patient profile.

The transactional system is the basic module of the entire system and functions at the operational level, managing the patient data recorded in the database. This system is designed for allow a simultaneous access to data, making it possible to expand the system's utilization to different professionals of an hospital, or even to the staff of many different hospitals. It has a web interface to the entire system with encryption mechanisms to secure patients confidential data.

The rehabilitation system consists mainly on a set of exercises for stimulate and train the residual patient vision and its creation was oriented by the need to train the eye-movements (saccadic and persecution) and the eye-hand co-ordination. A detailed description of this module can be found in [2] and [3].

4   Knowledge Acquisition System

The knowledge acquisition system is the module responsible for allow data rigorous and systematic analysis, helping in the studies concretisation. The knowledge acquisition client is responsible for receive users' requests and send them to knowledge acquisition server, and then retrieve its answers to users. On the other side, there is the knowledge acquisition server, which has two main functions: receive clients' requests and process them. The communication between these modules is made throw the Remote Method Invocation mechanism, and requests processing are done using knowledge discovery from databases techniques. The term knowledge discovery from databases is used to describe "the non-trivial extraction of implicit, previously unknown and potentially useful knowledge from data" [4].

In domains like low vision, the number of records is extremely reduced, but the number of attributes recorded for each patient isn't so little. The main goal of a knowledge acquisition system in such domains is to obtain compact descriptions of the information that is behind the data recorded in the database, in order to discover the existent relations between attributes of each entity.

In contrast with what is usual, it wasn't created a data warehouse. This is due essentially to the reduced number of patients in such domains, and over all, to its previsible evolution (it is perfectly expectable that in normal conditions, the consultation population doesn't grow substantially). Thus, the data repository to submit to the knowledge extraction process is the database used by the transactional system. However, like has been said the database is in the third normal form, and without any pre-processment it isn't possible to discover relations between different entities. In order to make it possible, the system provides some pre-processment tools to final users (such discretization and denormalization).

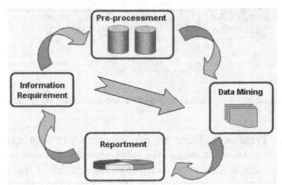

Fig. 2. Functioning cycle of the knowledge acquisition system

Other tasks like data enrichment are done automatically by the system, and at the moment the data mining mechanism that could be applied to data is the *Apriori* algorithm. [5]

The first step in the process is to read data from the database and maintains it in memory. The data reading is done based on the database meta-information (its schemes, entities, attributes and primary keys) and using the WEKA (Waikato Environment Knowledge Analysis) package, programmed in Java [6]. This package provides a set of data mining mechanisms and tools to support the knowledge acquisition process. Having the required data in memory, the next step is applying the enrichment techniques, in particular the addition of new attributes derived from old ones (for example patient age from his birthday). At this level, data is ready to be submitted to data mining mechanisms, and it is up to the user to decide if he invokes this mechanism or applies any pre-processment mechanisms (such those described in [7]) to data. If user chooses applying some pre-processment he has three choices: treating missing values, discretizing numeric values or denormalizing some tables.

Denormalization. Denormalization provides a way to re-structure the read data to make possible the discovery of relations between different entities (for example between personal data and pathologies) or between different instances of the same entity for the same patient (for example the relations between different treatments). Denormalization implementation depends on its nature: to relate two (or more) different entities, the system looks for the instances of each entity that refers to a same patient and join them in a new line of a new table; to relate different instances of a same entity (different lines in a table), the system looks for any instance of the entity that refers to a same patient and creates a new table with this data.

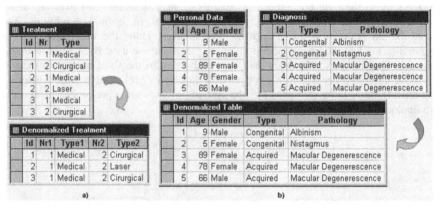

Fig. 3. Denormalization examples: a) to denormalize one table; b) to denormalize different tables

Missing Values Treatment. There are two approaches to treat missing values: the substitution by the *unknown value* and the substitution by *the most probable value for the class*. The first one reveals to be useless for data sets full of missing values, since discovered rules express the inexistence of information. The second approach could only be applied in supervised learning (when there is information about data classes). [8]

Numeric Values Discretization. Discretization is needed when the data mining mechanisms are not able to deal with numeric values. It consists in transforming a continuous domain in a discrete domain with nominal values.

After applying data mining mechanisms, discovered rules are reported to the final user with its confidence and support level.

5   Results

The data used by the knowledge acquisition system, is the data recorded in the low vision consultation of the Hospital de Santa Maria. There are few patients (around 150), and only 20% have historical and diagnosis data. On the other side, only 15% have visual functions and functional vision records. So, it was only considered the personal and diagnosis data as the source data to the knowledge acquisition system. Another important aspect is the high amount of missing values between data, and the inexistence of class information.

Nevertheless, the system had discovered some rules with reasonable confidence levels (higher than 75%), but with reduced support (10%) due to the few number of patients. For example, without any pre-processment it were discovered the following rules:

- Family clinical history = irrelevant => Prematurity = false (c=0.8, s=0.2)
- Impairment installation = sudden => Impairment evolution = stable (c=0.8, s=0.2)
- Pathology Name = Macular Degenerescence => Pathology Type = Acquired (c=1.0, s=0.1)

With table denormalization, it were rediscovered some rules, but also new ones. For example:

- Pathology Type#1 = Congenital => Pathology Type#2 = Congenital (c=0.9, s=0.2)
- Pathology Type#1 = Acquired => Pathology Type#2 = Acquired (c=0.8, s=0.1)
- Treatment Type#1 = Medical => Treatment Type#2 = Cirurgical (c=0.8, s=0.1)

These rules express some relations between different records of a same entity. With discretization, the system discovered another set of rules. For example:

- Impairment Age < 9 => Illness Age < 9 (c=1.0, s=0.1)
- Illness Age < 9 => Pathology Type = Congenital (c=0.6, s=0.2)

Although support levels of these rules are very low, they have significant confidence level and were already approved by low vision professionals.

6   Conclusion

This project began four years ago, with the creation of the first database and an application to manage it. In the following years, the focus had been centred in the improvement of the processes that compose the assessment of patients' situation, as well as in the creation of the first set of rehabilitation exercises. At the beginning of 2000, the system was fully integrated, to allow a distributed access to eye care professionals, allowing the support of all consultation steps. Now with the conclusion of the knowledge acquisition system, and beside the quantity and quality data problems that characterized the data, the system had discovered some interesting relations. These relations have high level of confidence but low support, since patients of the considered population are significantly different.

For the future, in rehabilitation it is urgent to formalize and record rehabilitation plans, then it would be useful to relate these plans with patients and situations. At the knowledge acquisition level it would be interesting discover patient profiles, using artificial intelligence techniques, like clustering. With this classification it would be possible to adjust rehabilitation exercises to patient needs, which would be a first step in rehabilitation optimisation.

References

[1] Colenbrander, A.: GUIDE for the Evaluation of VISUAL Impairment. Pacific Vision Foundation, San Francisco (1999)

[2] Antunes, C., Lynce,, I., Pereira, J.M., Martins, J.P.: Realidade Virtual em Subvisão. Actas do 9° Encontro Nacional de Computação Gráfica. Marinha Grande (2000)

[3] Neves, C., C.Antunes, I. Lynce, J.P. Martins, A.C. Dinis."A Computer-Based Assessment and Rehabilitation of Visual Function in Low vision Children", in Stuen, C., A. Arditi, A. Horowitz, M.A. Lang, B. Rosenthal and K. Seidman, Vision Rehabilitation, Assessment, Intervention, and Outcomes (pg. 376-379).Swets & Zeitlinger Publishers. 2000.

[4] Frawley, W.J., G. Piatetsky-Shapiro, C.J. Matheus. "Knowledge discovery in databases: An overview". AI Magazine, vol. 13 n°. 3 (pg. 57-70). 1992.

[5] Agrawal, R., Srikant, R.: Fast algorithms for mining association rules in large databases. Proceedings of International Conference on Very Large Databases. Morgan Kaufmann. Los Altos, CA (1994) 478-499

[6] Witten, I.H., Frank, E.: Data Mining Practical Machine Learning Tools and Techniques with Java Implementations. Morgan Kaufmann (2000)

[7] Adriaans, P., Zantinge, D.: Data Mining. Addison-Wesley. Harlow (1996)

[8] Quinlan, J.R. "Induction of Decision Trees", in Machine Learning, vol. 1 (pg 81-106). Kluwer Academic Publishers.1986.

Systematic Construction of Texture Features for Hashimoto's Lymphocytic Thyroiditis Recognition from Sonographic Images

Radim Šára[1], Daniel Smutek[2], Petr Sucharda[2], and Štěpán Svačina[2]

[1] Center for Machine Perception, Czech Technical University, Prague, Czech Republic
sara@cmp.felk.cvut.cz
[2] 1st Medical Faculty, Charles University Prague, Czech Republic
smutek@cesnet.cz, {petr.sucharda, stepan.svacina}@lf1.cuni.cz

Abstract. The success of discrimination between normal and inflamed parenchyma of thyroid gland by means of automatic texture analysis is largely determined by selecting descriptive yet simple and independent sonographic image features. We replace the standard non-systematic process of feature selection by *systematic feature construction* based on the search for the separation distances among a clique of n pixels that minimise conditional entropy of class label given all data. The procedure is fairly general and does not require any assumptions about the form of the class probability density function. We show that a network of weak Bayes classifiers using 4-cliques as features and combined by majority vote achieves diagnosis recognition accuracy of 92%, as evaluated on a set of 741 B-mode sonographic images from 39 subjects. The results suggest the possibility to use this method in clinical diagnostic process.

1 Introduction

Hashimoto's lymphocytic thyroiditis, one of the most frequent thyropathies, is a chronic inflammation of the thyroid gland [21]. The inflammation in the gland changes the structure of the thyroid tissue. These changes are diffuse, affecting the entire gland, and can be detected by sonographic imaging.

The advantages of using sonographic imaging are obvious. However, in clinical praxis the assessment of the diffuse processes is difficult [16,19] and the diagnosis is made only qualitatively from the size of the gland being examined, from the structure and echogenicity of its parenchyma, and from its perfusion. In making an overall evaluation of a sonogram, the physician uses her/his clinical experience without giving any quantifiable indexes which are reproducible.

Early studies of automatic texture analysis of thyroid gland [10] were limited to the comparison of grey-level histograms of different diagnoses. Later works involved mainly localised changes (e.g., nodules, tumours and cysts) in thyroid tissue [6,12,13]. Our final goal is quantitative assessment of the diffuse processes associated with chronic inflammations. This is facilitated by recent developments in imaging technology that considerably improved the quality of sonograms, mainly of subsurface organs such as thyroid gland.

S. Quaglini, P. Barahona, and S. Andreassen (Eds.): AIME 2001, LNAI 2101, pp. 339–348, 2001.

This paper focuses on diagnosis recognition problem rather than on finding quantitative indexes measuring the degree of inflammation. Classification is a much simpler task, since it requires less training data. If properly chosen, the classification methods generalise to regression methods.

In the first stage of our project we showed that local texture properties of sonographic B-mode images measured by the first-order texture statistic are independent of the location in the image and thus are suitable for tissue classification [15]. Further step of our research focused on the selection of a subset of co-occurrence matrix features suitable for classification [17]. In [18] we tried to use a large set of texture features based on co-occurrence matrices combined with features proposed by Muzzolini et al. [14]. As there was no way to systematically explore all possible features to find the best-suited, we turned our attention towards methods that do not require classical features.

This paper is concerned with the following principal questions: *What are the simplest texture features that are most efficient in distinguishing between normal tissue and the chronic inflammation process in thyroid gland by means of texture analysis? Can these features be found in a systematic way?*

The approach we take avoids the standard heuristic and non-systematic process of descriptive feature selection. The texture feature of our choice is nothing but a small subset of untransformed image pixels. All such possible features differ in how many pixels are involved. They are all parameterised by the separation vectors among the pixels. The search for the optimal feature can thus be done in a systematic way. It is implemented as a simple exhaustive search for the optimum separation distances in a clique of s sampling pixels. The search is performed in a space of dimension $2(s-1)$ and minimises the conditional entropy between class label and data. This *systematic feature construction* procedure is fairly general and does not require any assumptions about the form of the class probability density function.

2   Systematic Feature Construction

On the image grid we define a system of data sampling variables by a set of translation rules according to [8]. Each data sampling variable holds the value of an individual image pixel. Their range is thus a discrete set. The translation rules define the mutual positional relationship among the sampling variables and can be represented by a rectangular mask as illustrated in Fig. 1. Let C be class label variable and D be a system of s data sampling variables. We say certain vector $\mathbf{d}$ of dimension s is a data sample if it is obtained by placing a sampling mask at some position in the image and reading out the image values in the order defined by the order of the corresponding translation rules. The mask must only be placed such that no image pixel is used more than once in this data collection procedure. The position of the mask shown in Fig. 1 defines a data sample of $\mathbf{d} = [3, 7, 5]$.

Fig. 1. A system of three sampling variables (shaded) defined on image grid and represented by the sampling mask (thick rectangle). The triple has a base variable corresponding to translation rule $(0,0)$ (upper left corner of the mask) and two more variables defined by translation rules $(3,1)$ and $(1,2)$, respectively. Numbers are image values

1	0	0	3	0
1	3	3	23	15
0	3	0	5	18
3	12	3	8	0
11	2	7	0	30
9	0	5	5	2

Conditional entropy $H(C \mid D)$ tells us how much information in bits is missing in all image data about the class we want to determine:

$$H(C \mid D) = -\sum_{i=1}^{n} p(C, D) \log p(C \mid D), \qquad (1)$$

where n is the number of samples collected from all data, $p(\cdot)$ is probability, and $\log(\cdot)$ is the dyadic logarithm. If $H(C \mid D) = 0$ the data contain unambiguous information about the class, i.e. there is some (unknown) function f such that $C = f(D)$. If $H(C \mid D) = H(C)$ the data contain no information about the class. It is not difficult to prove that

$$B = \frac{H(C \mid D)}{c \log c} \qquad (2)$$

is an upper bound on Bayesian classification error (of a sample), where c is the number of classes. No classifier can achieve worse error. For the definition of Bayesian error see, e.g. [4].

A sampling system is equivalent to object feature in the classical recognition literature [4]. There is no known efficient way to systematically generate all possible object features. In sampling systems the situation is quite different. Since a sampling system of s variables is defined by $2(s - 1)$ parameters, it is possible to find an optimum system for a given recognition problem. We suggest the optimality of a sampling system should be measured by B. It is easy to evaluate B for given discrete data in $O(s\,n \log n)$ time, where n is the data size. The advantage of using entropy is that the resulting optimal sampling system is not biased by any systematic or random artefacts (patterns) in sonographic images.

3 Experiments

The principal goal of the experiments was not to design an efficient classifier with good generalisation properties, it was merely to estimate the sufficiency of our data for the classification task, estimate the smallest number of sampling variables needed, and obtain a good estimate of the classification accuracy that can be achieved. By classification we mean automatic diagnosis recognition given a set of sonographic scans collected for an individual.

We collected data from 37 subjects, 17 of them had normal thyroid (class N) and 20 had Hashimoto's lymphocytic thyroiditis (class LT). The diagnosis was confirmed by clinical examination, elevation of level of antibodies against thyroid gland and by fine needle aspiration biopsy, which are standard diagnostic criteria. Typically, 10 images of the longitudinal cross-section of the left lobe and 10 images for the right lobe were acquired. Twenty images per subject were found sufficient to suppress data acquisition noise. We did not distinguish between the left and right lobe scans in this experiment, since the observed changes are supposed to be diffuse, affecting the entire gland.

Sonographic imaging system (Toshiba ECCO-CEE, console model SSA-340A, transducer model PLF-805ST at frequency 8 MHz) was used to acquire input images. The system settings were kept constant during data collection. We reduced the original 8-bit image resolution to 5 bits. Reductions to 4 up to 6 bits showed very similar results but the computational time needed to compute B differed significantly, especially for large sampling systems.

Typical images of our two classes at full resolution are shown in Fig. 2. Note that the variability of the LT class is much greater. This is due to the fact that chronic inflammations of thyroid gland can be divided into several nosologic units [9].

Fig. 2. Typical longitudinal cross sections of the thyroid gland in four different subjects. Skin is the topmost white structure. The classes are N (normal) and LT (Hashimoto's lymphocytic thyroiditis). The outline roughly delineates the gland and is the region from which data was considered. Image size is 250 × 380 pixels

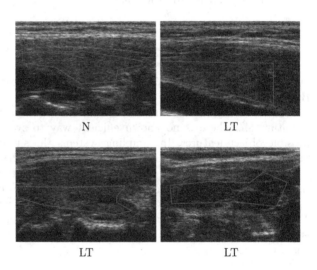

Since the changes in the gland are diffuse it is possible to use global textural characteristics within each image region corresponding to the thyroid gland tissue. Automatic segmentation of such regions is complex and is not the subject of this paper. An interactive tool was used to delineate the boundary of the gland. See Fig. 2 for the result of this manual segmentation.

3.1 Evaluation of B from Data

For a given sampling system, the maximum possible number of non-overlapping samples was collected from the thyroid region in each image. Each individual sample was assigned class label (N, LT). A collection of such samples from all images of a subject formed a data set representing that subject's thyroid. All data from all subjects together with the corresponding class labels in each sample formed one large data-system with s data variables D and one class variable C. This data system was then reduced to discrete probability function by aggregating equal states and estimating the probability $p(C, D)$ of each of the states as its relative frequency in the dataset [8]. The probability $p(C, D)$ was subsequently used to evaluate B using (2).

3.2 Full Search in Low-Dimensional Space

For given s we first constructed optimal sampling system by exhaustive search for the minima of B over the space of $s - 1$ separation variables. We have chosen only vertical and horizontal separations since these are the two natural independent image directions: Namely, the vertical direction is the ultrasonic wave propagation direction. In our experiments we always found a unique global minimum for B for given s. Within the separation search range of $[0, 30]^s$ there were other minima with close values of B as well, however.

Once the optimum sampling system was found, the corresponding probability density functions $p(C \mid N)$ and $p(C \mid LT)$ were used in a network of weak Bayes classifiers whose structure is shown in Fig. 3. All classifiers use the same two probability density functions. Each of them classifies *one* independent (i.e. non-overlapping) texture sample defined by the sample mask. Their outputs are then combined by majority vote to determine the final class label (i.e. the most probable subject diagnosis). The number of classifiers used to determine one final class label per subject is not constant and depends on the number of data available for each subject (the number of images and the size of the thyroid region). It generally decreases with increasing s as there are usually less independent samples that can be collected. In our case it varied between about 250 000 for $s = 1$ and 15 000 for $s = 8$.

For the networked classifier we evaluated the re-substitution error R, which measures the ability of features to describe the entire training dataset, and the leave-one-out error L, which is related to the generalisation capability of the classifier. Both errors are evaluated on the set of 37 subjects, not just individual images or samples (the resolution of the experiment is thus $100/37 \approx 2.7\%$). See [4] for the definition of R and L. Note that B is an upper bound on *sample* recognition error, not the diagnosis classification error. In a properly designed classifier, however, smaller sample recognition error results in smaller object recognition error [4] (as long as it is smaller than 0.5).

The experimental results are shown in Tab. 1. Each sampling system S_s is represented by the set of translation rules. Along with the Bayesian error upper bound B, the leave-one-out classification error L, and the re-substitution error

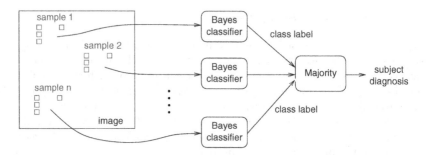

Fig. 3. Classifier structure

R we also show false negatives F^- (inflamed state not recognised), and false positives F^+ (normal state misclassified). It holds that $L = F^- + F^+$. We can see that the system for $s = 4$ is the first one in complexity that is able to fully describe the training set (its re-substitution error is zero). We can also see that the false negative rate F^- is always higher than the false positive rate F^+. This is probably related to the fact that the LT class has richer structure than the N class. The simplest explanation is that the LT class is represented by several subclasses in our data and has thus multi-modal probability distribution function. We observed this property in our earlier experiments as well [18].

Table 1. Recognition results for optimal sampling systems for given s. The experiment resolution is 2.7%

s	system S_s	B	L	R	F^-	F^+
1	$(0,0)$	25.3%	**8.1%**	8.1%	8.1%	0%
2	$(0,0), (11,0)$	19.9%	**10.8%**	8.1%	5.4%	5.4%
3	$(0,0), (11,0), (0,34)$	16.6%	**13.5%**	10.8%	8.1%	5.4%
4	$(0,0), (7,0), (15,0), (0,32)$	14.2%	**8.1%**	0%	5.4%	2.7%

We can see that the leave-one-out error L increases initially and then drops back to the 8.1% level. This suggests an important part of information about class is present in higher-dimensional features. The relatively good results in leave-one-out error L for the simplest sampling system may be due to the fact that the simplest classifier has a good generalisation property. This observation is consistent with reports of successful classification of sonographic textures using one-dimensional histograms [6,10].

Figure 4 shows images for the three misclassified cases using sampling system S_4. The sonographic texture in the two false negatives still exhibits some non-uniformity suggesting the model S_4 may not be sufficient. The false positive image (far right) seems to be influenced by acoustic shadows below the superficial hyperechogenic structures (arrow). In all three misclassifications, the assigned class label probability was near to the undecidability level of 0.5, namely it was

0.48 for the two LT cases and 0.498 for the N case. There were three more class label probabilities below 0.6 in the correctly classified diagnoses. Thus, with S_4 the total of just six cases belonged to the correct class with probability smaller than 0.6. For comparison, with S_1 there were nine such cases.

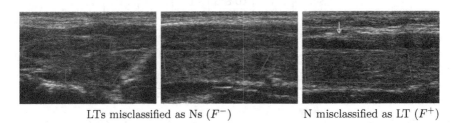

LTs misclassified as Ns (F^-) N misclassified as LT (F^+)

Fig. 4. Images misclassified using S_4

Sampling systems larger than $s = 4$ were not considered because of prohibitively long computational time needed to search through the high-dimensional space. For higher dimensions we used approximate search as described next.

3.3 Approximate Search in High-Dimensional Space

In this experiment we did not search the entire parameter space to find the optimum sampling variable configuration. Instead, a higher-order system $\widehat{S}_{n+1}$ was constructed from $\widehat{S}_n$ by adding one optimal translation rule at a time, while the translation rules in $\widehat{S}_n$ remained fixed. To distinguish systems found by optimal and sub-optimal search we denote them as S_i and $\widetilde{S}_i$, respectively.

Each new translation rule was found by minimising a one-parametric bound $B(x)$ for system $\widehat{S}_{n-1} \cup (x, 0)$, where x was the only free variable. The variable range was limited to the interval of $[0, 30]$. Since the full search experiment results suggest that sampling variables defined by vertical translations are more relevant for our recognition task and since it is also the principal direction in the sonographic image, we used only vertical translations in this experiment. The search begun with the simplest system $\widehat{S}_1 = \{(0, 0)\}$. The order in which the optimal translation rules were added was $(11, 0)$, $(17, 0)$, $(5, 0)$, $(20, 0)$, $(14, 0)$, $(7, 0)$, $(2, 0)$. The largest system we tested was thus $\widehat{S}_8$ comprising of all eight translation rules.

The results of the search are shown in Tab. 2. The first system that is able to fully describe the training set, $\widehat{S}_5$, has one variable more than the fully descriptive system in the previous experiment. This shows that the approximate search is quite efficient and finds systems close to those that are optimal. Note that the leave-one-out error is larger in this set of classifiers because of the false negative component of the error. This suggest the horizontal direction plays some role after all and should be accounted for as well.

Table 2. Recognition results for approximately optimal sampling systems $\widehat{S}_s$

system	B	L	R	F^-	F^+
$\widehat{S}_1 = S_1$	25.3%	**8.1%**	8.1%	8.1%	0.0%
$\widehat{S}_2 = S_2$	19.9%	**10.8%**	8.1%	5.4%	5.4%
$\widehat{S}_3$	17.3%	**10.8%**	8.1%	8.1%	2.7%
$\widehat{S}_4$	15.1%	**10.8%**	2.7%	8.1%	2.7%
$\widehat{S}_5$	12.2%	**10.8%**	0.0%	8.1%	2.7%
$\widehat{S}_6$	7.2%	**10.8%**	0.0%	8.1%	2.7%
$\widehat{S}_7$	2.8%	**8.1%**	0.0%	2.7%	5.4%
$\widehat{S}_8$	0.7%	**8.1%**	0.0%	0.0%	8.1%

The leave-one-out recognition accuracy remains at the 92% level for systems above 6 sampling variables. Larger systems would probably result in overfitting [4]. For completeness, in S_8, the total of four cases belonged to the correct class with probability below 0.6 (cf. the results reported in the previous section).

Note that the trend of the F^- error is exactly opposite to that of the F^+. The $F^- = 0$ means that the Hashimoto's lymphocytic thyroiditis was always recognised and $F^+ = 0$ means that normal condition was always recognised. This means that low-order features capture the N class well, while the high-order features capture well the structure of the LT class. The residual errors of 8.1% suggest the existence of partial class overlap in feature space, which is in agreement with observations made by Mailloux et al. [10].

Our next goal is to collect more data to see whether the achieved classification accuracy is low due to the small size of our dataset, due to large class overlap, or due to poor discriminability of our features.

3.4 Comparison with Other Sonographic Texture Recognition Results

We are not aware of any published results that would discriminate between normal and chronically inflamed thyroid parenchyma based solely on sonographic texture analysis. However, other types of tissue were discriminated successfully as shown in the following brief overview.

Hirning et al. report 85% success in detection of nodular lesions in thyroid using the 90-percentile of one-dimensional histogram as a feature [6]. Muller et al. report 83.9% diagnostic accuracy in distinguishing malignant and benign thyroid lesions based on three texture features [13]. Ariji et al. report 96.9% diagnostic accuracy in the diagnosis of Sjogren's syndrome in parotid gland using a combination of spectral feature and standard deviation features [1]. Cavouras et al. report 93.7% classification accuracy for distinguishing normal and abnormal livers (cirrhosis, fatty infiltration) using twenty two features [2]. Horng et al. report 83.3% classification accuracy for distinguishing normal liver, hepatitis and cirrhosis using two-dimensional histograms defined on sonographic image gradient [7]. Mojsilovic et al. report 92% classification accuracy in detecting early stage of liver cirrhosis using wavelet transform [11]. Sujana et al. report up to 100% classification accuracy in distinguishing liver lesions (hemangioma and malignancy) using run-length statistics and neural network [20]. Chan reports 94% classification accuracy in images of unspecified tissue [3].

Although the results of these methods are not comparable since they were applied to very different tissues and the classification error was evaluated using different statistical methods, the overview suggests our features have good discriminatory power as compared to features used in similar recognition problems using B-mode sonographic images.

4   Conclusions

Our results show that it is possible to achieve good discrimination (92%) of chronically inflamed thyroid tissue from normal thyroid gland by means of low-dimensional texture feature vector. The vector is constructed from a sample of just four pixel values. The four pixels are separated by certain translation vectors that are found by a simple optimisation procedure. Of all possible feature vectors it minimises the conditional entropy of class label given all collected data *and* is the smallest-dimension vector that achieves zero re-substitution error. This optimality property guarantees the best utilisation of available data and the best generalisation properties of a classifier using the features. Note that our features have no explicit intuitive meaning as standard features often do.

The results suggest that the information related to diagnosis can be extracted well from high-quality sonographic images. There is thus a possibility to calculate quantitative characterisation of the chronic inflammatory processes in thyroid gland, which the human visual system is not capable to achieve. In clinical diagnostic process this characterisation enables objective reproducibility of sonographic findings. This facilitates the assessment of changes in the thyroid tissue in follow-up examinations of the same subject made by different physicians.

Acknowledgements. This research was supported by the Ministry of Health of the Czech Republic under project NB 5472-3. The first author was supported by the Czech Ministry of Education under Research Programme MSM 210000012.

We would like to thank Mohamed Bakouri who implemented an efficient Matlab toolbox for computations involving discrete probability functions.

References

1. Y. Ariji et al. Texture analysis of sonographic features of the parotid gland in Sjogren's syndrome. *AJR Am J Roentgenol*, 166(4):935–941, 1996.
2. D. Cavouras et al. Computer image analysis of ultrasound images for discriminating and grading liver parenchyma disease employing a hierarchical decision tree scheme and the multilayer perceptron neural network classifier. In *Medical Informatics Europe '97*, vol. 2, pp. 522–526, 1997.

3. K. Chan. Adaptation of ultrasound image texture characterization parameters. In *Proceedings of the 20th Annual International Conference of the IEEE Engineering in Medicine and Biology Society*, vol. 2, pp. 804–807, 1998.
4. K. Fukunaga. *Introduction to Statistical Pattern Recognition*. Computer Science and Scientific Computing. Academic Press, (2nd ed.), 1990.
5. R. M. Haralick and L. G. Shapiro. *Computer and Robot Vision*, vol. 1. Addison-Wesley, 1993.
6. T. Hirning et al. Quantification and classification of echographic findings in the thyroid gland by computerized B-mode texture analysis. *Eur J Radiol*, 9(4):244–247, 1989.
7. M.-H. Horng, Y.-N. Sun, and X.-Z. Lin. Texture feature coding method for classification of liver sonography. In *Proceedings of 4th European Conference on Computer Vision*, vol. 1, pp. 209–218, 1996.
8. G. J. Klir. *Architecture of Systems Problem Solving*. Plenum Press, 1985.
9. P. R. Larsen, T. F. Davies, and I. D. Hay. The thyroid gland. In *Williams textbook of endocrinology*. Saunders (9th ed), 1998.
10. G. Mailloux, M. Bertrand, R. Stampfler, and S. Ethier. Computer analysis of echographic textures in Hashimoto disease of the thyroid. *JCU J Clin Ultrasound*, 14(7):521–527, 1986.
11. A. Mojsilovic, M. Popovic, and D. Sevic. Classification of the ultrasound liver images with the $2N$ multiplied by 1-D wavelet transform. In *Proceedings of the IEEE International Conference on Image Processing*, vol. 1, pp. 367–370, 1996.
12. H. Morifuji. Analysis of ultrasound B-mode histogram in thyroid tumors. *Journal of Japan Surgical Society*, 90(2):210–21, 1989. In Japanese.
13. M. J. Muller, D. Lorenz, I. Zuna, W. J. Lorenz, and G. van Kaick. The value of computer-assisted sonographic tissue characterization in focal lesions of the thyroid. *Radiologe*, 29(3):132–136, 1989. In German.
14. R. Muzzolini, Y.-H. Yang, and R. Pierson. Texture characterization using robust statistics. *Pattern Recognition*, 27(1):119–134, 1994.
15. R. Šára, M. Švec, D. Smutek, P. Sucharda, and Š. Svačina. Texture analysis of sonographic images for diffusion processes classification in thyroid gland parenchyma. In *Proceedings Conference Analysis of Biomedical Signals and Images*, pp. 210–212, 2000.
16. J. F. Simeone et al. High-resolution real-time sonography of the thyroid. *Radiology*, 145(2):431–435, 1982.
17. D. Smutek, R. Šára, M. Švec, P. Sucharda, and Š. Svačina. Chronic inflammatory processes in thyroid gland: Texture analysis of sonographic images. In *Telematics in Health Care – Medical Infobahn for Europe, Proceedings of the MIE2000/GMDS2000 Congress*, 2000.
18. D. Smutek, T. Tjahjadi, R. Šára, M. Švec, P. Sucharda, and Š. Svačina. Image texture analysis of sonograms in chronic inflammations of thyroid gland. Research Report CTU–CMP–2001–15, Center for Machine Perception, Czech Technical University, Prague, 2001.
19. L. Solbiati et al. The thyroid-gland with low uptake lesions—evaluation by ultrasound. *Radiology*, 155(1):187–191, 1985.
20. H. Sujana, S. Swarnamani, and S. Suresh. Application of artificial neural networks for the classification of liver lesions by image texture parameters. *Ultrasound Med Biol*, 22(9):1177–1181, 1996.
21. L. Wartfsky and S. H. Ingbar. *Harrison's Principles of Internal Medicine*, chapter Disease of the Thyroid, p. 1712. McGraw-Hill (12th ed), 1991.

Dynamic Adaptation of Cooperative Agents for MRI Brain Scans Segmentation

Nathalie Richard[1,2], Michel Dojat[1,2], and Catherine Garbay[2]

[1] Institut National de la Santé et de la Recherche Médicale, U438 - RMN Bioclinique, Centre Hospitalier Universitaire - Pavillon B, BP 217, 38043 Grenoble Cedex 9, France
{nrichard, mdojat}@ujf-grenoble.fr
[2] Laboratoire TIMC-IMAG, Institut Bonniot, Faculté de Médecine, Domaine de la Merci, 38706 La Tronche Cedex, France
(catherine.garbay@imag.fr)

Abstract. To cope with the difficulty of MRI brain scans automatic segmentation, we need to constrain and control the selection and the adjustment of processing tools depending on the local image characteristics. To extract domain and control knowledge from the image, we propose to use *situated cooperative agents* whose dedicated behavior, i.e. segmentation of one type of tissue, is dynamically adapted with respect to their position in the image. Qualitative maps are used as a common framework to represent knowledge. Constraints that drive the agents behavior, based on topographic relationships and radiometric information, are gradually gained and refined during the segmentation progress. Incremental refinement of the segmentation is obtained through the combination, distribution and opposition of solutions concurrently proposed by the agents, via respectively three types of cooperation: integrative, augmentative and confrontational. We report in detail our multi-agent approach and results obtained on MRI brain scans.

1 Introduction

Functional magnetic resonance imaging (fMRI) is a recent noninvasive neuroimaging technique that allows the detection of cortical activity in response to various types of brain stimulations. Conventionally, visual cortical maps are then produced as a set of two series, anatomical and functional, of planar slices through the measured brain volume. The projection on the surface of a 3D rendering brain displays advantageously all activations on a single image, but hides the exact topology of the brain. Neurons, the cells responsible of measured activity, are essentially located in the gray matter, a 2-D ribbon several millimeters thick, highly folded inside the skull. The primates cortex is divided into several functional areas that can be distinguished thanks to specific local neurons properties [1]. Retinotopic property for instance and fMRI allow the precise delineation of functional areas involved in human vision [2].

S. Quaglini, P. Barahona, and S. Andreassen (Eds.): AIME 2001, LNAI 2101, pp. 349–358, 2001.
© Springer-Verlag Berlin Heidelberg 2001

1.1   Context

There is no ways to study properly the complex spatial organization of cortical areas, intrinsically 2-D surfaces, with a 3-D representation. Thus, a rationale way to visualize and analyze cortical maps consists in unfolding the gray matter [3]. Boundaries of functional areas, determined in advance, can then be mapped to the unfolded surface allowing the precise localization of the set of cortical areas involved in a specific cognitive task [4]. Flattened or unfolded representation displays the activity across a large cortical region on a single plane, instead of a multi-slices image or a volume rendering brain, while preserving some aspects of spatial connections. It allows the visualization of activation buried in cortical sulci, whose anatomy is widely variable across individuals, and permits comparisons between individual and species 3,4]. The first step to create a flattened representation consists in the segmentation of the cortical gray matter. Segmentation is a crucial step for successfully unfolding: poor unfolding maps are usually caused by small errors in the segmentation phase [6]. For unfolding, the respect of topological relationships, no cavities (a tissue A is completely surrounded by a tissue B) or self-intersections, is more important that the precise determination of the boundaries between white matter (WM) and gray matter (GM) or gray matter and cerebro-spinal fluid (CSF) [7]. How this could be automatically achieved in a multi-agent environment is the main focus of this paper.

1.2   Rationale

The automatic segmentation of MR images is a difficult task. Image artifacts inherent to the acquisition procedure, such as partial volume effects (one voxel contains several tissues), magnetic susceptibility artifacts and the non uniformity of the gray level intensities for a given tissue, are difficult to tackle. To illustrate the latter

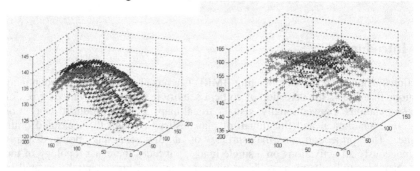

Fig. 1. A sphere (radius= 15 voxels) is moved to several positions along a regular mesh (5 voxels) for the MNI phantom (3% noise + 20% inhomogeneity) (at left) and for a real T1 weighted image (voxel size 1=mm^3) (at right). For each position of two axial slices (slice 1=++, slice 2=••), the gray level of the local histogram peak corresponding to white matter is reported. (x, y: coordinates of the sphere in the mesh for a given z in the mesh. z-vertical axis: WM peak gray level).

point, Figure 1 shows the non-uniformities of the gray levels for WM for a realistic phantom provided by the Montreal Neurological Institute (MNI) [8] and for a real T1 weighted image.

Several methods have been already proposed for MRI brain scans segmentation in the context of flattened representation [7, 9-12]. Segmentation process requires 1) the insertion of *a priori* knowledge, 2) the ability of adaptation to take into account of local gray level variations and 3) the control of the entire process. Several types of *a priori* knowledge, explicit (model based or symbolic approach) or implicit (data-based), about cortical anatomy or brain scans features can be inserted. However, the inter-subject variability of the human brain anatomy limits the utilization of general anatomic knowledge, such as the thickness of cortical ribbon or the position of the ventricles. Statistical methods are generally used to extract information from the images. The histogram plus a peak-finding algorithm determine the main modes present in the image, one for CSF, one for GM and one for WM, which are in conventional anatomical images (T1 weighted) ordered by gray intensity levels with highest intensity for WM (implicit knowledge). Prior probabilities and Bayes' rule can be used to maximize *a posteriori* probabilities [7]. Adaptability can be obtained via user interactions that refine preliminary results (additional knowledge). The user adjusts thresholds to obtain a visually satisfactory segmentation, checks topology relationships and removes holes or handles (generally, bridges across opposite sides of a sulcus) [7]. Specific filtering techniques (anisotropic smoothing [7], intensity normalization, skull-stripping, and non-linear filtering based on *a priori* knowledge [10] are introduced to refine a preliminary crude segmentation. The segmentation strategy (control) depends on the method used. Teo et al.[7] exploit the fact that intensity levels in WM have smaller intensity variability than in GM (in T1 weighted scans) and that GM necessarily surrounds WM. Then, a connected representation of GM is automatically created by a constrained growing-out from WM. In [10], the WM is also firstly segmented. At the opposite, in [12], morphological operators delineate fine structures labeled as sulci. From this mask, a region growing process determines the GM ribbon. In [11], the use of a deformable model allows to position accurately seeded-region-growing agents that firstly segment GM. From the GM ribbon, a second population of seeded-region-growing agents are then specialized for WM segmentation. Specialized fusion operators can be introduced to finely control the overall segmentation process [13]. In the cited examples, due to the sequencing nature of the process, the quality of the second tissue segmentation relies on the quality of the first tissue segmentation. Setting thresholds for each tissue classification remains the Achilles heel of these approaches. Starting from the global histogram, for each tissue T_i with a mean μ_i, we have the classification constraint C1:

C1: $\forall$ p with gray intensity level Ip, $p \in T_i$ if $\mu_i - k_i \leq I(p) \leq \mu_i + k_i$.

Depending on the k_i value, T_i could be over (k_i too high) or under segmented (k_i too low) at different positions in the volume. For two tissues T_i and T_j, four situations listed in Table 1 can be encountered.

To conclude, three points are central in brain scans segmentation:

1) the automatic extraction of knowledge from the intensity levels to limit *a priori* knowledge insertion

2)   the dynamically adaptation of the segmentation constraints based on local radiometric information to take into account of gray level inhomogeneities over the volume
3)   the control of the global process

Table 1. Several situations for two tissues Ti, Tj encountered during classification when using thresholds based on a global histogram.

	T_i under segmentation	T_i over segmentation
T_j under segmentation	incomplete global segmentation	T_i extended over T_j
T_j over segmentation	T_i extended over T_i	over segmentation for the first tissue segmented. In general, no re-classification via negotiation is allowed.

A multi-agent approach is advocated as a way to cope with these difficulties. In the remainder of the paper, we detail in section 2 our complete multi-agents system. In section 3 we evaluate the segmentation in using phantoms and real brain scans. Then, in section 4 we discuss several aspects of our work and point out work under development.

2   The Proposed Approach

Agents are meant to work locally, adaptively and cooperatively, thus coping with (i) the local variations in the image appearance, (ii) the lack of *a priori* knowledge and (iii) the weakness of the segmentation tools. An agent is defined as an autonomous entity, provided with some knowledge of the task at hand, together with processing resources and communication abilities. Agents are not meant to work in isolation, rather they cooperate to solve a problem that they are unable to solve alone. Information exchange takes place between their environment and the other agents, allowing the dynamic adaptation of their behavior.

2.1   Knowledge and Agent Models

To face the difficulty of image segmentation, a major issue is to constrain the processing tools selection and adjustment in a way that is context-dependent. In other words, some knowledge of the situation is needed to process it correctly. The notion of *situated agent* appears well adapted to face such an issue: an agent is situated with respect to a goal - segment GM, WM or CSF in our case - and with respect to a position - a zone in the image. It is provided with specific knowledge and dedicated resources, depending on its goal, and with the ability to self adaptation, depending on the zone under interest. Then it works under a collection of context-dependent constraints. Such agents are moreover defined as *cooperative* entities. Three cooperation modes are distinguished [11], according to which the solutions to a given problem are combined (*integrative cooperation*), distributed (*augmentative cooperation*) or opposed (*confrontational cooperation*). A kind of social constraint is therefore considered in addition. Domain knowledge is handled in our approach, and comprises knowledge about topographic relationships as well as radiometric information, most of which being gained dynamically by the agents themselves. Control knowledge has to be handled in addition, which comprises knowledge about the agent location, goal and behavior. Qualitative maps are used as a common framework to represent these various types of knowledge: they tie topographical knowledge about the image with agents locations and goals (see Figure 2). They also support a local description of the image properties.

2.2   Problem Solving Approach

The adequacy of the agents in processing the image directly depends on the adequacy of the constraints that drive their behavior (positioning as well as segmentation criteria). These constraints are very difficult to specify, due to the difficulty of the problem to solve and to the lack of *a priori* knowledge. We propose an incremental approach in which the agent constraints are progressively refined. Such strategy relies on three principles of cooperation. After preprocessing, two stages, rough segmentation and refinement, that exploit dedicated qualitative maps and dedicated agents, are successively undertaken (see Figure 2).

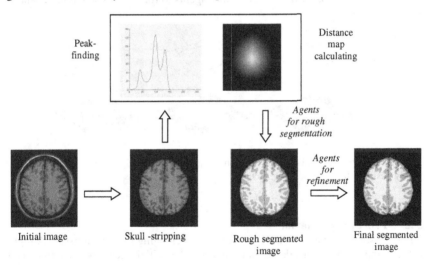

Fig. 2. All phases of segmentation process

Firstly, *a priori* topological knowledge and global statistics are used to compute initial qualitative maps (distance maps) and roughly situate the agents. Starting from this information, the agents evolve locally and concurrently according to augmentative (coordinated) cooperation. Then, the refinement stage is launched. For this purpose, a new qualitative map is created. New agents are launched at strategic positions i.e. around the WM to GM interface where segmentation errors are likely to take place. Confrontational cooperation is then used to negotiate the voxel labeling. The final segmentation is generated.

2.3   Rough Segmentation Stage

Any agent in the system undertakes two successive behaviors: a rooting behavior and a processing behavior.

2.3.1   Rooting Behavior

The rooting behavior exploits knowledge about the brain topography (distance to the cortical envelope of the major brain tissues), which is provided in the form of three initial qualitative maps. Each map gives information about the approximate location of the brain tissues (GM, WM and CSF) and provides a partitioning of the corresponding zones, in the form of an adaptive-size mesh (see Figure 3). Each map allows positioning each agent, depending on its type, roughly inside the brain. Then the purpose of the rooting behavior is to refine the initial agent's position, based on the fuzzy evaluation of the match between the current agent location features and the corresponding tissue characteristics (these characteristics are evaluated locally, for each agent, according to the procedure proposed in [14]). Self-regulation of the launching phase is obtained by constraining agents to root only where other agents do not already work.

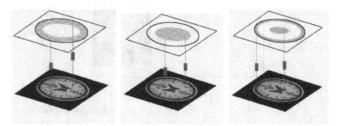

Fig. 3. Three initial qualitative maps for each tissue (from left to right : GM, WM and CSF) to roughly position the corresponding agents.

2.3.2   Processing Behavior

The processing behavior labels image voxels as belonging to a given tissue. A region growing approach is considered starting from the initial agent location (the seed). From this seed, neighboring voxels are evaluated one by one, based on their radiometry and on the topology of their neighborhood. This step is based on severe radiometric constraints, which are computed locally by the agent. Its purpose is to achieve reliable partial labeling of the tissue under consideration. Coordinated region growing is launched upon completion of the previous step (e.g. when no additional voxel can be aggregated). The purpose is then to relax the previous classification constraints in order to progressively label voxels that may appear at the frontier between two tissues. In order to avoid labeling errors, this process is engaged in a coordinated way: all agents wait for each other to relax their classification parameters.

Before relaxation, each agent recalculated the peak of the tissue it has already segmented. Several relaxation steps may take place successively.

2.4   Refinement Stage

The refinement stage is under development. Its purpose is to revise the labeling in places where labeling errors are likely to occur. Refinement agents are rooted along tissue frontiers. A second map is computed to this end, based on the previously obtained segmentation results, and using a mesh model of the 3D boundary between GM and WM. GM and WM agents are then launched on each part of the tissue frontiers. Their role is to negotiate the labeling of voxels situated along these frontiers; each labeling is re-evaluated to this end, with respect to the new agent zone characteristics. The two agents on both sides of the frontier evaluate, based on their own local histogram, a membership probability to each tissue for all voxels. The agent with the higher evaluation will finally "win", and label the voxel correspondingly. This moves the frontier, putting new voxels under consideration.

2.5   Implementation Issues

The agents are implemented as C++ objects. They run under control of a global scheduler, simulating concurrent resources allocation and processes execution. An abstract agent class contains data and abstract methods required for agent activation by the scheduler. An agent hierarchy is defined and two subclasses are created: rough segmentation agents and refinement agents. A task, the tissue to segment, and a localization inside the image volume are set at each agent's instantiation. Two behaviors, rooting and labeling, are provided to segmentation agents. A behaviors scheduler switches autonomously from the former to the latter behavior. When a tissue specific agent has no more voxels to aggregate, the scheduler deactivates it temporarily (removed from the active agents list), until it receives a specific event indicating that all agents for the same tissue have finished their tasks. Then, the agent is reactivated and pursues its task in relaxing its own classification constraints. All agents communicate through a shared environment composed by the image volume and the information accumulated by the agents across time and organized according to tissue type (see Figure 4).

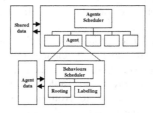

Fig. 4. Agent model and Control Architecture

3   Results

To quantitatively evaluate our segmentation we used a MNI realistic phantom [8] with 3% noise and 20% inhomogeneity. To test the adaptation capabilities of the system proposed, the evaluation was performed in two steps, firstly agents behaviors were defined with fixed constraints, and then the constraints relaxation was envisaged with and without coordination.

Fixed constraints: Table 2 shows the results obtained when the classification constraint varies for each tissue. Harder is the constraint (0.5 standard deviation), higher is the quality of the segmentation (higher true positive value) on a restricted volume (low completion). Looser is the constraint (3 standard deviation) higher is the completion and lower is the quality of the segmentation (lower true positive value)

Table 2: Variations of the classification constraint k for the three tissues. SD= standard deviation of the corresponding tissue estimated from the global histogram.

Initial constraint k	0.5SD	SD	2SD	3SD
TP (true positive)	99.72%	99.19%	95.3%	86.07%
Completion of the segmentation	53.89%	78.19%	97.49%	100%

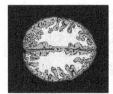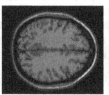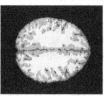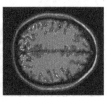

Fig. 5. Two couples of images. From left to right: segmentation with k=SD for all tissues and corresponding errors, segmentation with k=2SD for all tissues and corresponding errors.

Figure 5 displays the errors positions during the 3D segmentation process. Two types of errors occur: misclassification at the frontier between two tissues, essentially due to partial volume effect, and presence of cavities or self intersections for a tissue.

Constraints Relaxation: The constraints relaxation provides a complete segmentation. As showed in Table 3, it clearly requires the coordination of the concurrent agents: for each level of constraint, each agent waits for each other before relaxing its constraints. More precisely, Table 4 shows that constraints relaxation should be synchronized for each tissue to avoid the over segmentation of a tissue, i.e. less false negative and less true positive, and consequently, more true negative and more true positive for the other tissue.

Table 3. The classification constraint k is relaxed from the inferior (initial value) to the superior value of the interval both for GM and WM. Agents are or are not coordinated.

	TP (true positive)	
Relaxation of k	Not coordinated	Coordinated
k ∈ [0.5SD, 3SD]	87.89%	94.88%
k ∈ [1SD, 3SD]	91.30%	94.87 %
k ∈ [2SD, 3SD]	91.09%	94.15%

Table 4. Different constraints relaxations (a) WM agents with k ∈ [2SD, 3SD] and GM agents with k ∈ [1SD, 3SD] (b) WM agents with k ∈ [SD, 3SD] and GM agents with k ∈ [2SD, 3SD] (c) WM agents with k ∈ [1SD, 3SD] and GM agents with k ∈ [1SD, 3SD]. TP(FP) stand for true positive (false negative) respectively. For all situations for CSF agents k ∈ [1SD, 3SD].

	TP in WM	FN in WM	TP in GM	FN in GM	Global TP
(a) WM over-segmentation	91.21%	0.93%	94.51%	10.85%	93.24%
(b) GM over-segmentation	99.13%	8.98%	85.43%	1%	92.55%
(c)	96.54%	3.17%	92.75%	4.45%	94,89%

A trade off avoids to favor a tissue and a result for a real T1 image in shown in Figure 6.

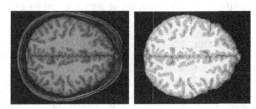

Fig. 6. Left: Real T1 image (3D Flash sequence, scanner Philips 1.5 T), Right: segmentation of WM, CSF and GM.

4   Discussion

In this paper we present a multi-agent environment to cope with the inherent difficulties of automatic MRI brain scans segmentation. In general, in the context of brain unfolding, tissues are segmented sequentially and user interactions refine the final segmentation. In our approach, tissues are segmented concurrently. We have introduced the notion of situated agent particularly well-suited to implement augmentative cooperation: several GM, WM and CSF agents, located at different positions in the image, work in a concurrent way. The main difficulties are 1) to correctly position the agents, 2) to define the adequate classification constraints and 3) to control the global process. This latter point is less crucial in standard sequential methods. Positions and classification constraints are roughly defined from the histogram on the global image and progressively adapted from local image characteristics and from the evolution of the segmentation process. Qualitative maps are introduced to gather all intermediate results obtained at a given time and control agents behaviors. Augmentation and integrative cooperation are envisaged under a coordinated viewpoint which leads to encouraging results on realistic phantom and real images. We will use the confrontation of each tissue segmentation and negotiation to improve the agents behavior. Fusion of information can be nicely introduced into our framework. The insertion of gradients information (gray levels discontinuities) can be used to refine, by negotiation between agents, the frontier between two tissues intrinsically difficult to delineate due to partial volume effects. A specific sulci maps obtained by morphological operators or genetic approach can be usefully added to improve the gray ribbon delineation. Information exchange between unfolding and segmentation can be used to dynamically improve the global process of MRI brain scans flattening.

References

1.   Zeki, S. and Shipp, S.: The functional logic of cortical connections. Nature 335 (1988) 311-314.
2.   Tootell, R. B., Hadjikhani, N. K., Mendola, J. D., et al.: From retinotopy to recognition: fMRI in human visual cortex. Trends Neurosci 2 (1998) 174-182.
3.   Van Essen, D. C., Drury, H. A., Joshi, S. et al.: Functional and structural mapping of human cerebral cortex: solutions are in the surfaces. PNAS USA 95 (1998) 788-795.
4.   Wandell, B. A.: Computational neuroimaging of human visual cortex. Ann Rev Neurosci 22 (1999) 145-173.
5.   DeYoe, E. A., Carman, G. J., Bandettini, P., et al.: Mapping striate and extrastriate visual areas in human cerebral cortex. PNAS USA 93 (1996) 2382-86.
6.   Wandell, B. A., Chial, S. and Backus, B. T.: Visualization and measurement of the cortical surface. Journal of Cognitive Neuroscience 12 (2001) 739-752.
7.   Teo, P. C., Sapiro, G. and Wandell, B. A.: Creating connected representations of cortical gray matter for functional MRI visualization. IEEE Trans Med Imag 16 (1997) 852-863.
8.   Collins, D., Zijdenbos, A., Kollokian, V., et al.: Design and construction of a realistic digital brain phantom. IEEE Trans Med Imag 17 (1998) 463-468.
9.   Drury, H. A., Van Essen, D. C., Anderson, C. H., et al.: Computerized mappings of the cerebral cortex: a multiresolution flattening method and a surface-based coordinate system. Journal of Cognitive Neuroscience 8 (1996) 1-28.
10. Dale, A. M., Fischl, B. and Sereno, M.: Cortical surface-based analysis I: segmentation and surface reconstruction. NeuroImage 9 (1999) 179-194.
11. Germond, L., Dojat, M., Taylor, C. and Garbay, C.: A cooperative framework for segmentation of MRI brain scans. Artif Intell in Med 20 (2000) 77-94.
12. Warnking, J., Guérin-Dugué, A., Chéhikian, A., et al.: Retinotopical mapping of visual areas using fMRI and a fast cortical flattening algorithm. Neuroimage 11 (2000) S646.
13. Bloch, I.: Information combination operators for data fusion: A comparative review with classification. IEEE Trans Systems, Man, Cybernetics 26 (1996)
14. Comaniciu, D. and Meer, P.: Distribution free decomposition of multivariate data. Pattern analysis applications 2 (1999) 22-30.

Numeric and Symbolic Knowledge Representation of Cortex Anatomy Using Web Technologies

Olivier Dameron[1], Bernard Gibaud[1], and Xavier Morandi[1,2]

[1] UPRES-EA "Intégration de données multimédia en anatomie et physiologie cérébrale pour l'aide à la décision et l'enseignement" Université de Rennes 1, F35043 Rennes cedex, France
[2] Laboratoire d'anatomie, Faculté de Médecine, F35043 Rennes cedex, France

Abstract. We propose an ontology of the brain cortex anatomy representing both numeric and symbolic knowledge. Implementation with web technologies facilitates the ontology's dissemination and reuse in different application contexts. This model references the main terminological sources and can be integrated into larger scale models. It was instantiated as an XML file encompassing anatomical features of the frontal, temporal and parietal lobes. A standalone Java application and an HTML based one have been developed in order to illustrate the knowledge base flexibility. They are both fully interactive with 3D VRML scenes representing the shapes of brain sulci.

Keywords: Brain atlas, knowledge representation, ontology, XML

1 Introduction

Brain cortex anatomy is usually described in terms of gyri and sulci. Their anatomical description proves very useful for neurosurgery procedures and for sharing neuro-imaging data, a key aspect in research on brain anatomy-function relationships. Interindividual variability highlights the need to refer to a model that describes the structures and the relations among them. However, there is still no sound model of cortex anatomy.

We propose a model of brain cortex anatomy that represents both numeric (i.e. derived from images) and symbolic (i.e. based on language descriptions) knowledge. This model extends existing symbolic models and references the main terminological sources. It should provide both human users and applications with grounds for semantic interoperability.

2 Background and Objectives

This section presents the main means of representing anatomical knowledge. We distinguish the trend based on pictures from the one based on symbolic descriptions. We then highlight the limitations of these applications, which led us to define a model of anatomical knowledge for the cerebral cortex encompassing both numeric and symbolic features.

S. Quaglini, P. Barahona, and S. Andreassen (Eds.): AIME 2001, LNAI 2101, pp. 359–368, 2001.
© Springer-Verlag Berlin Heidelberg 2001

2.1   Image-Based Approach

Historically, anatomical pictures and printed atlases were the first media used to represent anatomy. By providing *a priori* knowledge on anatomy, they can help interpret brain pictures. The shift from data to knowledge is specially far from being trivial in neuroscience because of the inter-individual variability. As for brain cortex anatomy, the widely accepted Ono and Duvernoy atlases [1] [2] describe sulci and gyri with statistical variation information. Talairach and Tournoux [3] proposed a 3D squaring system facilitating the matching of patient data against atlas knowledge. However, the printed support restricts (i) representations to static 2D pictures of 3D structures, (ii) extension as it is not possible to add information, and (iii) navigation because of the mostly linear framework.

Computerised atlases let us overcome these limitations. Nowinski's approach [4] consists in achieving a database of corresponding items from various traditional atlases and in reconstructing 3D pictures. A 3D visualisation tool lets the user match data against one of the atlases, and then match this atlas against another. Höhne's team in Hamburg presents a picture-oriented symbolic representation of anatomy. This "Intelligent Volume" model has two layers [5]. The data layer manages CT or MRI labelled volumes. The knowledge layer is a semantic net based on the "anatomical part of" relation. It contains 1000 objects for 2500 links in the domains of morphology, pathology, functional anatomy and the vascular system. Similarly, Kikinis et al. generated a 3D atlas for teaching, segmentation and surgery planning applications from a healthy volunteer [6]. Unlike Höhne's team work, their volumic model is accessible, they use various rendering techniques, and their symbolic model is used in various applications.

Image-based approaches consist in labelling pictures. Relations among labelled elements implicitly lay within the pictures. Other approaches discussed in the next section are based on an explicit description of abstractions of these elements.

2.2   Concept-Based Approach

Symbolic representation of anatomical knowledge consists in identifying abstractions of anatomical elements and shape or location properties. This approach is also implied by terminological issues involved in information sharing. Thus UMLS, a NLM initiative, attempts to facilitate the search for and integration of biomedical information by grouping terminology and nomenclatures of various languages [7]. A semantic net, the metathesaurus, models biomedical information and particularly anatomy. As for brain anatomy, UMLS integrated NeuroNames in 1992. NeuroNames is a hierarchical nomenclature of mutually exclusive structures that constitute a frame to reference neuroanatomic information for humans and macaques, used for teaching, indexation or as an atlas [8]. This terminology is available through the NeuroNames Template Atlas [9], an on-line atlas that visualises the hierarchical structure, locates a concept or retrieves the designation of a location.

Our goal to conceptualise gross anatomy is shared by the Digital Anatomist's (DA) team from the Washington University in Seattle [10]. Rosse et al. distinguish instantiated anatomy from canonical anatomy. The former contains anatomical data generated during clinical practice, and is explicit in clinical reports. The latter is the synthesis of generalisations based upon individual anatomical pieces and is often implicit in clinical reports [11]. The Digital Anatomist's goal is to achieve a symbolic canonical model based on the UMLS Metathesaurus and improved by partition and spatial localisation relations. This model was integrated within the UMLS Metathesaurus in 1998. The Digital Anatomist considers anatomy of the whole body. It is mainly focused on organs but it is scalable as description fields range from tissues to body parts.

The GALEN team stated that needs for medical terminology concern (i) the use of information in various contexts, (ii) the representation of complex and detailed descriptions, (iii) automation of information processing and (iv) maintenance and coherence. GALEN formal concept modeling is based on the GRAIL language. Thanks to this system, coherence rules can be generated and new concepts can be created by composition of other concepts. GRAIL is based upon a concept organisation in orthogonal taxonomies. Thus, specialisation ("is a kind of") can be distinguished from composition ("is a part of"), a prerequisite for processing transitivity problems. This formalism is used in an anatomy model [12][13].

2.3   Motivations

Picture-based approaches rely on the visual aspect of anatomy. Usually, these models are only directed to humans as they require an implicit understanding. Gibaud et al. proposed to re-evaluate the brain atlas concept according to the way content can be used and maintained [14]. They advocated that knowledge should be useable by both humans and applications. This implies a shift from anatomical structure 3D representation to explicit representation of anatomical knowledge. This shift appears in works based upon symbolic approach. However, few of them take advantage of the 3D possibilities offered by electronic support, although 3D representation is a major feature of anatomy. It seems important that a symbolic model should provide a conceptual structure for the actual 3D representation of anatomy, be it of numeric nature.

2.4   Objectives

The objective of this work was to propose a model of brain cortex anatomical structures. This model should explicit the major conceptual entities, their relations as well as 3D representation of their shapes and anatomical variations. Therefore it seemed interesting to enrich symbolic knowledge of cortical features such as sulci with 3D representations of their shapes. Such representations are essential to help clinical users apprehend the 3D shapes of the brain sulci, as well as their respective positions in the 3D space.

The idea is to be able to refer to and/or use this model in a variety of contexts such as decision support in neurosurgery, education, and research in the field of relationships between brain anatomy and functions. The general approach partly relies on Rosse and Brinkley's work with the Digital Anatomist. Particular care was devoted to the semantic definition of conceptual entities and relations in order to guarantee coherence over the whole knowledge corpus. This is essential with regards to the goal of semantic interoperability between independent data or knowledge bases that might use this model in the future.

As far as implementation is concerned, we chose to use technologies developed for the web. Actually, it is obvious that the Internet will constitute the primary vector for knowledge dissemination, be it of a symbolic or numeric nature (images, 3D surfaces, probability maps).

This paper reports the first results of this project. It focuses on a conceptual model of brain cortex anatomical features and explains relationships with other frameworks of modeling such as NeuroNames and Digital Anatomist. It shows that languages and data syntaxes such as XML, XSL, VRML and Java can advantageously be used to represent, browse and display symbolic and numeric data.

3   System Design

3.1   Methods

As we intended to model canonical knowledge, we relied on classical sources such as Ono [1] and Szikla [15] atlases and NeuroNames terminology [8] as well as discussions with clinicians and anatomists. We first identified the concepts involved in cortex anatomy and their relations. The modeling step was performed according to the UML method with class-diagram formalism. We then manually derived a Document Type Definition (DTD) from this diagram. Although it was achieved manually, it followed the principles advocated by Bosworth and al. [16]. Objects were expressed as elements. Properties were attributes. Relations were attributes whose values were IDREF. The Knowledge Base was produced as an eXtensible Markup Language (XML) file, valid according to the DTD.

The 3D models of the sulci shapes represent the median surface of each sulcal fold. They are generated from 3D MRI images by means of a method called "active ribbon method ", developed by Le Goualher and Barillot [17]. The sulci extraction itself involves two steps. The first extracts the sulci external traces on the brain surface, the second models the 3D shape of each sulcus. This process is achieved using an active curve (1D model) which moves from the external trace to the buried part of the sulcus down to the sulcus fundus. A 2D model is then computed from the successive positions of the 1D curve and encoded into a 3D VRML file.

3.2   Ontology of Cortical Anatomy

We present the major concept types and their relations as textual definitions. They are formalised in a UML class diagram (Figure 1).

Concept: A concept is an abstract entity that can be derived in subclasses such as AnatomicalConcept or FunctionalConcept. We only describe AnatomicalConcepts. It may have 0 or more *TextualDescriptions*.

Designation: A Designation is a sequence of symbols (string) relative to a *Terminology*. If the Terminology is UMLS, the designation can also hold CUI, LUI and SUI values (Concept, Label and String Unique Identifier).

AnatomicalConcept: An AnatomicalConcept is a *Concept* that belongs to anatomy as a domain. It has an *AnatomicalNature* and an *AnatomicalParity*. AnatomicalParity expresses the relation between a concept and the cardinality of its concrete instantiation(s). It lets you manipulate concepts without considering their materialisation, for example we could call "Central Sulcus" what is common to the left and right central sulci. AnatomicalParity is necessary to generate an "abstract" cortical anatomy model that holds CentralSulcus and from which a lateralised model is derived with left and right central sulci.

Hemisphere: A Hemisphere is an *AnatomicalConcept*. It is the top level concept for the "anatomical part of" relation in our model. It is composed of anatomical parts which are *Lobes*. We deliberately restricted our study to external cortical representation, excluding sub-cortical structures such as white matter or basal ganglia. Lobe delimitation by sulci is expressed at the *Sulcus* level.

Lobe: A Lobe is an *AnatomicalConcept*. Its anatomical parts are *GyriSet*, *Gyrus* or *Pars*.

GyriSet: A GyriSet is an *AnatomicalConcept*. It is a set of *Gyri*.

Gyrus: A Gyrus is an *AnatomicalConcept*. Its anatomical parts are *Pars*. A Gyrus may be involved in 0 or more *Delimitation* relations by a *Sulcus*. It may be connected to another Gyrus or *Pars* by zero or more *PliDePassage* or *Operculum*.

Pars: A Pars is an *AnatomicalConcept*. Like a *Gyrus*, it may be involved in 0 or more *Delimitation* relations by a *Sulcus*. It may be united with another *Gyrus* or Pars by zero or more *PliDePassage* or *Operculum*.

Sulcus: A Sulcus is an *AnatomicalConcept*. It is a fold of the cortex. It may delimit zero or more *Delimitations*. A Sulcus may be composed of segments that are other Sulci. It can bear branches on its sides that are also Sulci.

ConventionalDelimitation: A ConventionalDelimitation is an *AnatomicalConcept*. It connects two *Gyri* or *Pars* that show no anatomical disruption by *Delimitation*.

Delimitation: A Delimitation is a relation between one or two *Gyri* or *Pars* or *Operculum* or *PliDePassage* and one *Sulcus* or *ConventionalDelimitation*.

Operculum: An Operculum is an *AnatomicalConcept*. It is a bulge of tissue joining two *Gyri* or *Pars* and separating two *Sulci*.

PliDePassage: A PliDePassage is an *AnatomicalConcept*. It is a bulge of tissue joining two *Gyri* and separating two segments of a *Sulcus*.

These definitions were formalised in a UML class Diagram presented in figure 1.

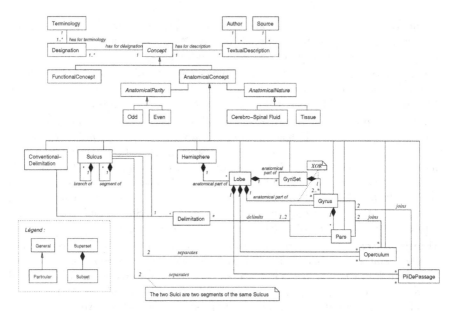

Fig. 1. UML class diagram of cortex anatomy

3.3 Compatibility with NeuroNames and Digital Anatomist

Like NeuroNames, our model defines mutually exclusive concepts. Whenever we found that one of our concept was referenced by NeuroNames, we added the matching *Designation* and specified the CUI, LUI and SUI values.

Our model attempts to represent specific structures of brain cortex that complete the organ-centred body model of Digital Anatomist (DA). Therefore, our "final" classes are specialisations of DA classes (Figure 2). CerebroSpinal Fluid is clearly a kind of DA's BodySubstance. *Sulcus* and *ConventionalDelimitation* are subclasses of AnatomicalSpatialEntity. The others (*Gyrus, Pars, Operculum* and so on) are rather subclasses of OrganSubdivision.

3.4 Knowledge Base Generation

From the UML class diagram, we manually developed a Document Type Definition. This file is a grammar that defines the structure of the knowledge base.

The knowledge base was then populated with the most significant sulci, gyri, pars, pli de passage and operculum of the frontal, temporal and parietal lobes. The structure of this base is a directed graph. The nodes are the concepts and the relations are the arcs. The XML file is a collection of anatomical concepts. Relations are represented by IDREFs references between them.

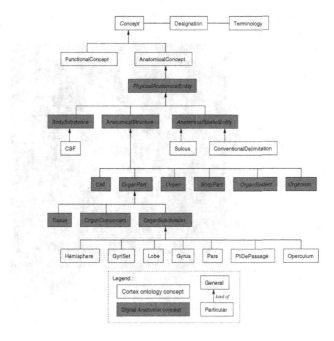

Fig. 2. Integration of cortex anatomical model with Digital Anatomist

4   Demonstration Software

Standalone Java and HTLM applications were developed to facilitate the knowledge base browsing and to demonstrate its flexibility.

4.1   XML Processing

Both applications rely on the XML knowledge base. Thanks to the DOM API, the Java application loads a representation of the XML file. Structure is then reorganised according to the "anatomical part of" relation, and displayed as a tree . With a right click on a concept, a contextual menu presenting the concept properties and relations pops up. The HTML application was generated thanks to XSL Stylesheets. These generate a hierarchy of concepts according to the "anatomical part of" relation and a page of description per concept. Relations between concepts were represented by hyperlinks (figure 3).

Both applications also perform simple inferences. For example, lobe contiguity relations are inferred from gyri. If a G_1 gyrus, anatomical part of a L_1 lobe and a G_2 gyrus, anatomical part of L_2 lobe are separated by a S sulcus, and if L_1 is different from L_2, then S separates L_1 from L_2.

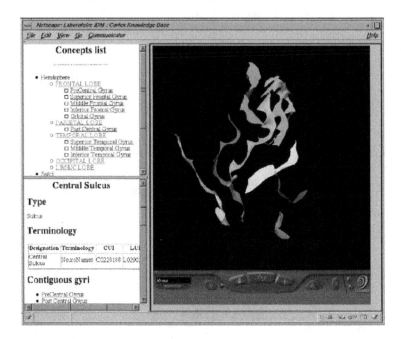

Fig. 3. XSL generated web application from the XML knowledge base file

4.2   3D Interactivity

As 3D representation is an important aspect of anatomy, we proposed an XML
interface to describe a 3D VRML scene and interact with it. We took advantage
of the VRML DEF field to provide an identifier for every shape in a scene. An
XML file can describe a scene by linking a concept identifier to zero, one or many
DEF values.

The Java standalone application is based on the Java3D API to display a
3D VRML scene. In the "*Examine*" mode, the 3D scene can be manipulated.
From the contextual menu in the tree, a concept can be highlighted in the scene
by colouring its shape(s) red. In the "*Select concept*" mode, clicking on a shape
selects the matching concept in the tree, provided the shape describes a concept.

The HTML-based application relies on a VRML plugin to display a VRML
scene. Thus, it is not the original VRML scene that is used, but an upgraded
scene with JavaScript code to manage concept selection by the user. This
JavaScript code performs the adequate changes of colour and updates the concept description in the lower left frame.

Both applications synchronise the conceptual view of anatomy and numerical
aspects.

5   Discussion

We experienced some difficulties when defining entities that were ill-formalised in the anatomical sources such as *Gyrus*, *Pars*, *Operculum* or *PliDePassage*. The choices we made were a compromise between a highly formalised model that wouldn't match the intuitive aspect of anatomy, and a model that would be a straightforward transcription of anatomists' discourse but would lack consistency. For example our model shows no structural difference between a *Lobe* and a *GyriSet*: both are a set of contiguous *Gyrus* entities. On the other hand, usual distinctions between primary, secondary and tertiary sulci were not taken into account.

GALEN could have been a solution for better formalisation and increased inference capabilities. However, our current goal is mainly descriptive whereas GALEN formalism and GRAIL are optimised to link pathological processes and functions with anatomy, which is out of our scope and would have led to an overcomplicated model. On the other hand, terminology such as NeuroNames provided a sound starting point but had to be extended with additional anatomical structures and relationships (in particular spatial relationships).

XML must be seen as a file exchange format rather than a storage format. Our knowledge base has to be accessible in various application contexts. Therefore, we used XML for implementation in order to benefit from both its capacity to deliver the information a client application has specifically requested, and its platform and application independence features. The applications we presented can be seen as client-sides that received the knowledge base as an XML file after a request to a server. We did not consider that our model should be stored as an XML file on the server side.

The XML file format is based on ASCII characters. It can specify the encoding mode, thus ensuring syntactical interoperability. We expect semantic interoperability to derive from our UML model and its integration in semantic nets such as UMLS.

6   Conclusion

We have presented a model that represents numeric and symbolic knowledge of cortex anatomy. The knowledge base was then populated with the most significant anatomical features of the frontal, temporal and parietal lobes. The use of XML combined with XSL or Java enabled us to quickly implement demonstration applications.

We plan to use this model in various application contexts. However, we still need to confirm that when used in different perspectives (neurosurgery or research on anatomy-function relationships for instance), our model is still adequate for each context or context-sensitive interpretation. Furthermore, one of our goals is to use it as a reference to federate neuro-imaging data from multiple sites. Our detailed model for concepts and relations may help to remove semantic conflicts that will certainly arise between site-specific representations. More complete formalisation may be required, such as that available within GALEN.

References

1. Ono M, Kubik S, Abernathey C. In : Atlas of the Cerebral Sulci. Georg Thieme Verlag ed. Thieme Medical Publishers, Inc. New-York. 1990.
2. Duvernoy HM. In : The Human Brain : Surface, Three-Dimensional Sectional Anatomy and MRI. Springer-Verlag, Wien New-York. 1991.
3. Talairach J, Tournoux P. In : Co-Planar Stereotactic Atlas of the Human Brain. Georg Thieme Verlag ed. Thieme Medical Publishers, Inc. New-York. 1988.
4. Nowinski WL, Fang A, Nguyen BT, Raphel JK, L Jagannathan, R Raghavan, RN Brian, GA Miller. Multiple Brain Atlas Database and Atlas-Based Neuroimaging System. Computer Aided Surgery. 1997 2:42-66.
5. Pommert A, Schubert R, Riemer M, Schiemann T, Tiede U, Höhne KH. Symbolic Modeling of Human Anatomy for Visualization and Simulation. In : Visualization in Biomedical Computing RA Robb ed., Proc. SPIE 2359, Rochester, MN. 1994. 412-423.
6. Kikinis R, Shenton ME, Iosifescu DV, McCarley RW, Saiviroonporn P, Hokama HH, Robatino A, Metclaf D, Wible CG, Portas CM, Donnino RM, Jolesz FA. A Digital Brain Atlas for Surgical Planning, Model-Driven Segmentation, and Teaching. IEEE Transactions on Visualization and Computer Graphics. Sept 1996 Vol2 Num3. 232-241.
7. National Library of Medicine.Overview of the UMLS Project. In : CDROM Documentation. 2-16.
8. Bowden DM, Martin RF. NeuroNames Brain Hierarchy. Neuroimage. 1995, 2. 63-83.
9. RPRC Neurosciences Division, University of Washington, Seattle (WA). NeuroNames Template Atlas Homepage. http://rprcsgi.rprc.washington.edu/neuronames/
10. Structural Information Group, University of Washington, Seattle (WA). The Digital Anatomist Project. http://sig.biostr.washington.edu/projects/da/
11. Rosse C, Mejino JL, Modayur BR, Jakobovitz R, Hinshaw KP, Brinkley JF. Motivation and Organizational Principles for Anatomical Knowledge Representation. JAMIA. Jan-Feb 1998 volume 5 number 1. 17-40.
12. Rector A, Gangemi A, Galeazzi E, Glowinski AJ, Rossi-Mori A. The GALEN Model Schemata for Anatomy : Towards a re-usable Application-Independant model of Medical Concepts. Proceedings of Medical Informatics in Europe MIE94. 229-233.
13. Rector A, Zanstra PE, Solomon WD, Rogers JE, Baud R, Ceusters W, Claassen W, Kirby J, Rodrigues JM, Rossi-Mori A, van der Haring EJ, Wagner J. Reconciling Users' Needs and Formal Requirements : Issues in Developping a Reusable Ontology for Medicine. IEEE Transactions on Information Technology in Biomedicine. Dec. 1998. Vol 2 Num 4. 229-242.
14. Gibaud B, Garlatti S, Barillot C, Faure E. Computerized brain atlases as decision support systems : a methodological approach. Artificial Intelligence in Medicine. 1998, 14. 83-100.
15. Szikla G, Bouvier G, Hori T, Petrov V. In : Angiography of the Human Brain Cortex. Spinger-Verlag ed. Berlin Heidelberg New-York. 1977.
16. Bosworth A, Layman A, Rys M. Serialising Graphs of Data in XML. The GCA XML Europe 99 Conference Proceedings Granada, Spain. May 1999. (http://www.biztalk.org/Resources/canonical.asp).
17. Le Goualher G, Barillot C, Bizais Y. Modeling cortical sulci with active ribbons. Int. J. of Pattern Recognition and Artificial Intelligence. 1997. Vol.11, num8. 1295-1315.

Depth-Four Threshold Circuits for Computer-Assisted X-ray Diagnosis*

A. Albrecht[1,2], E. Hein[3], K. Steinhöfel[4], M. Taupitz[3], and C.K. Wong[2]

[1] Dept. of Computer Science, Univ. of Hertfordshire, Hatfield, Herts AL10 9AB, UK
[2] Dept. of Computer Science and Engineering, CUHK, Shatin, N.T., Hong Kong
[3] Faculty of Medicine, Humboldt University of Berlin, 10117 Berlin, Germany
[4] GMD–National Research Center for IT, Kekuléstraße 7, 12489 Berlin, Germany

Abstract. The paper continues our research from [1]. We present a stochastic algorithm that computes threshold circuits designed to discriminate between two classes of CT images. The algorithm is evaluated for the case of liver tissue classification. A depth-four threshold circuit is calculated from 400 positive (abnormal findings) and 400 negative (normal liver tissue) examples. The examples are of size $n = 14161 = 119 \times 119$ with an 8 bit grey scale. On test sets of $100 + 100$ examples (all different from the learning set) we obtain a correct classification of about 96%. The classification of a single image is performed within a few seconds.

1 Introduction

The present study was performed to investigate the computer-assisted interpretation of CT scans of the liver. Forty cases with normal findings and 150 cases with liver pathology were selected from a total number of 735 abdominal and biphasic upper abdominal CT examinations. The abnormal findings were confirmed by histology in 83 patients and by follow-up in patients with known malignancy in 67 instances. Ten to fifteen slices were selected for the cases with normal findings and between one and five slices from the portal-venous phase for those with abnormal findings.

Representative areas from these slices depicting normal liver tissue as well as vessel cross-sections and cysts or one or more focal liver lesions surrounded by normal liver tissue were identified and recalculated for a matrix of 128x128. A total number of 500 ROIs showing normal liver parenchyma and another 500 ROIs with abnormal findings (hypodense lesions) were used in our study.

The paper describes a learning-based method of computing depth-four threshold circuits for classification purposes. The main features of the algorithm and first results for a smaller number of examples have been presented in [1] already. We are focusing on the comparison of classification results for circuits

* Research partially supported by the Strategic Research Programme at The Chinese University of Hong Kong under Grant No. SRP 9505, by a Hong Kong Government RGC Earmarked Grant, Ref. No. CUHK 4010/98E.

S. Quaglini, P. Barahona, and S. Andreassen (Eds.): AIME 2001, LNAI 2101, pp. 369–373, 2001.
© Springer-Verlag Berlin Heidelberg 2001

of a depth up to four, where the underlying set of learning examples consists of $400 + 400$ images. The test is performed on $100 + 100$ additional positive and negative examples.

To our knowledge, the first papers on learning-based methods applied to X-ray diagnosis are [3,8]. Recent work on AI methods in medical image classification is published in [4,6,7]. Usually, these methods require pre-processing and incorporate feature extraction from CT scans, cf. [6]. In our approach, we take the image information as the only input to the algorithm.

Our algorithm consists of two main steps: Firstly, linear threshold functions are calculated which are designed to approximate randomly chosen subsets S of fixed size out of $400 + 400$ learning examples. These functions are taken for the first layer of the threshold circuit. To minimise the error on the subsets S, we use a new combination of the Perceptron algorithm with simulated annealing. The cooling schedule is defined by a logarithmic decremental rule, while the neighbourhood is determined by the Perceptron algorithm. Secondly, the functions from the first layer are combined by a fixed structure to a depth-four threshold circuit. The threshold functions from the second layer were determined by computational experiments, while the functions (gates) from the third layer and the output gate (fourth layer) are simple majority functions.

2   The Learning Algorithm

We assume that rational numbers are represented by pairs of binary tuples of length d and denote the set of linear threshold functions by $\mathcal{F} := \cup_{n \geq 1} \mathcal{F}_n$ for $\mathcal{F}_n = \{ f(\boldsymbol{x}) \; : \; f(\boldsymbol{x}) = \sum_{i=1}^n w_i \cdot x_i \geq \vartheta_f \}$, where w_i and x_i are pairs $\pm(p_i, q_i)$, $p_i, q_i \in \{0, 1\}^d$. The functions from $\mathcal{F}$ are used to design circuits $\mathcal{C}$ of threshold functions, i.e., acyclic graphs where the nodes v are labelled either by input variables or threshold functions. The depth of $\mathcal{C}$ is the maximum number of edges on a path from an input node x_i to the output node v_{out}. In the present paper, the maximum depth of $\mathcal{C}$ is four.

We consider a sample set $S = \{ [\boldsymbol{x}, \eta] \}$ for $\eta \in \{+, -\}$ and $\boldsymbol{x} = (x_1, ..., x_n)$, where $x_i = (p_i, q_i)$, $p_i, q_i \in \{0, 1\}^d$. The objective is to minimise the number $| S \Delta f |$ of misclassified examples, $S \Delta f := \{[\boldsymbol{x}, \eta] : f(\boldsymbol{x}) < \vartheta_f \& \eta = +$ or $f(\boldsymbol{x}) > \vartheta_f \& \eta = - \}$, and we denote $\mathcal{Z}(f) := | S \Delta f |$. Given $f \in \mathcal{F}_n$, the neighbourhood relation $\mathcal{N}_f$ is suggested by the Perceptron algorithm [5] and defined by

$$(1) \qquad w_i(f') := w_i - y_j \cdot x_{ij} / \sqrt{\sum_{i=1}^n w_i^2}, \; j \in \{1, 2, ..., m\},$$

for all i simultaneously and for a specified j that maximises $| y_j - \vartheta_f |$, where $y_j = \sum_{i=1}^n w_i \cdot x_{ij}$. The threshold $\vartheta_{f'}$ is equal to $\vartheta_f + y_j / \sqrt{\sum_{i=1}^n w_i^2}$.

Given a pair $[f, f']$, $f' \in \mathcal{N}_f$, we denote by $G[f, f']$ the probability of generating f' from f and by $A[f, f']$ the probability of accepting f' once it has been generated from f. To speed up the local search for minimum error solutions, we take a non-uniform generation probability where the transitions are forced into the direction of the maximum deviation.

The non-uniform generation probability is derived from the Perceptron algorithm: When f is the current hypothesis, we set

$$
(2) \qquad U(\boldsymbol{x}) := \begin{cases} -f(\boldsymbol{x}), & \text{if } f(\boldsymbol{x}) < \vartheta_f \text{ and } \eta(\boldsymbol{x}) = +, \\ f(\boldsymbol{x}), & \text{if } f(\boldsymbol{x}) \geq \vartheta_f \text{ and } \eta(\boldsymbol{x}) = -, \\ 0, & \text{otherwise.} \end{cases}
$$

For $f' \in \mathcal{N}_f$, we set $G[f, f'] := U(\boldsymbol{x})/\sum_{\boldsymbol{x} \in S\Delta f} U(\boldsymbol{x})$. Thus, preference is given to the neighbours that maximise the deviation. Now, our heuristic can be summarised in the following way:

1. The initial hypothesis is defined by $w_i = 1$, $i = 1, 2, \ldots n$ and $\vartheta = 0$.
2. For the current hypothesis, the probabilities $U(\boldsymbol{x})$ are calculated; see (2).
3. To determine the next hypothesis f_k, a random choice is made among the elements of $\mathcal{N}_{f_{k-1}}$ according to the definition of $G[f, f']$.
4. When $\mathcal{Z}(f_k) \leq \mathcal{Z}(f_{k-1})$, we set $A[f_{k-1}, f_k] := 1$.
5. When $\mathcal{Z}(f_k) > \mathcal{Z}(f_{k-1})$, a random number $\rho \in [0, 1]$ is drawn uniformly.
6. If $A[f_{k-1}, f_k] := e^{-(\mathcal{Z}(f_k) - \mathcal{Z}(f_{k-1})/c(k))} \geq \rho$, the function f_k is the new hypothesis. Otherwise, we return to 3 with f_{k-1}.
7. The computation is terminated after a predefined number of steps K.

The crucial parameter $c(k)$ is defined by $c(k) = \Gamma/\ln(k + 2)$, $k = 0, 1, \ldots$ (for a theoretical justification, see [2]).

3   Implementation and Results

The heuristic was implemented in C^{++} and we performed computational experiments on SUN Ultra 5/270 workstation with 128 MB RAM under Solaris 2.6.

The input to the algorithm was derived from the DICOM standard representation of CT images. In Figure 1 and Figure 2, examples of input instances are shown in the DICOM format. From these 128×128 images we calculated 8-bit grey scale representations of size 119×119.

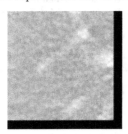

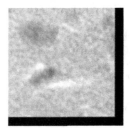

Fig. 1. An example of normal liver tissue (negative example).

Fig. 2. An example of tumour tissue (positive example).

From a total number of 400 positive (abnormal findings) and 400 negative examples (normal liver tissue) we computed 11 independent hypotheses of the type $f = w_1 \cdot x_1 + \cdots + w_n \cdot x_n \geq \vartheta$ for $n = 14161$. The parameter Γ was determined by computational experiments and set equal to 77.

Each particular function was trained on a random choice of $100 + 100$ examples out of $400 + 400$ examples. We used a combined termination criterion: The learning process terminates for a single function when either $k > L_{\max}$ or the percentage of correctly classified examples is larger than or equal to 99%.

A depth-two sub-circuit consists of 11 linear threshold functions (first layer gates). Due to the random choice of 200 out of 800 examples, the examples are learned in the average "2.75 times." The weights of the threshold functions at level two are normalised to 1, and the threshold values were determined by computational experiments. Three sub-circuits of depth two are calculated independently and taken together with an additional gate $x_1 + x_2 + x_3 \geq 2$ to form a depth-three threshold circuit.

Table 1

$n = 14161$	$|$POS$|=|$NEG$|= 100$ out of 400		$|$T_POS$|=|$T_NEG$|= 100$		
Depth of Circuits	Total Run-Time (Min.)	Errors on POS NEG		Errors on T_POS T_NEG		Percentage of Errors
2	2797	1	1	21	25	23 %
3	7813	0	1	9	13	11 %
4	23072*⁾	0	1	3	5	4%

From three independent, parallel computations of depth-three circuits we calculated the output of a virtual depth-four circuit (indicated by *⁾ in Table 1).

References

1. A. Albrecht, K. Steinhöfel, M. Taupitz, and C.K Wong. Logarithmic Simulated Annealing for Computer-Assisted X-ray Diagnosis. To appear in *Artificial Intelligence in Medicine*.
2. A. Albrecht and C.K. Wong. On Logarithmic Simulated Annealing. In: J. van Leeuwen, O. Watanabe, M. Hagiya, P.D. Mosses, T. Ito, eds., *Theoretical Computer Science: Exploring New Frontiers of Theoretical Informatics*, pp. 301 – 314, LNCS Series, vol. 1872, 2000.
3. N. Asada, K. Doi, H. McMahon, S. Montner, M.L. Giger, C. Abe, Y.C. Wu. Neural Network Approach for Differential Diagnosis of Interstitial Lung Diseases: A Pilot Study. *Radiology*, 177:857 – 860, 1990.
4. H. Handels, Th. Roß, J. Kreusch, H.H. Wolff and S.J. Pöppl. Feature Selection for Optimized Skin Tumour Recognition Using Genetic Algorithms. *Artificial Intelligence in Medicine*, 16(3):283 – 297, 1999.
5. M.L. Minsky and S.A. Papert. *Perceptrons*. MIT Press, Cambridge, Mass., 1969.

6. C.A. Pea-Reyes and M. Sipper. A Fuzzy-genetic Approach to Breast Cancer Diagnosis. *Artificial Intelligence in Medicine*, 17(2):131 – 155, 1999.
7. A.L. Ronco. Use of Artificial Neural Networks in Modeling Associations of Discriminant Factors: Towards an Intelligent Selective Breast Cancer Screening. *Artificial Intelligence in Medicine*, 16(3):299 – 309, 1999.
8. W.H. Wolberg and O.L. Mangasarian. Multisurface Method of Pattern Separation for Medical Diagnosis Applied to Breast Cytology. *Proceedings of the National Academy of Sciences U.S.A.*, 87:9193–9196, 1990.

Management of Hospital Teams for Organ Transplants Using Multi-agent Systems

Antonio Moreno, AïdaValls, and Jaime Bocio

Departament d'Enginyeria Informàtica i Matemàtiques
Universitat Rovira i Virgili
Carretera de Salou, s/n. 43006-Tarragona, Spain
{amoreno,avalls}@etse.urv.es

Abstract. In this work we have used Artificial Intelligence techniques to ease the management of hospital teams for organ transplants. We have designed and implemented a multi-agent system that provides a fast mechanism for having an operating theatre and a transplant medical team ready when an organ to be transplanted arrives to a hospital, thereby avoiding potentially fatal delays due to any mistake in the management of the necessary items for the operation. The experimental results made in the laboratory have been successful, both in the response time of the system and in the quality of its performance.

1. Introduction

Co-ordinating all the processes involved in an organ transplant operation is a very challenging problem. When an organ is available at a certain hospital, at least three issues must be sorted out:

- The most appropriate receptor must be found.

    This problem is quite difficult, since there may be many patients distributed around the country waiting for a certain type of organ. It is important to take into account factors such as the distance to the organ's donor (which determines the temporal and economic cost of the transport of the organ), the urgency with which the potential recipient requires the organ, and the adequacy of the available organ with the characteristics of the patients who are waiting for it.
- The organ must be sent to the hospital of the chosen recipient.

    Once the receptor has been chosen, the organ must be sent to his/her hospital as soon as possible. Finding a good solution to this problem may involve looking up several (spatially distributed) databases with timetables of means of transport, such as trains or planes, and making spatial and temporal reasoning to provide the most efficient route. Notice that, unlike other human components such as blood or tissues, that may be frozen and kept for days or weeks, there is a very short period of time (just some hours) in which an organ may be used for a transplant. Therefore, these two steps have to be performed as quickly as possible.
- All the necessary elements for performing the operation must be ready when the organ arrives.

S. Quaglini, P. Barahona, and S. Andreassen (Eds.): AIME 2001, LNAI 2101, pp. 374–383, 2001.
© Springer-Verlag Berlin Heidelberg 2001

While the organ is being transported to the recipient's hospital, everything must be set up there so that the operation may be performed as soon as the organ arrives. This is the problem considered in this paper. Note that this arrangement process must also be made very quickly, in parallel with the previous one.

In the rest of the article the reader should always bear in mind that the following simplifying assumptions have been considered:

- The first two issues (finding a receptor and an optimal way of transporting the organ) have already been sorted out. Thus, it is known which is the type of the organ and its arrival time to the receptor's hospital.
- There may be several operating theatres in the hospital. All of them are assumed to be identical, so any of them may be used for any kind of transplant operation.
- Each kind of transplant operation requires a certain amount of doctors, nurses and anaesthetists (we have not considered other kinds of medical personnel). The chosen doctors must be specialists in the particular type of organ; nurses and anaesthetists do not have any speciality, and may participate in all transplant operations. Each of these people has access to a personal computer.

The aim of the system is to find an operating theatre in which the transplant operation may be performed, and also find the medical team (doctors, nurses and anaesthetists) that will be assigned to that operation. It must detect those cases in which it is impossible to perform the operation (e.g. when there is not any available operating theatre). In these cases the system will tell the transplant co-ordinator that it is not possible to perform the operation at that hospital, and another waiting patient would be selected by the transplant co-ordinator of the donor's hospital.

The paper is organised as follows. First, it is argued why Artificial Intelligence techniques (in particular, Multi-Agent Systems, MAS) offer an appropriate framework for attacking this problem. After that, we describe the particular MAS that we have designed and implemented, and we describe with detail the co-ordination process that it supports. The paper finishes with a brief discussion and an outline of some future lines of work.

2. Multi-agent Systems

The design and implementation of MAS [1] is one of the main leading problems in Artificial Intelligence at the moment. A MAS may be defined as a collection of individual, communicating, intelligent, autonomous programs (agents) that co-operate to solve a task that may not be individually solved by any of them. Having a distributed MAS (instead of a single centralised program) that tries to solve a complex problem (such as the management of medical teams) is interesting for the following reasons:

- Each of the agents may be executing in a different computer. Therefore, all of them may be working at the same time, and this will lead to a faster solution to the problem. For example, all the agents that manage the schedule of an operating theatre may be checking at the same time whether it may be used for a transplant operation.

- Each agent may access resources that are available in the computer in which it is running. Thus, it is possible to solve inherently distributed problems, in which knowledge is spatially distributed. This is certainly the case in our problem, in which each member of the hospital staff is assumed to maintain his/her weekly schedule in a different personal computer.
- It is possible to add more agents into the system (or to remove some of them), without modifying the existing ones. In our case, it would be very easy to add more operating theatres or doctors to the running system.
- The system is more robust to failures, because there may be several agents that solve the same kind of problem; if the computer in which one of them is running goes down, the other agents in the MAS can notice this fact and solve the problem that had been previously assigned to that agent. For instance, if the personal computer of a nurse is not working, the transplant operation will be scheduled with the rest of the personnel.
- It is not necessary to write complex programs that solve difficult problems. It is easier to write simpler agents, specialised in particular tasks, and let them communicate and co-operate to solve larger problems. In section 4 the co-ordination process will be explained, and it will be seen how it involves simple decisions by each agent.

3. Architecture of the Multi-agent System

In the task of managing hospital teams for organ transplants, it is possible to assign one agent to each member of the personnel (doctor, nurse or anaesthetist). This program is continuously running on the person's computer, and it has the basic mission of keeping track of the user's schedule. Each day has been divided in 48 slots of 30 minutes. Each of these slots may be in three different states: *free* (the user is not busy at that moment, and could be assigned to an operation, if required), *occupied* (the user has to perform a certain task at that particular time), and *operating* (the user has been assigned an organ transplant operation in that slot). The user may access this schedule at any time, and may modify the days and hours in which he/she is *free* or *occupied*. When an agent notices that his/her associated user has been assigned to a transplant operation, it tells him/her by sending a message or showing an appropriate sign on the computer's screen.

The MAS also contains agents for maintaining the schedule of each operating theatre. The daily schedule is also divided in 48 slots; each slot may only be *free* (if that operating theatre is available at that time) or *occupied* (if there is an operation scheduled there at that time). These agents are running in the computer of the member of the personnel responsible of co-ordinating the activity of the operating theatres. This person may access the schedules and modify them appropriately, if necessary.

The architecture of the MAS that has been designed and implemented is shown in Fig. 1. In that figure the agents that take care of the different schedules (medical personnel, operating theatres) are represented by tables. The seven large boxes represent the other agents in the system.

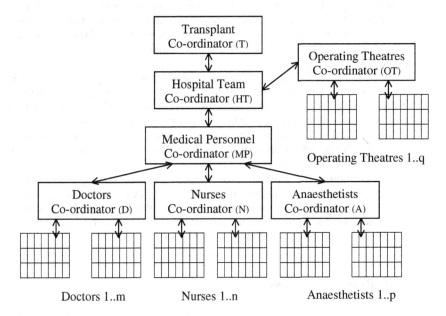

Fig. 1. Architecture of the Multi-agent System

We will now provide a brief description of each of the basic agents of the system. In the next section the co-ordinating process in which they engage will be carefully detailed. The main agents of the system are the following:

- Transplant co-ordinator (T)

    This agent presents the interface of the MAS with the environment. When it receives a message with the type of organ and its arrival time, it initiates the co-ordinating process by sending this information to the hospital team co-ordinator (HT). If the process is successfully completed, T will receive from HT a message with the elements selected to perform the operation (initial time, operating theatre, and medical personnel).

- Hospital team co-ordinator (HT)

    This is the central agent of the system. It receives from T the basic data necessary for arranging the operation (type of organ and arrival time), and passes it along to the operating theatres co-ordinator (OT) and the medical personnel co-ordinator (MP). When HT receives from these agents the times in which there are free operating theatres and there is enough personnel, it tries to match them to find an appropriate time for the operation. If this matching is successful, OT and MP will receive the confirmation of the selected operating theatre and medical team.

- Operating theatres co-ordinator (OT)

  This agent receives from HT the information about the time in which the organ is arriving. It gets in touch with the agents associated to the operating theatres to find out which of them are available in appropriate time intervals. After receiving the different possibilities in which the operation may be performed, it sends them to HT (which tries to match them against the times in which there is enough personnel available). HT will select one of the possibilities, and then OT will tell the selected operating theatre so that it can update its schedule.

- Medical personnel co-ordinator (MP)

  This agent receives from HT the information about the type of organ and its arrival time. It sends this information to the agents that co-ordinate the schedules of doctors (D), nurses (N) and anaesthetists (A). It will receive information from those agents about the personnel which may perform the operation, and it will try to form medical teams with the appropriate number of people of each of the three categories. The possible teams that may perform the operation will then be sent to the hospital team co-ordinator.

- Doctors co-ordinator (D), nurses co-ordinator (N), anaesthetists co-ordinator (A)

  Each of these agents is responsible of the communication with the agents that keep the schedule of each person in the hospital. When they receive a request, they collect the data of all available staff members of a certain type, and send this information to the medical personnel co-ordinator.

4. Co-ordinating Process

The co-ordinating process will be described with the aid of an example, in which a hospital with 6 doctors, 6 anaesthetists, 6 nurses and 3 operating theatres will be considered. Fig. 2 shows the initial timetables; the empty slots are *free*, whereas the filled slots denote intervals that are *occupied* or *operating*.

	D1	D2	D3	D4	D5	D6		A1	A2	A3	A4	A5	A6		N1	N2	N3	N4	N5	N6		O1	O2	O3
2:00							2:00							2:00							2:00			
2:30							2:30							2:30							2:30			
3:00							3:00							3:00							3:00			
3:30							3:30							3:30							3:30			
4:00							4:00							4:00							4:00			
4:30							4:30							4:30							4:30			
5:00							5:00							5:00							5:00			
5:30							5:30							5:30							5:30			
6:00							6:00							6:00							6:00			

Fig. 2. Timetables of doctors, anaesthetists, nurses, and operating theatres

The MAS contains 28 agents: the 7 basic co-ordinating agents, the 18 agents that control the schedule of each member of the staff, and the 3 agents that control the schedule of the operating theatres. Note that the latter 21 agents may be easily running in different computers, while the 7 former agents would probably be running in a single computer (e.g. in the office of the person in charge of organ transplants in the hospital).

When there is an organ available for transplant and it has been assigned to a patient of the hospital, the transplant co-ordinator (T) receives a message with four items: the arrival time of the organ, the final time in which the operation must have been already completed, the length of the operation and the type of organ. In the example, this initial message will be (02:00 06:00 01:00 heart). That means that the system must schedule a heart transplant operation, that this operation will last 1 hour, and that it must be made between 02:00 and 06:00. Thus, the first interval in which the operation may be performed is 02:00-03:00, while the last possible interval is 05:00-06:00. T will send the same message to the hospital team co-ordinator, HT, that will pass it along to the medical personnel co-ordinator (MP) and the operating theatres co-ordinator (OT). In the latter case, as the selected operating theatre does not depend on the type of organ to be transplanted, this information need not be sent to OT. MP will send the data to the co-ordinators of doctors (D), nurses (N) and anaesthetists (A). In the two latter cases the type of organ is not needed either (see Fig. 3).

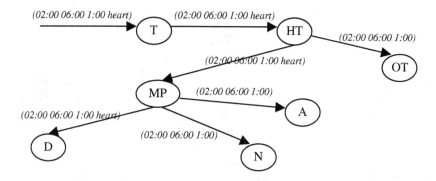

Fig. 3. First steps of the co-ordinating process

At this point of the process OT, D, N and A follow the same strategy. Each of them starts a *contract-net protocol* [2] in order to find out which operating theatres (doctors / nurses / anaesthetists) could participate in the transplant operation in the required time span. In a contract net protocol, an agent sends a *call for proposals* to a set of agents, asking them whether they are willing to give a certain service. The requested agents may reply with a *propose* (if they want to provide that service, under certain requirements) or with a *refuse* (if they are not interested in making any proposal). The initiator of the protocol evaluates the proposals and may send an *accept-proposal* message to the best offer and *reject-proposal* messages to the rest. In our case, OT will send a *call for proposals* to each of the agents that control the schedule of each operating theatre. Each of them will answer with a *proposal* (specifying the available time intervals) or a *refuse* to make a proposal, if there is not any available free interval of the required length (see Fig. 4 at the top of the next page).

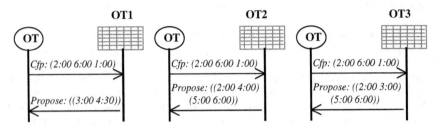

Fig. 4. Start of the contract net protocol between OT and the operating theatres

Following the same strategy, D, N and A receive the availability of each doctor, nurse and anaesthetist in the required time interval (i.e. free continuous spaces of at least 1 hour between 02:00 and 06:00). In the example it is assumed that the 6 doctors are heart specialists. Having received all this data, D, N and A send it to the medical personnel co-ordinator (MP). These messages are shown in Fig. 5.

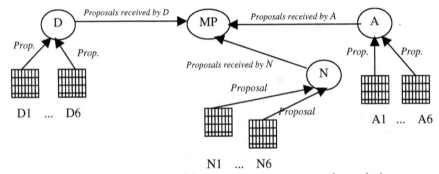

Fig. 5. MP receives the data of the available doctors, nurses and anaesthetists

MP knows how many people of each kind of staff is necessary for transplanting each type of organ. In this example it will be assumed that, in the case of heart transplants, it is necessary to have 2 doctors, 3 anaesthetists and 2 nurses. Therefore, MP finds out in which intervals (if any) is possible to join 7 people with the required characteristics. The hospital team co-ordinator receives from MP the intervals in which it is possible to join the medical team, and from OT the intervals in which there is an available operating theatre (see Fig. 6).

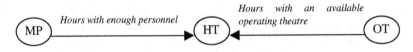

Fig. 6. HT receives time intervals from MP and OT

In the example followed in this section, the 1-hour intervals between 02:00 and 06:00 in which there are available operating theatres are ((02:00 03:00) (02:30 03:30) (03:00 04:00) (03:30 04:30) (05:00 06:00)). The 1-hour intervals in which it is possible to join 2 heart doctors, 3 anaesthetists and 2 nurses (which have been computed by MP from the information received from D, A and N) are ((03:30 04:30) (04:00 05:00) (05:00 06:00)). HT, after analysing these lists, notices that there are two possible intervals in which there is both an available medical team and a free operating theatre: (03:30 04:30) and (05:00 06:00). In order to decide which is the best possibility, the system follows the following criterion: it is interesting that the time intervals in which operating theatres are available are as long as possible, since that will leave the possibility of assigning more operations in the future. To achieve that goal, HT sends the possible intervals to OT, which forwards them to the agents that control the schedule of each operating theatre. Each of these agents replies to OT with an *score* for each possibility, that reflects how well the interval "fits" in the empty spaces in the operating theatre's schedule, and is computed as follows. If the operating theatre is not free in the given interval, the score is 0. If the given interval fits perfectly in a free space in the operating theatre's schedule (i.e. there are not free slots just before and after the interval), the score is 3. If there are empty slots right before and after the interval, the score is 1. If there is an empty slot in one side of the interval but the other side is not free, the score is 2. In the example, the scores obtained by the interval 03:30-04:30 are 2, 0 and 0, whereas the scores obtained by the interval 05:00-06:00 are 0, 3 and 3. Thus, OT would notice that the best option is to perform the operation from 05:00 to 06:00 in any of the two available operating theatres (2 and 3). All this process is shown in Fig. 7.

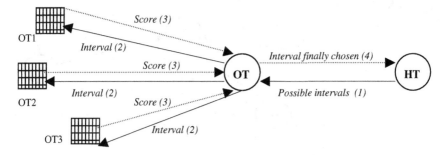

Fig. 7. Four steps in the selection of the best-fitting time interval

Assume that operating theatre 2 is selected. Then, OT would complete the previous contract-net protocol by sending an *accept-proposal* to operating theatre 2 and a *reject-proposal* to the other two operating theatres (see Fig. 8). Then, the agent in charge of the schedule of operating theatre 2 would update it by marking the interval 05:00-06:00 as *occupied*, and would inform OT of this updating. Then, OT can send the selected operating theatre and time interval to the hospital team co-ordinator, HT.

HT sends the interval of the operation to MP, who passes it to D, A, and N (along with the number of each type of staff members that have to be selected to perform the operation). Thus, in the example MP would tell D, A and N that the operation is going to take place from 05:00-06:00, and that 2 doctors, 3 anaesthetists and 2 nurses must be selected in that interval. Each of these three agents follows the same "scoring" procedure in order to make this selection: it will choose those staff members whose empty slots match better with the selected interval. In the example, the best scores are

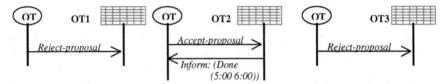

Fig. 8. Updating the schedule of the selected operating theatre

obtained by doctors 4 and 6 (3 points), anaesthetists 1 (3 points), 2 and 6 (2 points) and nurses 2 and 3 (2 points). Therefore, the schedule of these 7 people would be updated to reflect that they have been assigned to the transplant operation, and they would be told of this assignment by their personal agents. D, A, and N will tell MP which people have been chosen, and MP will send this information to HT. HT will then be able to send a message to T with the complete information: interval in which the operation is going to take place, operating theatre and medical personnel assigned to the operation. The final messages are shown in Fig. 9.

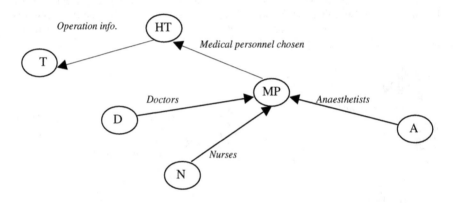

Fig. 9. Final messages in the co-ordination process

In the case in which it is not possible to set up the transplant operation with the given time requirements, HT will warn T of this failure and will explain its cause (lack of operating theatres, lack of medical personnel, impossibility of joining the medical team, or impossibility of matching the medical team with the available operating theatres).

5. Discussion and Future Work

The Multi-Agent System described in this paper has been implemented on Windows in standard PCs in Jade [3]. Jade is a collection of Java libraries that ease the implementation of FIPA-compliant multi-agent systems [4]. In the present stage the system has only been tested in the laboratory with toy examples. Another limitation in all the simulations that have been performed is that all the agents were running in the same computer. The response time of the system, in the case of trials of the size of the example used in this paper, is less than 10 seconds. This speed allows us to treat all the requests sent to a hospital separately, and not in parallel. In this way we can avoid many problems that should be tackled if several requests were being treated at the same time. The system could be easily extended to allow more types of organs or medical personnel.

The way of assigning operating theatres and people to the transplant operations, which tries to keep the empty spaces in their schedules as large as possible, is certainly quite rudimentary, and does not take into account other important factors (e.g. the work should be evenly distributed between all the members of the staff, or a doctor should rest for some hours between two transplant operations). The medical team co-ordinator (MT) should use different strategies in order to achieve these goals.

We are aware of previous works in which agents have been applied to the health-care domain, especially in the area of co-operative patient management [5],[6]. In [7] the use of an electronic institution (implemented with a MAS) to aid in a fair assignment of organs and tissues stored for transplant in human beings is proposed.

It is interesting to notice that the co-ordinating techniques developed in this work could be used in any other domain in which it is necessary to arrange the use of material resources (such as operating theatres) and different types of human resources (such as doctors or nurses) to solve a particular problem under given time constraints.

We are also developing MAS that tackle the issues of finding the most appropriate receptor of an organ and finding the most efficient route to send it to the receptor's hospital. We have also proposed a MAS that can co-ordinate the organ transplant operations among all Spanish hospitals [8].

Acknowledgments. This work has been supported by the CICYT project SMASH: Multi-Agent Systems applied to Hospital Services (TIC-96-1038-C04-04).

References

[1] Weiss, G. (Ed.) "Multiagent Systems. A Modern Approach to Distributed Artificial Intelligence". MIT Press, 1999.

[2] Reid, G., Smith, T. "The Contract Net Protocol: High Load Communication and Control in a Distributed Problem Solver". IEEE Transactions on Computers, Vol. C-29, No. 12, pp. 1104-1113, December 1980.

[3] Bellifemine, F., Poggi, A., Rimassa, G., "Developing multi-agent systems with a FIPA compliant agent framework", Software Practice and Experience, no.31, pp. 103-128, 2001.

[4] FIPA: Foundation for Intelligent Physical Agents (http://www.fipa.org).

[5] Decker, K., Li, J., "Coordinated hospital pacient scheduling", IV International Conference on Multi-Agent Systems, ICMAS-98, paris, 1998.

[6] Hannebauer, M., Geske, U., "Coordinated distributed CLP-solvers in medical appointment scheduling", XII Int. Conference on applications of Prolog, INAP-99, pp. 117-125, Tokyo.

[7] Cortés, U. Et al., "Carrel: an agent mediated institution for the distribution of human tissues". III Catalan Conference on AI. ACIA Bulletin, pp. 15-22. Vilanova, 2000.

[8] Aldea, A., López, B., Moreno, A., Riaño, D., Valls, A, "A multi-agent system for organ transplant co-ordination". VIII European Conference on AI in Medicine, AIME 2001, Cascais, Portugal, 2001.

An AI-Based Approach to Support Communication in Health Care Organizations

Diego Marchetti*, Giordano Lanzola, and Mario Stefanelli

Dipartimento di Informatica e Sistemistica, Università di Pavia, 27100 Pavia, Italy

Abstract. The increasing pressure on health care organizations to ensure efficiency and cost-effectiveness, balancing quality of care and cost containment, will drive them towards a more effective knowledge management. An appropriate information system will enable organizations to store, retrieve and apply all collective experience and know-how of its members, and to share it with other cooperating organizations. Information and communication technology provides effective tools for designing health care information systems and for supporting inter-organization communication. In this paper an organization is modeled starting from enterprise ontology and communication is supported through a KQML message-based representation; a conversation protocol explicitly defines cooperation modalities among communities of practice. A prototype of a communication broker has been designed and developed to assist health care professionals in scheduling activities within or across organizations; its implementation is based on the interchangeability between communication and computation tasks.

1. Introduction

The increasing pressure on Health Care Organizations (HCOs) to ensure efficiency and cost-effectiveness, balancing quality of care and cost containment, will drive them towards a more effective knowledge management derived from research findings. The relationship between science and health services has until recently been too casual. The primary job of medical research has been to understand the mechanisms of diseases and produce new treatments, not to worry about the effectiveness of the new treatments or their implementation. As a result many new treatments have taken years to become part of routine practice, ineffective treatments have been widely used, and medicine has been opinion rather than evidence based. This results in sub-optimal care for patients. Knowledge management technology may provide effective approaches in speeding up the diffusion of innovative medical procedures whose clinical effectiveness has been proved: the most interesting one is represented by computer-based utilization of clinical practice guidelines. Moreover, Information and Communication Technology (ICT) can provide effective tools to ensure a more efficient communication infrastructure. Observational studies assessed the size of the communication problem in HCOs [3,4,6,14] and prove that communication errors have a disastrous impact on safety in hospitals [2,10]. It can be tackled effectively if it is not separated from the problem of managing both medical and organizational knowledge [10].

---

* Corresponding author. *E-mail address:* d.marchetti@it.flashnet.it

S. Quaglini, P. Barahona, and S. Andreassen (Eds.): AIME 2001, LNAI 2101, pp. 384–394, 2001.

From a timing point of view, we can distinguish between synchronous communication (e.g., face-to-face, phone) and asynchronous (e.g., e-mail, fax, blackboard). In the former, the agent starting the communication act receives immediate attention interrupting the receiver's activity; in the latter, the receiver decides when to check and/or reply to the message. Clinical communication appears predominantly synchronous, face-to-face and phone calls [4, 6, 14], causing a heavily interrupt-driven working environment [2]. Interruption is necessary to obtain synchronous communication, but has powerful negative effects on *working memory* [9,10, 13] and therefore on the performance of individuals' activities.

However it seems very difficult to implement some kind of computer based communication as efficient as conversation, which is implicitly more fluid and interactive. Coiera points out that the informal nature of most conversations is essential, since many questions asked are poorly structured and become clear only through the act of conversation itself [2].

Our work was stimulated by the *'continuum'* view developed by Coiera [2]: he pointed out that communication and computation tasks are related, but drawn from different parts of a task space. We strongly believe that Artificial Intelligence may provide effective methods to overcome the false dichotomy between communication and computation tasks: workflow and software agents technologies have been used to make communication more efficient by supporting communicating agents in sharing the needed medical and organizational knowledge.

This paper proposes an organization ontology to model organizational and medical knowledge, describes health care processes through workflow models, and defines a communication protocol to support cooperation and interoperability within a single organization and between different organizations. Finally, it illustrates a service request manager complying with the developed models and protocols.

2. An Approach to Health Care Information Systems' Design

A Health care Information System (HIS) should enable collaboration between organizational agents, with a great impact on the efficiency and the effectiveness of their work. Effectiveness indicators allow to assess the efficacy and the quality of patient care management, while efficiency relates outcomes to the available resources.

We believe that a HIS should support organizational agent communication without introducing undesired rigidity. As pointed out before, conversation is the most flexible type of communication, which most medical staff members seem to prefer, but it could be too expensive. This powerful interaction should therefore be enforced for unstructured content communications, but avoided for sharing knowledge in some way already available within the organization. For example, to identify an individual playing a specific role it is not efficient to interrupt colleagues with synchronous phone calls, increasing overall call traffic. However, some clinical decisions could require to interact with clinical experts throughout a conversation, in order to acquire their opinion and to clarify the problem to be solved.

The challenge is to model HCO's knowledge, both medical and organizational, in order to support cooperative work and inter-agent communication maintaining the work flexibility needed in patient care management. To achieve so, it is necessary to create a common ground between organization members and their information system. All organization's knowledge must be formally modeled starting from a sound, coherent and complete HCO ontology.

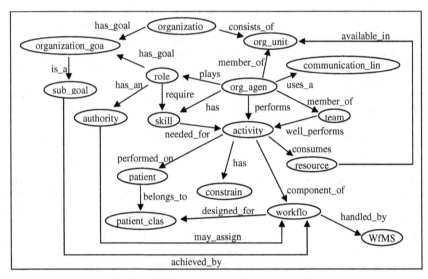

Fig. 1. An ontology for health care organizations.

Figure1 shows the basic elements of the organization ontology on which our model of HCO is based on. It represents an adaptation of the organization ontology developed within the TOVE project [7]. We consider a HCO as a set of constraints on the activities performed by agents. In particular, a HCO consists of a set of organizational units (department, wards, laboratories, etc.), a set of organizational agents (members of an organizational unit), a set of roles that the members play in the organization, and a tree of organizational goals that the members are trying to achieve.

An organizational agent plays one or more roles according to her/his personal skills (medical knowledge and professional expertise). Each role defines goals that it must fulfill, and is given enough authority to achieve them. An agent can also be a member of a team created to best perform a specific activity. Each agent can rely on a set of communication links defining the protocol with which it communicates with other agents inside and outside the organization.

At the heart of the proposed organization ontology lies the representation of an activity which is considered as the basic atomic action with which processes can be represented (workflow models). Activities are performed by agents, and consume resources such as materials, labs, and tools. Constraints set performances to be achieved on activities (time needed, cost specifications, etc.).

Workflow processes model organization services and achieve organization subgoals when carried out successively. Workflow models are used by a Workflow Management System (WfMS) to coordinate execution of activities and to monitor their results, both in terms of resource usage and clinical outcomes [11].

3. Workflow Models and Workflow Management System Process Modeling

A workflow management system (WFMS) is a software system that manages the flow of work between participants or users according to formal specifications of processes called workflows [1]. A workflow specifies activities to be performed and their execution order. Any workflow builder, such as the Oracle Workflow Builder we adopted, allows to define each activity specifying resources and agents needed for its execution, and handles their scheduling. Workflow implementation well adapts to the organization ontology described above, in which group of activities concur to develop a patient care process. Clinical practice guidelines very often suggest how to organize activities to accomplish the most effective clinical outcomes.

Guidelines (GLs) are defined by the National Institute of Health of the United States as "systematically developed statements to assist practitioner and patient decisions about appropriate health care for specific clinical circumstances". Their development process usually involves authoritative teams of experts, who reach a consensus after a complex process, encompassing literature reviews, epidemiological studies, meta analyses, personal communications and possibly a Consensus Conference. On these grounds GLs embody medical knowledge with the aim of providing a uniform and effective way of delivering health care services, and are seen as powerful tools for simplifying the decision process in medicine.

We believe an efficient HCO could comply with guideline intention by implementing a workflow process for each health care service it wants to offer, possibly according to public and certified guidelines. Furthermore any sequential process should be formalized throughout a workflow, including patient handling within the organization's structure.

A workflow is formalized throughout a visual representation, in which each block stands for an elementary activity or another workflow in a recursive manner. The bottom-most expansion of each block is always a set of activities, which represent real world tasks.

Figure 2 shows the top-level structure of the patient management workflow inside the organization's hospital. It starts with the *Patient Admission* activity, in which patient's anagraphic and anamnestic data are stored in the Electronic Patient Record (EPR). The *Information Acquisition* activity collects any already available clinical information, seeking for existing medical records stored in linked organizations' memories. The *Diagnosis* activity is necessary to determine the patient's health state. The *Treatment* block represents the execution of specific patient care processes throughout other workflows, possibly implementing existing evidence-based guidelines. Workflow execution may be triggered by clear and unambiguous symptoms and/or diagnosis, or else by an authorized expert's decision.

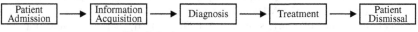

Fig. 2. Patient management workflow

In this last case, when the authorized clinician is ready to receive the patient, she/he will be able to access all the patient's information retrieved throughout the

Information Acquisition and *Diagnosis* activities. This can help to evaluate the patient's clinical status. Finally, the clinician may schedule care activities to be executed on the patient, according to the subgoals she/he wants to achieve. An example could be a blood exam shown in figure 3.

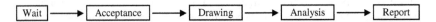

| Wait | ⟶ | Acceptance | ⟶ | Drawing | ⟶ | Analysis | ⟶ | Report |

Fig. 3. Blood exam workflow example. This process model represents one of the services offered by the organization.

The first activity is to wait until the scheduled start time; the *Acceptance* activity will end when the patient will be taken in the blood exam laboratory. The blood test results will follow the blood *Drawing* and *Analysis*, and finally the *Report* activity stores the results in the EPR.

Clinicians are supported by the workflow management system which automatically allows only non-overlapping scheduling, avoiding significant time loss and intensive traffic communication for process planning. After a clinician has planned workflows for a patient and must wait for their execution and reports, she/he can turn his attention to other patients.

When the clinician will reconsider the same patient, she/he will examine the reports of the committed clinical processes (if the workflows have completed execution), and decide whether to plan other workflows or to dismiss the patient. Patient dismissal expressed by authorized clinicians causes the patient management workflow (figure 2) to resume and to complete its execution.

The described scheduling policy requires all organization staff members to frequently consult their activity timetable, because while they are executing an activity, more work could have been scheduled for them. To be efficient this behavior must be enforced by the organization just like a professional skill.

4. The Communication Model

A distributed HCO could somehow partition itself into many sub-organizations, according for example to geographic location, setting up autonomous systems able to communicate with each other. We define inter-organization communication as any form of interaction between distinct organizations or sub-organizations. Inter-organization communication is bi-directional, implying that each system must act both as client and server, and must also support concurrent and simultaneous interactions.

To achieve inter-organization communication, we followed the Knowledge Query Manipulation Language (KQML) specifications proposed by Finin et al [5]. KQML is a direct consequence of Searle's Speech Act Theory [15]; each communication act is associated with a performative name, which expresses a communicative intention (illocutionary act) without depending on the message content. The minimum set of speech acts, necessary for communication request and replies to take place, includes query (i.e. ask-if) and informative (i.e. reply, reject) performatives.

For example, to request a patient record to another organization the query performative ask-if may be employed, while the other fields of the message will help understand what is being requested and how (content, language, ontology fields).

In the example below, organization ORG1 requests ORG2 to provide any information on Freeman Andrew contained in ORG2's database.

```
ask-if
    :content        Freeman Andrew all
    :language       patient record
    :ontology       organization
    :reply-with     12
    :sender         ORG1
    :receiver       ORG2
```

If ORG2 supports KQML, it will identify the ask-if performative as a request. In order to correctly interpret the meaning, it must also support the same language and ontology. This cost represents pre-emptive common ground, because it is knowledge prior to the communication.

ORG2 will return a reply performative with the requested records if the information is present, a reject performative otherwise. An example of the former would be:

```
reply
    :content        record1 attrib11 val11 attrib12 val12…recordN
                    attribN1 valN1…attribNM valNM
    :language       patient record
    :ontology       organization
    :in-reply-to    12
    :sender         ORG2
    :receiver       ORG1
```

The reject performative message would instead be:
```
reject
    :in-reply-to    12
    :sender         ORG2
    :receiver       ORG1
```

The advantage of this communication formalism is that even if the content of a message is incomprehensible, its receiver may react actively, for example forwarding a request message to other subcontracting candidates.

5. Conversation Protocol

To encourage collaborative work among different organizations, negotiation must be supported by the underlying systems. Negotiation can be defined as an interactive mechanism for agreeing on some sort of cooperation. Each organization modeled as above may be seen as an autonomous entity treating proper patients and able to perform clinical processes. To be able to share these services, organizations must communicate with each other, using a conversation protocol to keep track of negotiation steps known as states. The actual state and the incoming KQML performative determine together the subsequent state.

To model a conversation protocol, an Augmented Transition Network (ATN) seems the most appropriate formalism to adopt, in which circles identify states, while words near an arrow represent incoming performatives. When a negotiation takes place, we identify a contractor as the request sender and a subcontractor as the receiver. Since during negotiation the involved parties share the same protocol, we map a single ATN for both (figure 4), where the thick arrows represent messages sent by the contractor, the thin ones by the subcontractor [8].

A negotiation always begins with a contractor's *propose* message, including request specifications and other qualifying parameters (constraints). The next state transition will occur throughout the subcontractor's subsequent message, according to three possible alternatives. In the simplest case the subcontractor is not able to satisfy the request and returns a *reject* message. If the request can be fulfilled, an *accept* message will be sent along with parameters which define the offer. In the last case the subcontractor may issue a *counter-propose* message, expressing its willingness to satisfy the request, although with some deviations from the constraints initially specified in the propose message. This causes the conversation to enter the top-left box of the diagram, in which several negotiation steps may occur. The box will be exited either with a *reject* performative sent by one of the two parties, or with an *accept* performative sent by the subcontractor.

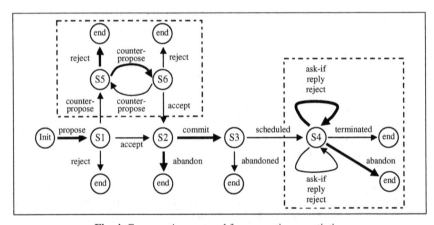

Fig. 4. Conversation protocol for supporting negotiation.

At this point the contractor may decide whether to *commit* the accomplishment of the request to the subcontractor or to interrupt the negotiation with an *abandon* performative. In the first case a *scheduled* message will be returned acknowledging that the request will be satisfied (*abandoned* performative otherwise).

Reaching state four the communication becomes totally unstructured, since it is unpredictable who will send the next message. In fact, the subcontractor may ask the contractor for additional information, or the contractor may probe for partial results.

Two more state transitions may occur, both leading to the end of the negotiation act. The contractor may believe the accomplishment of the request is no longer useful and decide to abandon the conversation (*abandon* performative message). Otherwise the subcontractor will communicate the end of his cooperative action returning execution information and data (*terminated* performative message).

Conversation protocols are content-independent and define a communicative interaction domain. Each conversation requires a protocol instance, along with state and other additional information; this is necessary for allowing multiple simultaneous negotiations even with the same partner.

6. Service Request Manager

In such inter-organizational context we now wish to focus our attention on the Service Request Manager (SRM) we designed and built. SRM requires communication interaction among cooperative organizations and defines a strategy to engage the subcontractor which *best* accomplishes a desired request (for example a specific health care service). The communicating participants must rigorously follow the conversation protocol showed above, or else no interaction may take place.

Figure 5 shows an SRM block scheme complying with the conversation protocol of figure 4. The first step is to define the request explicitly representing what is being asked and what constraints should be met for satisfying the proposal. To characterize a request three different types of constraints must be specified:

- a *name constraint* identifying the requested service,
- *numeric constraints* expressing intervals for desired attribute values,
- *symbolic constraints* listing keywords describing the requested service.

The resulting request representation will be put in the *propose* message content field, since it encloses only the semantics of the communication.

In the subsequent step, the contractor must determine a set of receivers, with which the contractor will instance a new dedicated conversation protocol. Then the messages will be sent, throughout an appropriate communication protocol.

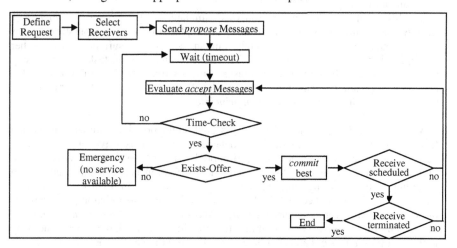

Fig. 5. Service Request Manager (SRM). Italic words represent message performatives.

At this point the contractor must wait for replies and hope to engage as many subcontractors as possible. To avoid stall, the message receiving wait time must be an appropriate fraction of the defined deadline (one of the numeric constraints). In the mean time all incoming replies will be stacked in a queue. A subcontractor receiving a *propose* message with additional constraint information, should find convenient to send the offer which best matches the constraint specifications or try to counter-

propose some valid alternative if unable to satisfy the proposed request (name constraint). The subcontractor's reply will be sent throughout an *accept* message, along with all information concerning the offer (symbolic and numeric constraints).

In the next step every newly received reply will be examined individually, and given a score. It will be evaluated testing the numeric constraints, and matching the symbolic ones, associating a final number to each subcontractor's offer.

A time check must then occur, to decide if a choice must be immediately taken. If the request deadline is not oppressive, a loop will start repeating the sequence: Wait, Evaluate *accept* Messages and Time-Check. When the check test returns a positive answer, the best-evaluated offer will be chosen. This will happen if the contractor has received at least one offer, otherwise some recovery procedure must be activated.

A *commit* message will be sent to the corresponding subcontractor. If the offer has remained valid, a *scheduled* performative message will be returned to the contractor, confirming scheduling, and a final *terminated* performative message will notify successful completion.

In waiting both the *scheduled* and *terminated* message an appropriate timeout is considered for avoiding indefinite delay and, while waiting for the latter, some informative interaction may occur (ask-if, reply, reject; see figure 4). Only at the step labeled *"End"* all resources allocated for the conversation protocol and negotiation overhead may be released.

The SRM described above may work autonomously or under the control of a human agent, with different and predictable communication traffic outcomes. We should note that the diagram in figure 5 is a combination of computation and communication tasks.

The SRM software implementation was stimulated by the Coiera's *"principle of identity"*, for which communication tasks are replaceable with computational tasks [2]. On the other hand, a completely human negotiation surrenders to another principle, the *"exclusivity principle"*, for which communication tasks are necessary and not replaceable by computational tasks. Any possible mixed solution reveals that communication and computation tasks are related, but drawn from different parts of a task space according to the *"continuum principle"*.

We believe a HIS should adhere to the continuum principle, allowing to switch from communication to computation whenever desired. This way, mixed solutions may be sought at run time, according to unpredictable necessities and work burden. Furthermore this flexibility allows best work distribution between man and system according to time-varying working conditions. For example in a particularly intense workday a clinician may commit an SRM agent to initiate a negotiation process in his place, freeing him for more urgent work. According to the *"continuum principle"* such a solution has the needed flexibility for allowing the clinician to re-enter actively in the negotiation process and conclude manually only the last and decisive steps.

7. An Application

We are developing a HIS for management of patients suffering from stroke [12]. The organization ontology discussed above has been formalized throughout tables of a relational model database, using Oracle platform (release 8.0.5). Procedures written in PL/SQL interact with the database, and implement the user interface via commercial browser. The resulting Web pages allow patient registration throughout a new patient management workflow instance (figure 2). Clinicians have a personal user interface for collaborating with other health professionals, which allows them to retrieve all available patients' information, and to commit services according to a well defined workflow process. Any inter-organizational communication passes through a Java Server, which handles information requests and replies, throughout KQML specifications and the conversation protocol of figure 5. Service requests are handled by a software SRM integrated in the server and implemented with a Java thread.

8. Conclusions

HCOs must be able to rely on HIS for improving their knowledge management and clinical outcomes. Organizational and medical knowledge modeling is essential for designing efficient and effective systems to enable knowledge management and communication among all organization agents. The HIS should assist and sometimes substitute human agents in performing tasks to achieve organization subgoals, especially for well structured activities, in order to reduce their work load. Inter-organization communication may efficiently be supported throughout KQML specifications, while complex negotiations require also a conversation protocol definition.

References

1. Bussler C. J. *Policy Resolution in Workflow Management System,* Digital Equipment Corporation 1995.
2. Coiera E. *When communication is better than computation,* J Am Med Inform Assoc 2000;7:277-286.
3. Coiera E,Tombs V. *Communication behaviours in a hospital setting: an observational study,* BMJ. 1998;316:673-676.
4. Covell DG, Uman GC, Manning PR. *Information needs in office practice: are they being met?* Ann Intern Med. 1985; 103:596-599.
5. Finin T., Fritzon R. *KQML as an Agent Communication Language,* The Proceedings of the Third International Conference on Information and Knowledge Management (CIKM'94). ACM Press.
6. Fowkes W,Christensen D, Mckay D. *An analysis of the use of the telephone in the management of patients in skilled nursing facilities,* J Am Geriatr Soc. 1997;45:67-70.
7. Fox M.S., Barbuceanu M. and Gruninger M. *An organization ontology for enterprise modeling, preliminary concepts for linking structure and behaviour,* Computers in Industry 1995; vol 29, pp 123-134.
8. Lanzola G., Gatti L., Falasconi S., Stefanelli M. *A framework for building cooperative software agents in medical applications,* Artificial Intelligence in Medicine 16 (1999) 223-249.

9. Logie RH. *Working memory and human machine systems*, Proceeding of the conference on Verification and Validation of Complex systems. 1993:341-53.
10. Parker J,Coiera E. *Improving Clinical Communication.* J Am Med Inform Assoc 2000;7:453-461.
11. Quaglini S., Saracco R., Dazzi L., Stefanelli M., Fassino C.. *Information technology for patient workflow and guidelines implementation.* Abstract book of the 14th Annual Meeting of the Association for Health Services Research 1997, june 15-17 1997, Chicago.
12. Quaglini S., Stefanelli M., Cavallini A., Micieli G., Fassino C., Mossa C. *Guideline-based on Careflow Systems,* Artificial Intelligence in Medicine 2000, 20 (1) 5-22.
13. Reitman JS. *Without surreptitious rehearsal, information in short-term memory decays,* J Verbal Learning Verbal Behav. 1974:13:365-377.
14. Safran C, Sands DZ, Rind DM. *Online medical records: a decade of experience*, Methods Inf Med 1999; 38: 308-312.
15. Searle JR. Speech Act. *An Essay in the Philosophy of Language*, Berkely:Cambridge University Press.
16. Stefanelli M. *The socio-organizational age of artificial intelligence in medicine*, to appear on Artificial Intelligence in Medicine.

TAME

Time Resourcing in Academic Medical Environments

Hans Schlenker[1], Hans-Joachim Goltz[1], and Joerg-Wilhelm Oestmann[2]

[1] GMD – German National Research Center for Information Technology
FIRST Institute, Kekuléstr. 7, 12489 Berlin, Germany, {hs,goltz}@first.gmd.de
[2] Humboldt University, Charité-Campus Virchow, Augustenburger Platz 1,
13353 Berlin, Germany, joerg.oestmann@charite.de

Abstract. Personnel planning in academic medical departments has to be extremely sophisticated to mobilize all reserves and arrange them in a fashion that permits sufficient and cohesive times for academic activities. We use Constraint Satisfaction in order to cope with problem structure on the one hand and problem complexity on the other. TAME, the current prototype for doing assistant planning, generates optimal plans within seconds of computing time.

1 Introduction

Constraint Logic Programming (CLP) over finite domains is a rapidly growing research field aiming at the solution of large combinatorial problems. For many real-life problems, the Constraint Logic Programming approach has been applied with great success (see e.g. [12,8,3]).

Our research is concerned with the development of methods, techniques and concepts for a combination of interactive and automatic timetabling. These are applied to various real-world problems. The automated solution search is implemented in such that it normally allows a solution to be found in a very short time, if such a solution exists at all. The systems are flexible enough to take into account special user requirements and allow constraints to be modified easily, if no basic conceptual change in the timetabling is necessary. An essential component is an automatic heuristic solution search with an interactive user-intervention facility. In the area of hospital logistics, we already used our techniques for course timetabling ([4]), nurse scheduling ([1]), and medical appointment scheduling ([5]).

Personnel planning in academic medical departments has to be extremely sophisticated to mobilize all reserves and arrange them in a fashion that permits sufficient and cohesive times for academic activities. This makes it an ideal problem to be solved with our methods. In this paper, we describe the approaches and the prototype and give an evaluation of its quality. We can show that the system generates good solution within seconds of computing time.

Section 2 gives a brief description of the problem. This is followed by a discussion of Constraint Logic Programming, problem modelling and search methods. Some remarks on the implementation and results are also given.

S. Quaglini, P. Barahona, and S. Andreassen (Eds.): AIME 2001, LNAI 2101, pp. 395–404, 2001.
© Springer-Verlag Berlin Heidelberg 2001

2   Problem Description

Clinical care for patients, teaching of medical students, training of specialists and scientific research are all different functions that have to be filled in academic medical departments. The functions are very different in character: time of day, duration, frequency, importance, required skills and interests vary a great deal. For excellent clinical care it is mandatory that physicians with adequate training are available for specific functions and that supervisors are present where necessary. For first line on-call service outside standard working hours a sufficient number of trainees with adequate capabilities need be ready in time. The teaching of students in small groups also requires rather large numbers of teachers that need to be far enough advanced in their training. Also the training of specialists should be completed within the time frames alotted. Cohesive research slots need to be established and be staffed with those physicians that have shown sufficient interest, activities and expertise whenever possible. All of this needs to be accomplished under increasing financial restrictions while keeping motivation of the employees high: A task that is impossible to solve with known planning tools. For that reason the rate of planning failures and the disenchantment of the employees is growing. Sophisticated planning tools are necessary.

Given this practical situation, TAME should fulfil at least the following requirements:

- Over a planning period of, say, one or two weeks, each working place has to be staffed each day.
- Some working places are driven by only one standard shift each day, others must be supplied a longer period each day. We therefore need some shift working model.
- Since there are situations where there is not enough personnel available to staff all working places all shifts, we need to assign priorities to the working places and shifts. Higher prioritzed places must be assigned to personnel more likely than less prioritzed ones.
- Each staff member has its own qualification profile. We need to have qualifiers that describe the qualification of each person. On the other hand, we need to assign the same qualifiers to working places, so that we can express conditions like: *A physician to work on CT1 must have at least 10 weeks CT experience.*
- There are some *natural* conditions like:
  - No one may be assigned to more than one working place at a time.
  - No one may work more than one shift a day.
- There are, additionally, some legal regulations like:
  - No one may work in the morning shift the day after she worked in the night shift.
  - No one may work more than ten consecutive days.
- Assistants should be able to express wishes for, say, days off. These should be taken into account as far as possible.
- The number of unassigned working places should be kept minimal.
- There should be as few changes as possible in the type of shifts and the working places for each person on consecutive days.

- Education plans for personnel should be taken into accout: if certain physicians have to make certain experiences during some time, they have to be assigned to the appropriate working places within that time.

For the further treatment of the planning problem, we divide these requirements into two main categories: *hard* requirements that *must* be fulfilled, and *soft* requirements that *should* be fulfilled (as far as possible). Roughly speaking, the first part of the above mentioned requirements are hard conditions (up to the *legal regulations*) and the rest of them are soft ones.

This problem is of course somehow similiar to the ones described above, that we already have solutions for. But, it differs in two central optimisation criteria, that are even a bit contradictory:

- The working places need to be staffed with personnel that has enough experience to fulfil its requirements. Hence, personnel should work on one (type of) working place for a long time.
- The personnel (or at least parts of it) are in an educational state. These have to work in different working places in order to get all their required certificates. Hence, they should work on one and the same place for not longer than at least needed.

These two criteria (in addition to a number of smaller ones) make the problem a challenging *new* one.

3   Constraint Logic Programming

Constraint Logic Programming (CLP) is a generalization of Logic Programming. It combines the declarativity of Logic Programming with the efficiency of constraint-satisfaction algorithms. Constraints are generated incrementally during runtime and passed to a constraint solver which applies domain-dependent constraint satisfaction techniques to help find a feasible solution for the constraints.

Formally, a Constraint Satisfaction Problem (CSP) consists of a basic domain D, a set of variables V, and a set of relations C, the constraints (see e.g. [11]). Each constraint $c \in C$ relates to a set of variables and describes a set of feasible value combinations of the according variables. Therefore, a constraint $c \in C$ is a tuple $\langle I, J \rangle$ with $I \subset V$ being the set of variables, the constraint relates to, and $J \subset \{j | j : I \to D\}$ being the set of all feasible variable assignments. An assignment $f : V \to D$ maps each variable onto a value out of the basic domain. A solution to the CSP is an assignment that fulfills all the constraints C, i.e.[1] $\forall c = \langle I, J \rangle \in C : f \downharpoonright I \in J$.

Constraint Logic Programming over Finite (integer) Domains, CLP(FD) ([6, 7]), is a well-known implementation of the underlying theories and has been established as a practical tool in the research community. Above all, it implements

---

[1] If $f : A \to B$ and $C \subset A$, then $g := f \downharpoonright C$ is the *reduction* of f on C, i.e. $g : C \to B$ and $\forall c \in C : g(c) = f(c)$.

arithmetic formulas as *basic constraints*: *equality*, *disequality*, and *inequalities* can be applied over linear terms built upon domain variables and natural numbers. *Symbolic constraints* can be used for more complex conditions concerning the relation between several domain variables. A change in the domain of one variable may have an effect on all other variables occurring in the constraint. A very useful symbolic constraint is `element(N,List,Value)`. It specifies that the Nth element of the nonempty list `List` of domain variables or natural numbers must be equal to `Value`, where `Value` is a natural number or a domain variable. The first element in `List` has index number 0^2.

A more application oriented system with substantial enhancements over the former implementations is COSYTEC's CHIP system ([2,10]). Its main improvement is the introduction of very powerful *global constraints*. Global constraints use domain-specific knowledge to obtain better propagation results and can be applied to large problem instances. Examples of global constraints are `cumulative`, `among` and `sequence`. The `cumulative` constraint was originally introduced to solve scheduling and placement problems. This constraint ensures that, at each time point in the schedule, the amount of resources consumed does not exceed the given overall limit. The `among` constraint can be used in order to express that exactly n variables among a list of variables take their value in a given list of values. Complex conditions about the way values can be assigned to variables can be specified by the `sequence` constraint. This constraint can be seen as an extension of the `among` constraint, where a variable is replaced by a group of consecutive variables and a value by a pattern.

4   Problem Modelling

A timetabling problem can be suitably modelled in terms of a set of constraints. Since constraints are used, the problem representation is declarative. In this section, the problem modelling is described briefly. The method chosen for problem modelling has a considerable influence on the solution search. The success of the search often depends directly on the model chosen. Furthermore, the modelling options depend on the chosen contraint solver. We use the constraint solver over finite domains of the Constraint Logic Programming language CHIP.

Let X be the set of days to be scheduled, Y be the set of working places to be staffed, and Z be the set of personnel to be assigned. All these sets are finite subsets of $\mathbb{N}$: $X = \{1, ..., |X|\}, Y = \{1, ..., |Y|\}, Z = \{1, ..., |Z|\}$. We additionally define $X' := X \cup \{0\}, Y' := Y \cup \{0\}, Z' := Z \cup \{0\}$. The additional value 0 serves for handling the assignments of *nothing*. Y contains an element for each working place *and* for each shift, the working place has to be run. If, for example, some working place must be occupied in a morning and an evening shift, this is represented by two according elements in Y. If the working place only has to be run in one shift a day, it is represented by only one element in Y. You can think of the elements of Y relating to some *virtual* working places. We additionally

---

[2] CLP(FD) actually uses 1 as number of the first element. Using this numbering would, however, complicate our presentation. We therefore fiddle a bit.

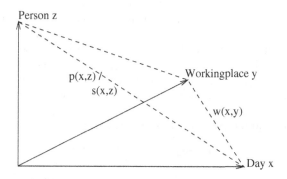

Fig. 1. The basic sets and variables.

need the set $A = \{1, ..., |A|\}$ of shifts, e.g. $\{1, 2, 3, 4\}$ for morning-, evening-, day-, and night-shift, respectively. We also define $A' := A \cup \{0\}$. We need the shift types for specifying some special rules: to exclude shift combinations, according to legal regulations. Each $y \in Y$ matches some $a \in A$. This property is used in the variable usage below.

Let $W = \{w_{x \in X, y \in Y}\}$ be domain variables for the working places, $P = \{p_{x \in X, z \in Z}\}$ be domain variables for the personnel, and $S = \{s_{x \in X, z \in Z}\}$ be domain variables for the shifts. Figure 1 depicts how the basic sets and the variables are related to each other. X, Y, and Z span a three-dimensional space. For each point in the X/Y-plane, we define a variable that takes its value out of Z. For each point in the X/Z-plane, we define $p_{x,z}$ to take its value out of Y and $s_{x,z}$ to take it out of the set of shift types A. A does not make up a dimension since the shift types are related to (virtual) working places and are therefore implicitly coded into Y. The usage of the variables is as follows:

- Each $w_{x,y}$ takes its value out of Z'. If $w_{x,y} = z$, then assistant z is assigned to working place x on day y; if $w_{x,y} = 0$, then no assistant is assigned to this shift.
- Each $p_{x,z}$ takes its value out of Y'. If $p_{x,z} = y$, then assistant z is assigned to working place x on day y; if $p_{x,z} = 0$, then assistant z has day x off.
- Each $s_{x,z}$ takes its value out of A', according to the following rule:
  - if $p_{x,z} = 0$, then $s_{x,z} := 0$
  - if $p_{x,z} = y$, then $s_{x,z} :=$ shift type of y

We notice that the variables are strongly connected: assigning a value z to some $w_{x,y}$ directly leads to appropriate values for $p_{x,z}$ and $s_{x,z}$. The CLP scheme gives us the possibility to express these relationships directly through constraints. We use the above described **element** constraint:

- $\forall x \in X, y \in Y : \mathtt{element}(w_{x,y}, [y, p_{x,1}, ..., p_{x,|Z|}], y)$
- $\forall x \in X, y \in Y : \mathtt{element}(w_{x,y}, [\text{shift type of } y, s_{x,1}, ..., s_{x,|Z|}], \text{shift type of } y)$

Note that the first element in each list is equal to the **Value**-part of the element-constraint since if $w_{x,y} = 0$, then (e.g.) $y = y$ and no other variable is envolved. A nice side-effect of this modelling is that it also implies that one person cannot work on more than one working places one day: if $y \neq y'$, $w_{x,y} = c$, and $w_{x,y'} = c$, then $p_{x,c} = y$ and $p_{x,c} = y'$ and therefore $y = y'$ in contradiction to the assumption. The same holds for the $s_{x,z}$: no one can be assigned to more than one shift a day.

Additional requirements can easily be stated:

- If a working place y has *definitely* to be staffed on day x, we state that $w_{x,y} > 0$.
- To eliminate certain shift combinations for each person, we use CHIP's **sequence** constraint. This global constraint allows the specification of feasible or infeasible value combinations for variable tupels. We state this constraint on the $s_{x,z}$.
- We use **cumulative** to express the number of unassigned working places each day. This value can then be minimzed (see section 5) to find optimal solutions. As a side-effect, **cumulative** increases propagation, i.e. further prunes the search space.
- The domains of the $w_{x,y}$ are reduced such that only persons that fulfil all the according working place's requirements, can be assigned to it.

Since the variables that make up the model are closely connected through the **element**-constraints, it suffices to label (i.e. assign values to) only a subset of the variables to get a complete assignment, i.e. timetable. We actually label only the $w \in W$.

5   Search Methods

A solution of the problem is an assignment of the given variables to values such that all hard constraints are satisfied. The soft constraints should be satisfied as far as possible. A constraint solver over finite domains is not complete because consistency is only proved locally. Thus, a search is generally necessary to find a solution. Often, this search is called "labelling". The basic idea behind this procedure is:

- Select a variable from the set of problem variables considered, choose a value from the domain of this variable and assign this value to the variable.
- Consistency techniques are used by the constraint solver in order to compute the consequences of this assignment; backtracking must be used if the constraint solver detects a contradiction.
- Repeat this until all problem variables have a value.

The search includes two kinds of nondeterminism: *selection of a domain variable* and *choice of a value of the domain* concerning the selected variable. It is well known that the heuristic used for variable selection exerts a considerable influence on the solution search. We use a static ordering for variable selection based on the given priorities of the working places and the number of persons available for this working place. During this search we also try to satisfy the soft constraints. The number of unassigned working places, for example, can be seen as a cost function. We use the *branch and bound* method in order to minimise this cost function. Other soft constraints, related to e.g. wishes, can be directly integrated into the choice of values.

Our experience has shown that in many cases either a solution can be found within only a few backtracking steps, or a large number of backtracking steps are needed. We therefore use the following basic search method: *the number of backtracking steps is restricted, and different orderings of variable selections are tried*. This means that backtracking is carried out on different heuristics.

The generation of a solution can also be controlled interactively by the user. The following actions are possible with the help of the graphical interface:

- to assign a value to an individual working place
- to assign values to a set of marked working places automatically
- to remove the value assignments of a set of marked working places
- to assign values to the remaining working places automatically

These actions can be perfomed in any order or combination, and no automatic backtracking is caused by such user actions. The user can, however, only alter a timetable in such as way that no hard constraints are violated. The constraint solver always ensures that no hard condition is violated.

The interactive component is very important. It greatly improves the practical usability. The interactive component makes step-by-step generation of a solution possible. Modifications of generated timetables are often required for different reasons. Special wishes that are not represented by constraints can often be integrated by modifying an automatically generated or partially generated solution. The human planner retains planning control.

6   Implementation

The Constraint Logic Programming language CHIP was selected as the implementation language. The global constraints and the object oriented component built into CHIP are particularly useful for problem modelling. The main components of our timetabling system are

transformation: transformation of a problem description into an internal representation and transformation of a state into an external description
graphical interfaces: graphical representation of timetables and interactions of the user with the system
search: generation of constraints and solution search

For representation of a timetabling problem, we used two phases: definition of the problem, and the internal object-oriented representation. For the first phase, definition of the problem, we developed a declarative language for problem description. All the components of a timetabling problem can be easily defined using this declarative language. In the second phase, the internal object-oriented representation is generated from the problem definition. This representation is used for the solution search and the graphical user interface. The problem description language is also used for saving states of scheduling. Thus, incomplete timetables can be saved. The search-component includes the generation of constraints and all strategies, methods and options of solution search. All the components of our timetabling system are implemented in CHIP.

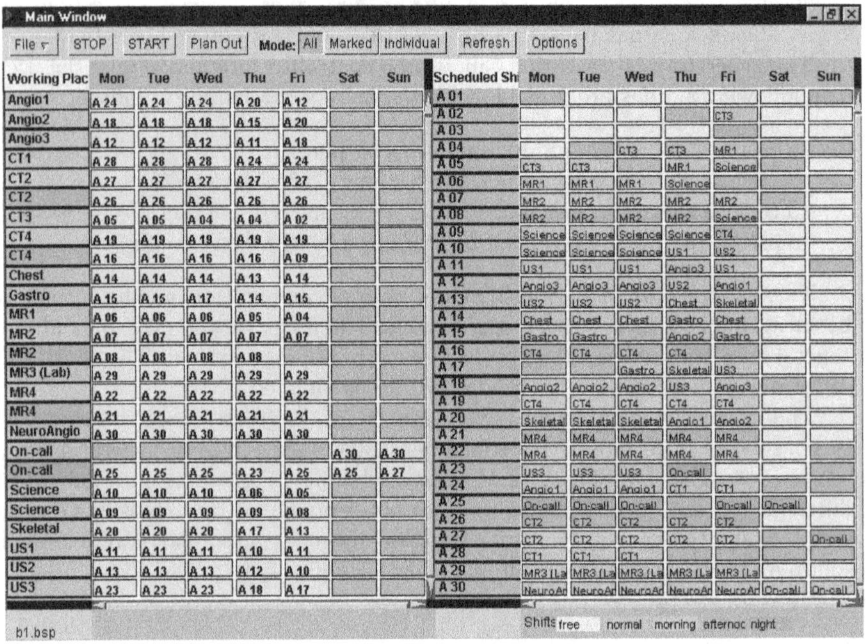

Fig. 2. Automatically generated complete roster.

Figure 2 shows TAME's user interface. It mainly consists of two tables: the *working place table* on the left hand side shows each working place in a row and each day in a column, the *personnel table* on the right hand side shows the personnel in the rows (they do not carry names here but numbers like *A 10*) and the days in the columns. There are (for example) two CT2 working places since it is to be run two shifts every day. All the unassigned dark cells in both tables were initially specified to remain unassigned. The bright ones in the personnel table were specified to be available, but were left free according to available redundant staff. The second *On-Call* working place is a *night-shift* working place. We can see that *A 23* has friday off since she had to do the night shift on thursday. *A 25* also has days off after night shifts. Thus, the above mentioned legal regulation is kept. TAME's GUI allows the user to graphically edit the problem specification, i.e. the qualification and available days of the personnel, the requirements and runnig times of the working places, priorities, and so on. Plans can be generated automatically and by hand, while TAME always ensures correctness of generated plans.

7   Results

Once the system is configured for the department, the time needed for workforce scheduling is greatly reduced from hours to minutes. Our experience within several weeks of system use in our medical department show reductions of about 80%. Senior staff is thus available for other professional activities. The rate of staff misplacements is reduced. The quality of clinical care, the efficacy of student teaching should increase significantly. The number of violations of the legal working hour ramifications is minimized. Finally the motivation of employees should rise and sick leave should decrease. In total, we can anticipate a productivity increase for the whole department in all its fields of activity.

We are, unfortunately, not able to directly compare plans generated by TAME with existing hand-made ones since the latter are unavailable. Thus, we are bound to give an estimation of the overall quality of the tool. We can, however, evaluate the computing time of the system and give some scalability results.

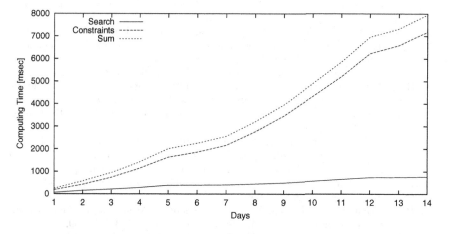

Fig. 3. Computing time in relation to problem size (in days).

Figure 3 shows them, generated on a 143MHz Sun UltraSparc-I, using CHIP 5.3 under Solaris 2.5.1. The results are based on our tests: for a typical ward (see Figure 2) with 30 persons, 26 working places and 14 qualifiers, we generated a number of plans. We altered the problem size in that we generated the plan for 1 up to 14 days. Each problem was solved a couple of times. We measured the time for setting up the constraints and that for searching a solution. Figure 3 shows the average values. We notice that the time to generate the constraints (which is kind of independent from the actual problem specification) exceeds the search time. The knicks on days 5 and 12 result from the weekends (days 6, 7, 13, and 14) being easier to plan according to less personnel requirements. Over all, (manually proven) good solutions for reasonable problem sizes are found within seconds of computing time.

8   Conclusions

The initial application of our system TAME was proven successful and demonstrates the suitability of the methods used. The importance of a combination of interactive and automatic search was shown. Future development of our system will include investigations of heuristics for variable selection and continued study of the influence of different modelling techniques on the solution search. Moreover, we will improve the possibilities of the user to control the soft constraints to be satisfied. This will include new optimization techniques.

References

1. S. Abdennadher and H. Schlenker. Nurse scheduling using constraint logic programming. In *Proc. of the Eleventh Annual Conference on Innovative Applica tions of Artificial Intelligence (IAAI-99)*. AAAI Press, 1999.
2. M. Dincbas, P. van Hentenryck, H. Simonis, A. Aggoun, T. Graf, and F. Berthier. The constraint logic programming language CHIP. In *Int. Conf. Fifth Generation Computer Systems (FGCS'88)*, pages 693–702, Tokyo, 1988.
3. C. Gervat, ed. *Proc. PACLP 2000*. The Practical Application Company Ltd, 2000.
4. H.-J. Goltz and D. Matzke. University timetabling using constraint logic programming. In G. Gupta, editor, *Practical Aspects of Declarative Languages*, volume 1551 of *Lecture Notes in Computer Science*, pages 320–334, Berlin, Heidelberg, New York, 1999. Springer-Verlag.
5. Markus Hannebauer and Ulrich Geske. Coordinating distributed CLP-solvers in medical appointment scheduling. In *Proc. of the Twelfth International Conference on Applications of Prolog (INAP-99)*, pages 117–125, Tokyo, Japan, 1999.
6. P. Van Hentenryck. *Constraint Satisfaction in Logic Programming*. MIT Press, Cambridge (Mass.), London, 1989.
7. P. Van Hentenryck, H. Simonis, and M. Dincbas. Constraint satisfaction using constraint logic programming. *Artificial Intelligence*, 58:113–159, 1992.
8. J. Little, ed. *Proc. PACLP 99*. The Practical Application Company Ltd, 1999.
9. K. Marriott and P. J. Stucky. *Programming with Constraints: An Introduction*. The MIT Press, Cambridge (MA), London, 1998.
10. H. Simonis and E. Beldiceanu. The CHIP System. COSYTEC, 1997.
11. E. Tsang. *Foundations of Constraint Satisfaction*. Academic Press, 1993.
12. M. Wallace. Practical applications of contraint programming. *Constraints, An International Journal*, 1:139–168, 1996.

A Conceptual Framework to Model Chronic and Long-Term Diseases

Ana Maria Monteiro and Jacques Wainer

Institute of Computing - Unicamp - Campinas - Brazil
Caixa Postal 6176, CEP: 13083-970
{anammont|wainer}@ic.unicamp.br

Abstract. The aim of this paper is to present a conceptual framework to help build modular and extensible knowledge-based systems to support care providers and physicians in the management of patients suffering from long-term or chronic diseases.

Keywords: Medical Assistant Systems; Patient's Health Management, Knowledge Representation.

1 Introduction

Considering the complexity of health care management, its economic and human importance, systems that assist in this work can help to accomplish a better and more economical work. Most medical systems consider only the problem of disease diagnosis although patient's management is concerned with much more than that. Diagnosis accounts for less than five percent of a physician's time [1], most visits to doctors are related to the evolution of previously diagnosed problems [2,3,4].

We developed a general framework for constructing modular and extensible knowledge-based systems to support health care providers in managing patients suffering from long-term or chronic diseases, and we developed an instance of this framework for the management of hepatitis. The support is viewed as a collaborative effort between health care providers and an intelligent assistant that uses medical knowledge and the patient's information in order to 1) monitor the patient's progress, 2) recommend a therapy or suggest modifications to the current one based on the current patient's status and clinical guidelines, and 3) predict the future development of the patient's health condition.

2 The Proposed Framework

The management of a patient is a process in wich the evolution of a disease is observed and an appropriate therapy is chosen in order to restore a patient's health or minimize the disease consequences.

The challenge to care providers is in following up those patients that are seen in periodical visits. We propose a conceptual framework to help building computational systems to support health care providers so that they can take the correct actions and cope with the patients' information fragmented along long periods of time.

S. Quaglini, P. Barahona, and S. Andreassen (Eds.): AIME 2001, LNAI 2101, pp. 405–408, 2001.
© Springer-Verlag Berlin Heidelberg 2001

2.1   States of the Framework

As a result of our interaction with specialists in long term or chronic diseases, we identified a set of states, each one defining a context with a specific set of data and relevant knowledge which reduces the complexity of patient's management along the disease evolution. The states we identified are characterized by the following attributes:

The events that cause a state change: some events, such as the presentation of the results of a certain test, induce state changes in the patient's management. In our framework, a logic expression determines the transition from one state to another.

The tests that each state demands: a set of tests and examinations have to be done at each state. These tests have a specific periodicity that depends on the state. Sometimes, a test may be asked only if certain conditions are met; therefore each test is associated with a set of preconditions.

What should be controlled: in each state of the patient's management, facts have to be controlled to guarantee the best results. As in the case of tests, the facts to be controlled are associated with periodicities and sets of preconditions. For example, patients with active hepatitis have to be inquired about a possible contact with drugs whenever their level of hepatic enzymes rises.

What actions should be taken: besides asking for certain tests, some actions should be taken to improve the patient's health status. These actions come associated with a set of preconditions.

A default period of time between appointments.

A default period of time for each state.

A set of explanations about the state.

As time passes, patients go through different states; the states discriminated in our framework are discussed below. Figure 1 depicts these states showing the possible transitions between them.

Disease diagnostic: at this stage the presence or absence of a specific disease is detected based on the patient's signs and symptoms as well as on some tests. If the disease is confirmed the management moves to a state where the therapy feasibility is assessed.

Therapy feasibility assessment: after the disease is confirmed, patient data is collected and examined in order to establish the feasibility of a treatment. If there are no contraindications, a particular therapy is chosen. Whenever a contraindication restricting the use of a therapy is found, it must be handled. If, on the other hand, it is considered that the patient still does not need therapy, the patient moves to the control management state.

Initial therapy management: once a therapy is chosen, the patient has to be monitored in order to check the impact of the therapy on his/her health status and quality of life. The patient's adherence to therapy, the physical and psychological side effects, and the remission, stability or worsening of the symptoms must also be supervised. Whenever the patient responds, the treatment goes on. Otherwise the side-effects and/or non-responsiveness are handled.

Management of responsive patients: patients are regularly monitored to check if the therapy should be modified or ended.

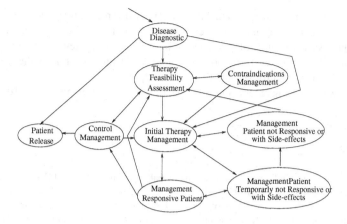

Fig. 1. Management States

Management of a patient temporarily not responsive or showing side-effects: a patient may not respond temporarily to a therapy or may present side-effects. The latter case has to be specially monitored until the unwanted effects disappear and the therapy proceeds, or until their presence causes suspension of the therapy and the management system switches to the management of a patient not responsive or showing side-effects.

Management of a patient not responsive or showing side-effects: in this case the patient is monitored until the effects dissapear and a new therapy may be assessed.

Management of contraindications: if any contraindication prevents the application of a therapy, it must be handled in order to reduce its effects. Whenever this goal is reached a therapy begins or the feasibility of a therapy is assessed.

Control management: the patient is not following any particular therapy. Whenever the reasons for control disappear the patient is released. Otherwise, after a significant change in the patient's status, the feasibility of a therapy is assessed once more.

It is important to note that in order to model a particular disease, not all the states need to be used.

We note that our system considers only knowledge specific to each state when issuing a recommendation or making a decision about moving to another state, we think that this caracteristic is positive since it allows for a more precise understanding of the managing process and consequently an easier and less error prone instantiation of our framework.

3 Validation of the Framework

We developed an instance of this framework for the management of hepatitis [5]. In order to validate these instance we developed a prototype that was tested with 10 randomly selected real patient histories. In each of the patients' visits to the hospital, we ran our system and compared its recommendations and decisions with those recorded in the patient's history. The system agreed in 94% of the recorded recommendations for drugs, tests and actions and did not make any recommendation that was classified as doubtful by a specialist. As an example of discrepancy, in one case the system's suggestion was to stop giving Interferon after forth months of high ALT values whereas in the real case the patient took Interferon for six month before stopping.

We are now developing other instances of the framework for tuberculosis and diabetes management.

References

1. R. B. Altman. AI in Medicine: The Spectrum of Challenges from Managed Care to Molecular Medicine. *AI Magazine*. Fall 1999. 67-77.
2. P. Lucas. Prognostic Methods in Medicine. 1999. *http://www.cs.ruu.nl/people/lucas*.
3. V. Moret-Bonillo, M. M. Cabrero-Canosa, E. M. Herandez-Pereira. Integration of data, information and knowledge in intelligent patient monitoring. *Expert Systems With Applications* 15(1998): 155-163.
4. G. K. McFarland, E. A. McFarlane. *Nursing Diagnosis & intervention: Planning for Patient Care*. Third Editon. Mosby. 1992.
5. Management, Control and Prevention of Hepatitis C. Guidelines for Medical Practitioners. *http://hna.ffh.vic.gov.au/phb/9609007/manage.htm*.

Modelling of Radiological Examinations with POKMAT, a Process Oriented Knowledge Management Tool

K. Faber[1], D. Krechel[1], D. Reidenbach[1], A. von Wangenheim[2],
and P. R. Wille[3]

[1] University of Kaiserslautern, Research Group Artificial Intelligence and
Knowledge-based Systems, Postfach 3049,
D-67618 Kaiserslautern, Germany
{faber, krechel, reidenba}@informatik.uni-kl.de
http://wwwagr.informatik.uni-kl.de
[2] Universidade Federal de Santa Catarina (UFSC), Department of Computer
Sciences - INE, 88049-200 Florianopolis S.C. Brazil
awangenh@inf.ufsc.br
http://www.inf.ufsc.br
[3] Radiologische Gemeinschaftspraxis Dr. Blasinger, Dr. Buddenbrock, Dr. Benz in
Mainz, Rheinstrasse 4A-C, D-55116 Mainz Germany
Paulo-Roberto.Wille@epost.de

Abstract. Medical knowledge grows exponentially. Thus the improvement of patient care by capturing this knowledge in a computable environment is a decisive challenge of medical informatics. In the German-Brazilian cooperation project Cyclops we try to build an integrated solution in order to cope with this task. In this paper we describe the POKMAT system, a process oriented knowledge management tool and its application to medical examination guidelines. The system is developed in close cooperation with private radiological hospitals in Germany and Brazil. We try to improve the daily work of our medical partners by the integration of the tool into the hospitals environment via DICOM interfaces. Another aim is an easy knowledge exchange between the medical partners in both countries. POKMAT should act as an Organizational Memory of the practice.

1 Introduction

Many problems occurring in an *Health Care Organizations (HCO)* are connected with "knowledge"[1]. When an experienced radiologist or other employee leaves an HCO, normally his or her knowledge about best practices, typical patient cases, or special skills of colleagues is lost for the organization. But this knowledge is very valuable and it takes a long time until a successor has recollected it. Problems also arise because processes and recurring tasks are not standardized. For instance, the *Results Report* which has to be written for every examination performed is not uniform in most HCOs. So every physician has to concern

S. Quaglini, P. Barahona, and S. Andreassen (Eds.): AIME 2001, LNAI 2101, pp. 409–412, 2001.

about it by his or her own. This circumstance also aggravates the development of systems like experience or knowledge databases which could be used by the medical staff and for the purpose of training.

From the view of a computer scientist, the work of physicians, especially radiologists, can be supported by computers in manifold manner. The basic approach is always to analyze and model recurrent processes, to support their execution and to optimize them on occasion. Therefore, a careful knowledge acquisition is necessary. Three different kinds of such recurrent processes are important in the context of private radiological hospitals. The first ones are organizational processes which mainly cope with patient management. The second and third kinds of process correlate with the actual examination process, thus the evaluation and analysis, e.g., of images. These processes are executed by a computer and can be distinguished in "automatic" ones and "interactive" ones.

Within the scope of this paper, a general architecture is presented [2] to model and execute the three kinds of process. On the one hand existing components of the Cyclops-System [3], a knowledge based image processing tool, are joined and on the other hand a large scale for future developments is created.

2   POKMAT System

In this section, the architecture of the *Process Oriented Knowledge Management Tool (POKMAT)* which supports the modelling and execution of automatic and interactive examination processes as well as organizational processes is introduced. POKMAT is tailored for the use in radiological practices, that means the examination processes correspond with the interpretation of images.

The system consists of three main components: the *Modeler*, the *Workflow Enactment Service*, and the *Information Assistant*. The system architecture is demonstrated in figure 1.

2.1   The Modeler

The Modeler is the knowledge acquisition tool. In contrast to the process definition tool specified by the Workflow Reference Model [4] it is not only responsible for constructing the process definitions, but also for the modelling of ontologies which represent, for instance, anatomical or organizational knowledge. It is possible to model different kinds of process:

Guidelines. Guidelines depict a good way for modelling the medical knowledge and provide standards of practice.

One has to differentiate between *examination guidelines* and *organizational guidelines*. Examination guidelines describe special examinations. These process models contain all examination steps, as well as textual descriptions and suitable example cases for different lesions. An ontology representing anatomical knowledge is used to model these processes. Organizational guidelines imitate organizational processes like the patient management process, e.g., defined by IHE [5].

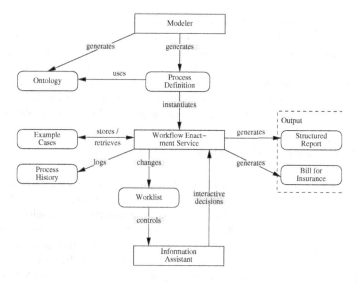

Fig. 1. POKMAT System Architecture

Image Processing Sequences. In order to perform special examination steps, a radiologist often has to applicate sequences of image processing operators. The finding of suitable parameters and the best possible order of operators is a complex and knowledge intensive task. One assignment of the Modeler is the creation and test of these sequences. The resulting process definition is an independent and complex operator which can be applied directly. This part of the Modeler is called Visual Cyclops [6].

2.2   The Workflow Enactment Service

The Workflow Enactment Service instantiates a process definition and controls the execution of the resulting process. During the execution of guidelines it administrates and documents all occurring data, creates one or more worklists at the beginning of the process execution, updates it/them according to the user's decisions, and produces output data. Output data of examination guidelines is a structured report; the execution of an organizational guideline produces a bill for the health insurance.

The technical implementation of the Workflow Enactment Service is a goal-operator configuration system, enhanced by a petri net based dataflow engine.

2.3   The Information Assistant

The Information Assistant is a combination of the workflow client application and the user interface defined by the Workflow Reference Model [4]. It is integrated in our existing DICOM software and supports the physicians during the daily work. The different kinds of process are supported variably.

In case a physician wants to perform a special kind of examination, he or she chooses the corresponding examination guideline which leads to the presentation of a worklist. The work items can be handled arbitrarily until all necessary structures are checked. Besides the images, supporting documents and graphics are presented and typical example cases can be retrieved, thus the Information Assistant can be used to teach students or unexperienced radiologists. Output is a structured report of the findings that is sent to the referring physician.

3   Conclusion and Outlook

In this paper we introduced the POKMAT system, a general architecture for process oriented knowledge management in the field of radiology. The knowledge acquisition is the most critical point in the development of knowledge management systems. The main work in the first project phase was the implementation of the modelling tools and the development of an acquisition methodology.

To be accepted by the practitioners a direct benefit for the user, in our system the automatic generation of the results report, is necessary. We modelled the MR knee examination as a first example. Now a young radiologist is trying to model a second examination guideline without the help of a tool expert. From this experiment we hope to get additional feedback to improve our tools.

In the future we must also deal with the organizational workflows in small radiological practices. We want to analyze the processes in the daily routine and try to improve their performance. With the help of case based reasoning techniques, we want to expand POKMAT to a real Organizational Memory of our partner hospitals.

References

1. M. Stefanelli: Artificial Intelligence for Building Learning Health Care Organizations. In: W. Horn at al., AIMDM'99. Springer-Verlag, Berlin Heidelberg (1999)
2. Kerstin Faber: The Process Oriented Knowledge Management Tool POKMAT, with an Application to Radiological Knee Examinations. Diplomarbeit, Universität Kaiserslautern (2001)
3. Aldo von Wangenheim: Cyclops: Ein Konfigurationsansatz zur Integration hybrider Systeme am Beispiel der Bildauswertung. Dissertation, Universität Kaiserslautern (1996)
4. David Hollingsworth: The Workflow Reference Model. Workflow Management Coalition, 2 Crown Walk, Winchester, Hampshire, UK. January 19, 1995.
5. IHE Technical Framework: Year 2. Integrating the Healthcare Enterprise. March 28, 2000.
6. Klaus Mandola: Visual Cyclops – Ein interaktives System zur Modellierung von wissensbasierten Bildverarbeitungsapplikationen. Diplomarbeit, Universität Kaiserslautern (1998)

A Multi-agent System for Organ Transplant Co-ordination

A. Aldea[1], B. López[2], Antonio Moreno[1], D. Riaño[1], and A. Valls[1]

[1]Research Group on Artificial Intelligence
Departament d'Enginyeria Informàtica i Matemàtiques
Universitat Rovira i Virgili (URV)
Ctra.Salou s/n, 43006 Tarragona, Spain
{aaldea,amoreno,drianyo,avalls}@etse.urv.es

[2] Departament d'Electrònica, Informàtica i Automàtica
Universitat de Girona (UdG)
Campus Montilivi , 17071 Girona, Spain
blopez@silver.udg.es

Abstract. The co-ordination of human organ transplants is a difficult task that involves legal, clinical, organisational and human aspects within a complex distributed environment of hospitals and governmental institutions. We propose a Multi-Agent Architecture that is the kernel of an Intelligent Decision Support System to co-ordinate the Spanish activity in organ transplants.

1 Introduction

Nowadays, there is an important success of organ transplants in Spain. This is due to two main reasons: the advances of Medicine and the appearance of an organisational structure that coordinates all the stages of the donation and transplant process according to the local, regional, national, and international norms and laws. This structure is supported by the figure of a transplant co-ordinator, which is a person that controls the transplant tasks of a particular hospital. This hierarchical structure defines the *Spanish model* [5], which is considered to be one of the most effective models in the world.

Organising and co-ordinating transplants are complex tasks that require several clinical activities involving many people or working teams, and also an administrative process which is parallel to the clinical process. The main activities of the transplant process are [4]: detection of the potential organ donors, clinical examination of the organ donor, brain-death confirmation, maintenance and handling of the organ donor, legal brain-death confirmation, securing the family consent and the legal authorisation, arrangement of the organisational factors, organisation of the organ extraction and transplant, and clinical examination of the evolution of the recipient. The different people involved in these tasks must bring the administration tasks into line with the clinical tasks and follow the norms and legislation established by the healthcare authorities and organisations: the *Organització Catalana de Transplantaments* (OCATT) in Catalonia, the *Organización Nacional de Trasplantes*

S. Quaglini, P. Barahona, and S. Andreassen (Eds.): AIME 2001, LNAI 2101, pp. 413–416, 2001.

(ONT) in Spain, the *United Network for Organ Sharing* (UNOS) in the USA, *the Eurotransplant International Foundation* for some countries in the EU, etc.

Recent studies published by the ONT [2] show that the number of people who die while waiting for a heart, liver, or lung transplant in Europe fluctuates between the 15% and the 30%. In order to improve the process, once the family consent and the necessary authorisations have been obtained, we are designing an information system to be used as a decision support system in the organisation of the extraction and implantation of the organ, which includes the process of deciding which patient should receive the organ. This information system must guarantee a secure distributed communication, maintain historical files, and extract new knowledge from the results (evolution of the recipient). In this work we present the architecture of a Multi-Agent System (MAS) that will support the communication and negotiation layers of this Transplant Co-ordination System. This MAS is designed to be compatible with the current Spanish organisational structure.

2 Applying Multi-agent Systems to Organ Transplant Co-ordination: Justification and Motivation

Health care authorities impose some structures in human organisations that cannot be violated [1][6]. The organisation of the transplant co-ordination in Spain is structured in four levels: national, *zonal*, regional and hospital level. At the hospital level all the data of patients is kept locally in the database of each hospital unit.

The type of data that the hospital keeps for each patient is quite diverse: electronic information such as clinical analysis results, images, signals, traditional X-ray photographs, ultrasounds and nurse recordings. All these data must be localised and kept at the level of the hospital unit(s) where the patient has been treated because every unit of the hospital is responsible of their own patients. As a result, a distributed approach is needed to maintain the current existing organisational structure. Multi-agent systems offer a platform for a distributed approach in which every agent is responsible of a given process, as units or hospitals are specialised on a given branch of Medicine. Moreover, a MAS approach is particularly suitable for the organ transplant co-ordination problem as a great amount of information related to donor and receptor is required during the transplant co-ordination process. Therefore, agents of different hospitals must communicate and co-operate to provide support to the transplant co-ordinator. These agents must follow some norms and laws and must respect the Spanish co-ordination structure, in which they play different roles and have restricted permissions. Special negotiation protocols will be defined in order to respect the Spanish model.

Finally, the use of a Multi-Agent approach makes the system easy to be adapted to structural changes in the organisational protocol, and to be extended to an European framework.

3 General Architecture of the Multi-agent System

In order to co-ordinate organ transplants among Spanish hospitals we propose the construction of a MAS such as the one shown in figure 1. This architecture reflects the organ transplant co-ordination structure that is employed in Spain. The national territory is partitioned into six zones. Each of these zones groups some of the nineteen Spanish autonomous regions.

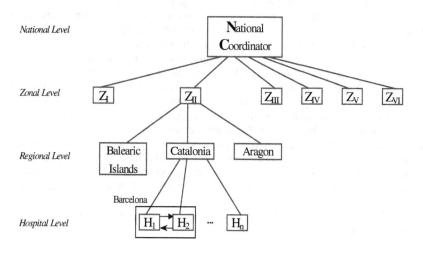

Fig. 1. Hierarchical dependencies among co-ordinators.

All these agents have different knowledge and play different roles, and they have to co-ordinate their activities to offer an efficient way of dealing with organ transplant management at the national level. There are two other agents in the global MAS, which have not been shown in figure 1 because they do not belong to the hierarchy:

- An agent called *Emergency Co-ordinator* (EC), which is the national co-ordinator of the 0-emergency cases. This is the name given to those patients that are waiting for an organ and have reached a very critical condition, in which their life is at high risk if the transplant is not performed in a very short period of time.
- An agent called *Historical Agent* (HA), which receives the data of all transplants made in Spain. With this information it can keep historical files, elaborate statistics, apply data mining techniques in order to gain useful knowledge, etc.

It is important to stress the fact that, as argued in section 1, all the agents of the system must behave in accordance with the regulations imposed by regional and national transplant organisations (OCATT and ONT). For instance, if it has not been possible to find a receiver in the organ's zone, the national co-ordinator will search in the other zones following an order that depends on the transplants made in the past.

4   State of the Work and Future Lines

We have studied the transplants co-ordination process in Catalonia, with the help of some doctors and transplant co-ordinators of nearby hospitals. With their information we have designed an initial architecture for a Multi-Agent System, which has been presented in section 3. This architecture maintains the current Spanish organisational structures and informs about the performance of the overall system by employing an agent that keeps up to date the history of the transplant procedures.

The automation of the co-ordination tasks allows the acceleration of the organ transplant process, which is crucial because organs degrade quickly, so there is a very brief period of time to perform the surgical operation (hours).

Currently there are several research groups investigating the use of multi-agent systems for hospital management [1]. However, this approach is different to ours as their main goal is to create a more profitable hospital system by decreasing the time that a patient stays in hospital and increasing the number of external patients.

The architecture presented in this paper focuses on the organ transplant co-ordination task. Two other research lines that we are going to study are the reasoning mechanism behind the decision making process for each agent and the incorporation of learning methods. Works on decisions with multiple criteria as the ones in [3] will be considered for decision making. The historical information gathered by HA will be used as input to learning methods that will improve the MAS and the co-ordination process itself.

After the building of a prototype, user needs and interests will be more clearly defined, and then security constraints and medico-legal issues will be studied in detail.

Acknowledgements. We are very grateful to the referees of the paper for their suggestions. We also acknowledge the support of the CICYT project SMASH: Multi-agent Systems applied to Hospital Services, TIC-96-1038-C04-04.

References

1. Decker, K., Li, J. *Coordinated Hospital Patient Scheduling*. Proc. ICMAS'98.
2. *Informes y documentos de consenso*. Organización Nacional de Trasplantes (Ed.), 2000.
3. Keeney R.L., Raiffa, H. *Decision with Multiple Objectives: Preferences and Value Tradeoffs*. Cambridge University Press, 1993.
4. López-Navidad, A., Domingo, P., Viedma, M.A., *Professional characteristics of the transplant co-ordinator*. Transplantation Proceedings, 29, pp. 1607-1613, Elsevier Science Inc., 1997.
5. Matesanz, R., Miranda, B., *Coordinación y Trasplantes: El modelo español*. Editorial Aula Médica, ISBN 84-7885-060-0, 1995.
6. So, Y., Durfee, E.H. *Designing Organisation for Computational Agents*. In: Simulating Organisations: Computational Models of Institutions and Groups. Edited by M.J. Prietula, K.M. Carly, L. Gasser. AAAI/Press/The MIT Press, 1998.

A Platform Integrating Knowledge and Data Management for EMG Studies

Julien Balter[1], Annick Labarre-Vila[2], Danielle Ziébelin[3], and Catherine Garbay[1]

[1]Lab. TIMC-IMAG, Grenoble, France
[Julien.Balter, Catherine.Garbay]@imag.fr
[2]Lab d'EMG – CHU, Grenoble, France
ALabarre-Vila@chu-grenoble.fr
[3]Action ROMANS - INRIA Rhône-Alpes, Grenoble, France
Danielle.Ziebelin@inrialpes.fr

Abstract. A multi-agent framework for data mining in EMG is presented. This application based on a Web interface provides a set of functionnalities allowing to manipulate one thousand medical cases and more than twenty five thousands neurological tests stored in a medical database. The aim is to extract medical informations using data mining algorithms and to supply a knowledge base with pertinent information. The multi-agent platform gives the possibility to distribute the data management process between several autonomous entities. This framework provides a parallel and flexible data manipulation.

1   Introduction

Electromyography (EMG) covers a set of electrophysiological techniques allowing to diagnose neuromuscular diseases. The domain is broad, covering more than a hundred diagnoses, and including thousands tests of nerve or muscle structures. Several computerized systems have been developed in this field, to support, facilitate and assist data collection, analysis and intepretation [1, 2, 3, 4, 5]. There is nowadays a growing demand for disseminating and sharing the medical expertise in this field, for building consensual databases and for sharing tools for their exploitation. This is the major goal of the EMG-Net project[1]. The guiding principle of this work was to design a web-based system integrating knowledge and data management facilities, thus benefiting from a coupling between knowledge-based representation of medical expertise and data-centered mining of the available cases.

   Data mining nowadays encompasses a large number of tools and methods, stepping from pure statistics to learning and visualization: the accuracy and interpretability of this step are known to be key features in medicine [6]. It implies considering data mining as a complex process whose main features are (i) to be grounded in medical knowledge, (ii) to support multistrategy methodologies [7] and (iii) to be carefully controlled: combining knowledge-centered modelling with agent-centered design is advocated in this paper as a way to cope with the above-mentionned issues [8, 9].

---

[1] European Inco-Copernicus project EMG-net n°977069

S. Quaglini, P. Barahona, and S. Andreassen (Eds.): AIME 2001, LNAI 2101, pp. 417–420, 2001.

2   Description of the Platform

The platform architecture follows a client-server approach (Fig. 1) ; it inherits from previous projects a significant amount of partially standardised knowledge and data. The database is implemented under SQL as a general data structure covering all anatomical structures, examination techniques and test parameters used by the physicians. Several computer programs have been implemented to allow the transfer of data from different EMG machines, the local sampling and interpretation of EMG examinations, the exchange of EMG examinations between laboratories and the transfer of EMG examinations to and from different decision support systems. The knowledge base formalises the EMG expert knowledge: it is expressed in a formal language carrying a precise semantics, under AROM[2] [10], and defines the elements that the different Data Mining modules will operate on. The World-Wide server allows to disseminate the results and provide friendly user interface.

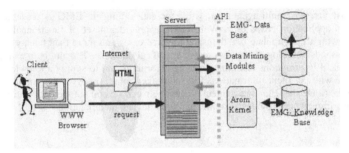

Fig. 1. The EMG platform.

3   An Agent-Centered Design for Data Management in EMG

Information retrieval and data mining tools have been added to WEB-AROM under the JSP technology. A nice coupling between knowledge-centered and data-driven analysis is obtained as a consequence, since the AROM knowledge model is used to assist request formulation and to drive the data exploitation process; data exploitation in turn is considered as a way to potentially enrich the knowledge base. As a consequence, information retrieval and data mining is approached at the "knowledge level", thus bridging the gap between statistical knowledge and medical expertise. Three types of agents have been designed to support these activities (Fig. 2). The Task-Agent plays the role of an interface between the user and the retrieval/mining processes; its role is (i) to receive the user query and transmitt the results back to the user, and (ii) to translate the query in terms of sub-tasks to be performed by sub-agents and to recover their results. The Sub-Agent is coupled with a specific type of information, eg information related to the anatomical structures or to the patient examination. Its role is (i) to manage the part of a query addressing a given type of information and (ii) to distribute this query, which may imply several kinds of information for a given type, to corresponding Data-Agents. Each Data-Agent is

---

[2] http://www.inrialpes.fr/sherpa/pub/arom

coupled with a specific table in the database; its role is to process a "simple" request, ie a request involving one parameter and one field of information.

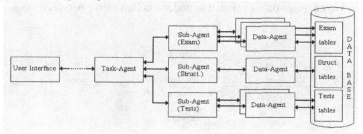

Fig. 2. Agent roles and coordination.

Data management is organized into successive layers, which ensure the circulation of information, and its progressive transformation, from data to knowledge and vice-versa, under dedicated agent control. Each agent is thus meant to work in a rather focalized way, under specific goals and assumptions. The agents (Java object) communicate through message sending and with the databases via JDBC (Java DataBase Connection). They execute under control of an administrator as an endless message waiting cycle. Data mining performs mere association rule computation. The system may for example look for associations beetween two nerve structures, eg Tibialis and Peroneus nerves : the request is first of all distributed to the corresponding data tables, the results being joined in a second step (Fig. 3). The request is formulated under the WebArom interface, as shown in Fig. 4.

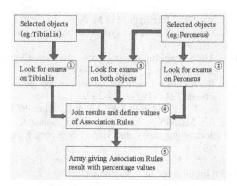

Fig. 3. Data mining process: functional pattern example.

4   Conclusion

Agent-centered design has been advocated as a way to cope with the specificities of data management in medicine, specifically in EMG. A working system has been presented. Information retrieval as well as data mining processes have been designed at the interface between data and knowledge, thus rendering the system usage more easy to the physician but also considering the extraction of knowledge as the ultimate goal of data exploitation. The agent-centered approach ensures processing efficiency, and allows to envisage data exploitation under a collaborative perspective.

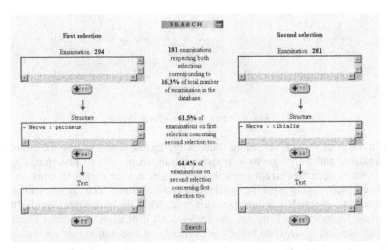

Fig. 4. A view of the user interface, request formulation step.

References

[1] Fuglsang-Frederiksen A., Ronager J., Vingtof S.: PC-KANDID - An expert system for electromyography. Artificial Intelligence in Medicine 1 (1989) 117-124.
[2] Ziébelin D, Vila A, Rialle V,: Neuromyosys a diagnosis knowledge based system for EMG. Proc. Conf. MIE 94 (1994).
[3] Schofield I,: HINT High Level Inferencing Tool : An Expert System for the Interpretation of Neurophysiologic Studies, Proc. Conf. MIE 94 (1994).
[4] Cruz J., Barahona P.: A causal functional model for applied to EMG diagnosis, Lecture notes in computer science 1211 (1997) 249-260.
[5] Andreassen S., Jensen F.V., Andersen S.K., Falck B., Kjærulff U, Woldbye M., Sorensen A.R., Rosenfalck A.: MUNIN - An expert EMG assistant. In : Desmedt, J.E. (eds): Computer-Aided Electromyography and Expert Systems, Elsevier Sciences Publishers, Amsterdam, 21 (1989).
[6] Zupan, B., Lavrac, N., Keravnou, E.: Data mining techniques and applications in medicine. Artificial Intelligence in Medicine 16 (1999) 1-2.
[7] Agre G.: A multifunctional platform for EMG studies. In: Agre, G., Ziébelin, D. (eds): Application of Advanced Information Technologies to Medicine (2000) 1-17.
[8] Stolfo, S., Prodromidis, A.L., Tselepis, S., Lee, W. & Fan, D.W.: JAM: Java Agents for Meta-Learning over Distributed Databases, Technical Report, Departement of Computer Science, Columbia University (1997).
[9] Kergupta, H., Hamzaoglu, I. & Stafford, B.: Scalable, Distributed Data Mining Using An Agent Based Architecture (PADMA), Proc. High Performance Computing'97 & Knowledge Data Discovery and Data Mining'97 (1997).
[10] Page M, Gensel J, Capponi C, Bruley C, Genoud P, Ziébelin D: Représentation de connaissances au moyen de classes et d'associations : le système AROM, Actes LMO'00 (2000) 91-106.

Using OncoDoc as a Computer-Based Eligibility Screening System to Improve Accrual onto Breast Cancer Clinical Trials

Brigitte Séroussi[1], Jacques Bouaud[1], Éric-Charles Antoine[2],
Laurent Zelek[3], and Marc Spielmann[3]

[1] Service d'Informatique Médicale, DSI/AP–HP & Département de Biomathématiques,
Université Paris 6, Paris, France
{bs,jb}@biomath.jussieu.fr
[2] Service d'Oncologie Médicale, Groupe Hospitalier Pitié-Salpêtrière, Paris, France
antoine.eric-charles@wanadoo.fr
[3] Département de Pathologie Mammaire, Institut Gustave Roussy
Villejuif, France

Abstract. While clinical trials offer cancer patients the optimum treatment approach, historical accrual of such patients has not been very successful. OncoDoc is a decision support system designed to provide best therapeutic recommendations for breast cancer patients. Developed as a browsing tool of a knowledge base structured as a decision tree, OncoDoc allows physicians to monitor the contextual instanciation of patient characteristics to build the best formal equivalent of an actual patient. Used as a computer-based eligibility screening system, depending on whether instanciated patient parameters are matched against guideline knowledge or available clinical trial protocols, it provides either evidence-based therapeutic options or relevant patient-specific clinical trials. Implemented at the Institut Gustave Roussy and routinely used at the point of care, it enhanced physician awareness of open trials and increased of 17% patient enrollment onto clinical trials. However, the analysis of the reasons for non-accrual of potentially eligible patients showed that physicians' psychological reluctance to refer patients to clinical trials, measured during the experiment at 25%, may not be resolved by the simple dissemination of personalized clinical trial information.

1 Introduction

Evidence-based clinical practice guidelines (CPGs) are currently edited and disseminated by medical associations and state organisms to provide physicians and patients with state-of-the-art knowledge to help them making more informed medical decisions [1]. However, if guideline-based treatments can be recommended to improve the quality of life or the survival of cancer patients, no curative solutions exist yet for such patients.

Randomized clinical trials (CTs) represent the most definitive method to evaluate the effectiveness or ineffectiveness of new therapies. Meta-analysis of randomized CTs provide the grades of evidence that support guideline recommendations. As a consequence, cancer CTs are imperative to improve the outcomes for cancer patients. However, only 2-3% of cancer patients, which represents less than 50% of eligible patients [2], are

S. Quaglini, P. Barahona, and S. Andreassen (Eds.): AIME 2001, LNAI 2101, pp. 421–430, 2001.
© Springer-Verlag Berlin Heidelberg 2001

actually enrolled in such trials. Low enrollment in cancer CTs is usually attributed to physician factors such as lack of knowledge about CTs, patient factors such as lack of patient-oriented information regarding trials, organizational barriers and health care system obstacles [3]. As lack of knowledge is often advocated, knowledge-based systems, designed to provide the right information to the right person at the right moment, should be able to improve CT accrual.

ONCODOC is a guideline-based decision support system for breast cancer patient therapy [4]. Designed as a browsing tool of a knowledge base structured as a decision tree, it allows the physician to monitor the contextual instanciation of patient parameters, thus offering the mandatory flexibility in the interpretation of guideline knowledge. When selecting the best patient-centered path during the hypertextual navigation, the physician is provided with the most appropriate therapeutic options, either as evidence-based guideline recommendations or candidate CTs. ONCODOC has been implemented at the Institut Gustave Roussy (IGR), known as the first European cancer research center, and routinely used at the point of care during a 4-month period study. The observed increase of accrual rate before and after using the system proved that physician awareness of available trials could indeed improve patient enrollment. However, when collecting the reasons for non-accrual, and when analysing the answers, it appeared that simply disseminating CT knowledge even withing the clinical workflow would not solve some physician's reluctance to refer breast cancer patients to CTs.

2   Decision Support for Eligibility Screening

Enrollment into CT protocols is a chronic problem for many clinical research centers. First, CTs are still today inefficient paper-based operations [5]. In medical oncology departments, new CTs are usually presented once by clinical researchers, during staff meetings, where physicians are given descriptive leaflets that remain in their pocket, or worst, on the shelves of their consultation office. Poor physician awareness of open clinical trials at the point of care could be then advocated to explain the low accrual rates commonly observed. Electronic versions of these leaflets, even when disseminated over networks, did not prove to be more efficient when classically displayed in a CT-centered view as the alphabetically ordered list of all open CTs. The National Cancer Institute's CancerNet system lists more than 1,800 open clinical trials in oncology alone. Eligibility determination is then difficult to assess [6].

Computer-based eligibility screening systems have been developed to automatically match patient characteristics and medical history information against available clinical trials protocols [7]. In the domain of breast cancer, Ohno-Machado et al. [3] have structured open clinical trials of the PDQ database (Phase II and Phase III trials) as collections of eligibility criteria using XML. For any new patient entered into the system, trials that the new patient is not eligible for are ruled out and relevant clinical trials are displayed in order of likelyhood of match. Gennari and Reddy [8] proposed to use participatory design to develop a decision support tool for eligibility screening. The user enters minimal patient information and gets a list of matching protocols, any of them could be viewed in detail when selected. In both cases, when the number of returned trials is too high, additional patient data can be input to narrow the search.

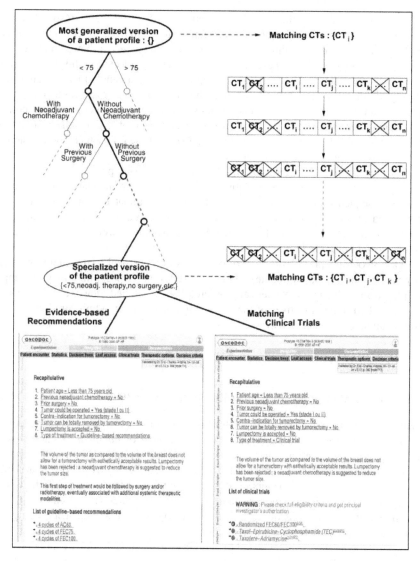

Fig. 1. Representation of the process underlying eligibility criteria screening.

ONCODOC [4] has been developed as a guideline-based decision support system to provide best treatment recommendations. Applied to breast cancer, it relies on a knowledge base structured as a decision tree where decision parameters aim to describe the patient state. As a result, the complete expansion of the decision tree is a patient-centered nosological repository of all theoretical clinical situations that could be met within breast cancer pathology. Therapeutic recommendations are displayed at the leaf level. They are suited to the clinical situation represented by the corresponding path through the decision tree. Therapeutic recommendations may be either evidence-based and have thus the value of clinical practice guideline statements or they could be chosen among "appropriate" CTs. These "appropriate" CTs are selected within the list of all open trials according to the screening of eligibility criteria handled by the navigation through the decision tree. Figure 1 illustrates the whole process. From the set $\{CT_i\}_{i=1,n}$ of all open CTs a priori appropriate to the most generalized version of a patient profile, the incremental specification of a given patient clinical profile gradually restricts the initial set of all CTs to the subset $\{CT_i, CT_j, CT_k\}$ of the CTs which are a posteriori potentially relevant for the given patient.

As a conclusion, ONCODOC follows the principle of using patient characteristics to discriminate between alternative treatments. However, the formalization of the patient state in a sequence of instanciated parameters is not automated from patient data but controlled by the physician on the basis of his contextual interpretation. Then, this approach serves the selection of the best guideline to apply as well as the determination of the relevant matching CTs.

ONCODOC also provides the list of open CTs in a classical trial-centered view independently of any patient context. For documentation purpose, they may be simply displayed in a classical alphabetically ordered list. A detailed view, *i.e.* the synopsis of the trial with the objectives of the study, eligibility criteria, administration scheme, follow-up modalities, is then available.

3   Method

3.1   Organization of Breast Cancer Encounters at the IGR

With 10 225 new patients per year, the IGR is the first European cancer research center. Breast cancer patients are managed by the department of mammary pathology in a two-steps process. They are first received by a breast specialist during a "reception" consultation. When the breast specialist experiences no difficulty to establish what should be the right treatment for a patient, he decides by himself of the therapy, and there is no second check. When it is not the case, there is a second encounter with a multidisciplinary committee of physicians, involving a medical oncologist, a radiotherapist, and a surgeon. Committees operate three times a week.

ONCODOC has been implemented for a life-size evaluation during a 4-month period. The system has been installed at the second step of the process, in the committee's consultation office. This choice was first driven by medical reasons, as committees were involved in the therapeutic decision of more complex cases that could benefit of ONCODOC's recommendations. In addition, it was also simpler for organizational reasons.

3.2   Experimentation Protocol

The objective of the study was to identify and to quantify physician factors for low accrual rates. As a consequence, only physicians used the sytem and the experimental protocol of use was implemented as follows. For each new incoming patient, IGR clinicians were asked *(i)* to register their initial therapeutic decision, *(ii)* to use ONCODOC and then *(ii)* to record their final therapeutic decision. While using the system, they had to proceed through the hypertextual navigation to reach the leaf level and the system's recommendations where guideline-based recommendations were provided as well as the CTs potentially suitable to the given patient, when existing.

To test the impact of physician awareness about open trials on the accrual rate, treatment decisions of clinicians have been compared before they used the system and after they used the system. When a given patient was potentially eligible, *i.e.* when eligibility criteria of open CTs were matching the patient characteristics instanciated by the navigation, but when physicians chose not to recruit the patient, the declined clinical trials were displayed. Figure 2 shows the experiment form that clinicians had to fulfill.

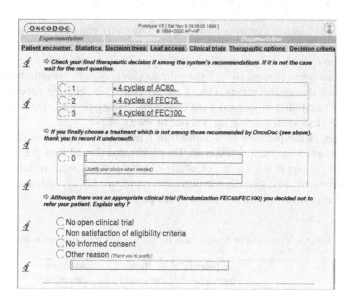

Fig. 2. Experiment form to be fulfilled by physicians with reasons for non-recruiting potentially eligible patients.

When the patient was potentially eligible but was actually not recruited, physicians had to acknowledge that there were appropriate CTs for the patient although they decided not to refer her and they had to justify why. Three main reasons were proposed to be checked off : "Non satisfaction of eligibility criteria", aside from those already checked by the navigation, "No informed consent" of the patient, "Other reasons" that should be specified. When there was no open trial for a given patient, the same experiment form had to be fulfilled by checking "No open clinical trial" answer.

At the end of the study, we sent a questionnaire to the involved committee clinicians. Among more than 150 questions, 12 items were about clinical trial management to evaluate (i) clinicians' estimation of IGR CT accrual rate (ii) impact of ONCODOC use upon CT accrual rate, (iii) estimated distribution of non accrual reasons.

4   Results

During the 4-month period of the experiment, 13 physicians were involved, 12 committee physicians and the head of the department. There were 9 breast cancer CTs but only 4 were open at the time of the study. Only 127 treatment decisions were usable for the survey out of the 141 recorded cases. Questionnaires were sent to all the physicians that participated to the experiment but only 7 were returned (54% of response).

4.1   IGR Accrual Rates: Observations and Estimations

Out of the 127 cases, 27 patients were a priori potentially eligible for CTs. However, it appeared that during the experiment, 2 clinical trials were temporarily suspended, and 4 patients initially found potentially eligible were finally classified as non potentially eligible. As a consequence, 18% of the patients (23/127) were potentially eligible for clinical trials during the survey. Out of the 23 potentially eligible patients, 12 were actually recruted after physicians used ONCODOC leading to a relative accrual rate of 52% (12/23) and to an absolute accrual rate of 9% (12/127).

The study of the questionnaires showed that IGR physician estimations of potentially eligible patients were rather optimistic. They estimated that 54% of the patients were potentially eligible, that 49% of potentially eligible patients were recruited, and that 34% of all patients were actually recruited. Table 1 reports CT accrual rates as observed during the experiment and as estimated by the physicians.

Table 1. Clinical trial accrual rates for breast cancer patients at the IGR.

	% of potentially eligible patients	Relative accrual rate	Absolute accrual rate
Observations	18%	52%	9%
Estimations	54%	49%	34%

4.2   Impact of Using ONCODOC upon Accrual Rate: Observations and Estimations

ONCODOC's contribution is to take advantage of the physician-controlled instanciation of patient characteristics during the hypertextual navigation to provide, at the point of care, relevant CTs along with evidence-based therapeutic recommendations. When comparing accrual rates before and after using the system, we could then measure the weight of physician unawareness of available trials in poor observed accrual rates.

At the IGR, the use of ONCODOC lead to an increase of 50% of the number of recruited patients : 8 patients were recruited before physicians used the system as 12 patients were recruited after. The corresponding increase of the accrual rate, 17% (4/23), measures the frequency of the situations where physicians, when being informed, finally referred a potentially eligible patient to a CT while they didn't think of it initially.

Table 2. Impact of using ONCODOC upon CT accrual rate : qualitative and quantitative measures.

	Trend of the impact	Measure of the impact
Observations	Increase	+17%
Estimations	No impact (50%)	0%
	Increase (50%)	+27%

When analyzing the questionnaires, it was interesting to notice that among the 7 received answers for the question about the impact of using ONCODOC upon CT accrual rate, 1 physician "didn't know", 3 physicians thought that the system had no impact, and 3 thought that ONCODOC had a positive impact leading to an estimated increase of CT accrual rate of 27% in average (see Table 2).

4.3   Reasons of Non-accrual: Observations and Estimations

When physicians decided not to recruit a potentially eligible patient, they had to justify their decision as a deliberate choice, and to explain why by determining the appropriate reason among 3 categories: (1) the patient was not satisfying CT eligibility conditions, (2) the patient did not consent to participate to a CT, (3) any other reason that should be specified. Out of the 11 potentially eligible patients that were not actually recruited, 64% (7/11) were not verifying eligibility conditions, none refused to give her consent, and 36% (4/11) were not recruted for other reasons.

When further analyzing the reasons given by physicians, within the category (1), 3 patients were not satisfying eligibility criteria but no additional explanation was given, 3 patients had particular clinical profiles (bilateral breast cancer or additional gyneco-logical cancer) excluding them from participating to CTs, and for the last patient, the maximum delay between surgery and chemotherapy as specified in the trial was ex-ceeded. In the last category, 2 patients were coming for a second medical advice, and the last 2 patients were not proposed to enter a CT for "psychological reasons".

Table 3. Reasons of non accrual: observations and estimations.

	Non satisfaction of eligibility criteria	No informed consent	Other reasons
Observations	64%	0%	36%
Estimations	50%	27.5%	22.5%

When considering the estimated distribution of non accrual reasons recorded in the questionnaires, we found that IGR physicians thought that 50% of the patients were not satisfying eligibility criteria, 27.5% did not give their informed consent, and "other reasons" reached 22.5%. Table 3 shows the distributions of non accrual reasons given by physicians, during the experiment and evaluated in questionnaires.

5 Discussion

Among questionnaires sent to physicians at the end of the study, the response rate was only 54% which can be explained in two ways. First, with more than 150 questions, questionnaires were rather long. Then, among the 13 physicians involved in the experiment, there were the chief of the department, 4 surgeons, 4 clinical oncologists, and 4 radiotherapists. The chief of the department did not return his questionnaire, as well as one medical oncologist and one radiotherapist, i.e. 75% of response for these two medical specialities. However, only one surgeon answered, i.e. 25% of response, pointing out the fact that surgeons did not really invest ONCODOC, a system they reasonably considered to be chemotherapy and radiotherapy oriented.

The percentage of potentially eligible patients was evaluated by physicians at 54%, which was quite optimistic as compared to the 18% actually measured. On the other side, they correctly evaluated the relative accrual rate. As a consequence, they seemed to over-estimate the number of open CTs for breast cancer during the experimentation.

When studying the results of the experiment, we found that among the 23 potentially eligible patients, 35% were initially recruited, i.e. before using ONCODOC, 17% were finally recruited, i.e. after using ONCODOC, 30% were not recruited because they were not completely matching eligibility criteria of pruned CTs, and 17% were not recruited for "other" reasons.

As a decision support system designed to deliver at the point of care the best therapeutic recommendations, ONCODOC provided physicians with relevant matching CTs for any patient found to be potentially eligible. The approach proved to be effective in increasing CT accrual rate of physicians although only half of them recognized the fact.

However, 30% of the patients were not recruited because they were not completely matching eligibility criteria. The corresponding 7 patients were found a priori potentially eligible but they were not actually eligible after completely checking CT eligibility criteria. ONCODOC has been designed as a guideline-based decision support system that could use the instanciation of patient parameters performed to get CPG recommendations to provide, as well, relevant matching CTs for breast cancer patients. The compromise adopted between the depth of the decision tree and the discriminating power of instanciated parameters along the path, if appropriate to provide guideline-based recommendations, was not adequate for efficiently selecting CTs.

Currently, there is no electronic patient record at the IGR. Although computer-based and disseminated over the HIS, medical reports are expressed using natural language and no automatic extraction of patient data to check eligibility criteria can be performed. For the moment, the hypertextual navigation through ONCODOC's knowledge base is handled interactively within the course of a medical consultation by a physician. No data is re-inserted. Only mouth clicks are performed to instanciate decision parameters modalities and thus identify potentially eligible patients. But to actually recruit a patient in a CT, complementary checkings are manually operated by clinical researchers.

When coupled with an electronic patient record, once the physician-controlled navigation would have identified the best formal equivalent of the actual patient and when the option of participating in a CT is considered, additional developments of ONCODOC should allow the system to provide automatic checking of CT eligibility criteria and display actual CTs a patient is eligible for. Although there could be a negociation on borderline eligibility criteria with the CT coordinator, this automation has been required by physicians. To preserve this negociation, though alleviating the burden of the task, a semi-automated approach could be designed with pre-instanciated default values that could be accepted as such or modified according to physicians interpretation depending on the case.

A complete computer-aided approach with a physician-controlled instanciation of decision parameters to identify the best formal equivalent of a given patient coupled with the automatically performed checking of CT eligibility criteria should thus display actually matching CTs. This optimal system would increase the rate of enrollment to reach 75% of potentially eligible patients : there were indeed 16 truly potentially eligible patients and 12 were actually recruited. It remains 25% of patients who were not recruited for "other" reasons. These "other" reasons can be interpreted as evidences of physicians' reluctance to refer patients to CTs [9]. Patients that came for a second advice as well as those excluded from CTs for psychological reasons could indeed have been enrolled if physicians were likely to make referrals. With a reflective, patient-centered, supportive and responsive behavior, physicians should have convinced patients seeking for the best treatment (why do they want a second advice ?) to participate in a CT. In the same way, although being in a physiological state of shock [10] just after being informed of a cancer diagnosis, a patient could be approached about CTs.

6 Conclusion

Treatments offered to control groups in a randomized CT ought to represent the current best standard treatment, while those allocated to the new treatment are receiving a treatment hypothesized to be at least similarly effective or at best better. Therefore well designed randomized CTs offer patients the optimum treatment approach. They should thus be recognized as the "standard" of care for cancer patients.

ONCODOC is a guideline-based decision support system designed to provide best therapeutic recommendations for breast cancer patients. Relevant CTs are thus displayed with CPG options for any patient described in terms of decision parameters instanciated by a physician-controlled hypertextual navigation. In oncology, CTs are rapidly evolving, new open trials substitute to old closed or suspended trials within very short periods of time (a few months). To be of effective use, ONCODOC has to be updated at the same rythm. As treatments are implemented at the level of the leaves of the decision tree, it is easy to maintain the knowledge base by adding a new trial or by closing an old one. It should be noticed that closed trials are never removed from the knowledge base. They continue to be provided to the user with an appropriate colour code indicating they are closed, for documentation purpose.

Implemented in a life-size experiment at the IGR, ONCODOC has been used to awake physician awareness of open CTs. While displaying within the clinical workflow matching CTs for any given patient, it proved to increase CT accrual rate. Although the relative increase of recruited patients is impressive (+50%), the corresponding absolute increase is low (+4), because it has been measured on a small size sample. These preliminary results need to be confirmed on a larger scale evaluation.

In addition, the experiment allowed to collect reasons for non recruiting potentially eligible patients. The feeling that CT participation was not worth the effort was perceived to be the major reason. Therefore, efforts to increase physicians' participation in randomized CTs need to overcome a reluctance of some doctors to recommend/propose patients to enter CTs. A way to prove this assumption should be to implement the system in waiting rooms of oncology departments to be used by patients, and to measure when and why the demand for participating in CTs could come from patients.

References

[1] Shiffman, R. N., Liaw, Y., Brandt, C. A., Corb, G. J.: Computer-based guideline implementation systems: a systematic review of functionality and effectiveness. JAMIA 6/2 (1999) 104–114.

[2] Ellis, P. M.: Attitude towards and participation in randomised clinical trials in oncology: A review of the literature. Ann Oncol 11/8 (2000) 939–945.

[3] Ohno-Machado, L., Wang, S. J., Mar, P., Boxwala, A. A.: Decision support for clinical trial eligibility determination in breast cancer. J Am Med Inform Assoc 6/suppl (1999) 340–344.

[4] Séroussi, B., Bouaud, J., Antoine, É.-C.: OncoDoc, a successful experiment of computer-supported guideline development and implementation in the treatment of breast cancer. Artif Intell Med (2001). *To appear*.

[5] Afrin, L. B., Kuppuswamy, V., Slatter, B., Stuart, R. K.: Electronic clinical trial protocol distribution via the world-wide web: A prototype for reducing costs and errors, improving accrual, and saving trees. J Am Med Inform Assoc 4/1 (1997) 25–35.

[6] Rubin, D. L., Gennari, J. H., Srinivas, S., Yuen, A., Kaizer, H., Musen, M. A., Silva, J. S.: Tool support for authoring eligibility criteria for cancer trials. J Am Med Inform Assoc 6/suppl (1999) 369–373.

[7] Carlson, R. W., Tu, S. W., Lane, N. M., Lai, T. L., Kemper, C. A., Musen, M. A., Shortliffe, E. H.: Computer-based screening of patients with hiv/aids for clinical trial eligibility. J Curr Clin Trials 179 (1995) –.

[8] Gennari, J. H., Reddy, M.: Participatory design and an eligibility screening tool. J Am Med Inform Assoc 7/suppl (2000) 290–294.

[9] Benson, A. B., Pregler, J. P., Bean, J. A., Rademaker, A. W., Eshler, B., Anderson, K.: Oncologists' reluctance to accrue patients onto clinical trials : an illinois cancer center study. J Clin Oncol 9/11 (1991) 2067–2075.

[10] Epping-Jordan, J. E., Compas, B. E., Osowiecki, D. M.: Psychological adjustment in breast cancer: processes of emotional distress. Health Psychol 18 (1999) 315–326.

Using Critiquing for Improving Medical Protocols: Harder than It Seems

Mar Marcos[1], Geert Berger[1], Frank van Harmelen[1], Annette ten Teije[2], Hugo Roomans[1], and Silvia Miksch[3]

[1] Vrije Universiteit Amsterdam, Dept. of Artificial Intelligence
De Boelelaan 1081a, 1081HV Amsterdam, Netherlands
[2] Universiteit Utrecht, Institute of Information and Computing Sciences
P.O. Box 80.089, 3508TB Utrecht, Netherlands
[3] Vienna University of Technology, Institute of Software Technology
Favoritestraße 9-11/188, A-1040 Vienna, Austria

Abstract. Medical protocols are widely recognised to provide clinicians with high-quality and up-to-date recommendations. A critical condition for this is of course that the protocols themselves are of high quality. In this paper we investigate the use of critiquing for improving the quality of medical protocols. We constructed a detailed formal model of the jaundice protocol of the American Association of Pediatrics in the Asbru representation language. We recorded the actions performed by a pediatrician while solving a set of test cases. We then compared these expert actions with the steps recommended by the formalised protocol, and analysed the differences that we observed. Even our relatively small test set of 7 cases revealed many mismatches between the actions performed by the expert and the protocol recommendations, which suggest improvements of the protocol. A major problem in our case study was to establish a mapping between the actions performed by the expert and the steps suggested by the protocol. We discuss the reasons for this difficulty, and assess its consequences for the automation of the critiquing process.

1 Introduction and Motivation

During the last years a high number of medical practice guidelines or protocols have been produced from systematic evidence-based reviews [9]. Protocols developed in this way provide clinicians with valid and up-to-date recommendations, and thus have a beneficial influence on quality and costs of medical care [2]. A critical condition for this is that the protocols are clearly and correctly defined. However, medical protocols are often ambiguous or incomplete [5]. If ambiguity or incompleteness (intended or not), or even inconsistency, occur in protocols the risks of being neglected in the delivery of care will be high. We are concerned with methods to uncover such apparent anomalies.

The critiquing approach has been adopted in many systems since Miller's first work [4]. Their common feature is that a problem specification and a solution proposed by the user are given as input, and a series of comments aimed at improving the solution is generated as output. Critiquing has proved to be a very suitable approach for decision support in domains like Medicine, where there is a high variability on what can be considered an acceptable solution. It usually implies identifying points where the proposed

S. Quaglini, P. Barahona, and S. Andreassen (Eds.): AIME 2001, LNAI 2101, pp. 431–441, 2001.
© Springer-Verlag Berlin Heidelberg 2001

solution is suboptimal and studying what are the explanations, if there are any, so as to produce an appropriate critique of unjustified choices. This is the usual view of critiquing, in which standards are used to give feedback on the user's behaviour. However, another possibility is to reverse these two roles, and to use the user's solution and its justification to refine the standards.

This paper presents the work we have done to explore this possibility in the framework of protocol quality improvement. It has consisted in: (1) modelling a protocol using a specific protocol language, (2) manually critiquing the solutions given by an expert to a set of predefined cases by comparing them against the prescriptions of the protocol, and (3) drawing conclusions about the utility of critiquing for protocol improvement.

As working example we have selected the jaundice protocol of the American Association of Pediatrics (AAP). We will briefly give its background in section 2. The protocol language that we have chosen, Asbru, is briefly explained in section 3. The rest of the paper presents the Asbru model of the jaundice protocol, the critiquing exercise and its results, and our conclusions on the utility of critiquing for the improvement of medical protocols.

2   The Jaundice Protocol

The illness. Jaundice (or hyperbilirubinemia) is a common disease in new-born babies. Under certain circumstances, elevated bilirubin levels may have detrimental neurological effects. In many cases jaundice disappears without treatment but sometimes phototherapy is needed to reduce the levels of total serum bilirubin (TSB), which indicates the presence and severity of jaundice. In a few cases, however, jaundice is a sign of a severe disease.
The protocol. The jaundice protocol of the AAP [1] is intended for the management of the disease in healthy term[1] new-born babies. The reasons for choosing this protocol were that, firstly, it is considered a high-quality protocol[2] and that, secondly, data corresponding to a set of test cases were available[3].

The protocol consists of an evaluation (or diagnosis) part and a treatment part, to be performed in sequence. During the application of the protocol, as soon as the possibility of a more serious disease is uncovered, the recommendation is to abort without any further action. The rationale behind this is that the protocol is exclusively intended for the management of jaundice in healthy new-borns. An important part of the protocol is the table used to determine the adequate treatment from the TSB value and the age of the infant.
The test cases. The data from the test cases were limited to a set of initial facts and lab test results, and they did not include a concrete solution to the case they illustrate. Therefore, we had to resort to a pediatrics expert to provide us with the necessary input for our critiquing exercise.

---

[1] Defined as 37 completed weeks of gestation.
[2] The jaundice protocol of the AAP is included in the repository of the National Guideline Clearinghouse (see http://www.guideline.gov/).
[3] In http://www.ukl.uni-heidelberg.de/mi/research/dss/sisyphus/

3   The Asbru Language

Asbru is a semi-formal language intended to support the tasks necessary for protocol-based care [8]. It is a time-oriented, intention-based, skeletal plan specification language. Asbru is an interesting language in a case-study on critiquing because it is much more detailed and formalised than other protocol representation languages, such as PROforma [3] or GLIF [6]. This makes Asbru in principle an attractive candidate for protocol improvement because the additional details in an Asbru representation will help to expose potential problems in the original protocol.

In Asbru, protocols are expressed as plan schemata defined at various levels of detail, precise enough to capture the essence of clinical procedures but leaving space for flexibility during their application. Major features of Asbru are:

- explicit intentions and preferences can be stated for plans.
- intentions, conditions, and states are temporal patterns.
- uncertainty in temporal patterns and parameters can be flexibly expressed.
- plans can be executed in different compositions, e.g. in parallel (TOGETHER), in sequence (SEQUENCE), in any order (ANYORDER), or every certain time (CYCLICAL); it can also be defined whether all the steps should be executed (ALL) or not (SOME).
- conditions can be defined to control plan execution, e.g. to set applicability conditions (FILTER) or to determine when execution should be interrupted (ABORT).

Some of the above elements need some explanation for the purposes of this paper, namely intentions and temporal patterns. Intentions are high-level goals that support special tasks such as critiquing and modification. They are patterns of states or actions to be achieved, maintained, or avoided (ACHIEVE, MAINTAIN or AVOID), during or after the execution of the plan (INTERMEDIATE or OVERALL).

Temporal patterns are crucial in Asbru. The time annotations used in Asbru allow the representation of uncertainty in starting time, ending time, and duration with intervals, as well as the use of multiple reference points. A time annotation is written in the form ([EarliestStarting,LatestStarting] [EarliestFinishing,LatestFinishing] [MinDuration,MaxDuration] REFERENCE). Thus, the temporal pattern (TSB-decrease=yes any [4 hours,_] [_,6 hours] [_,_] *self*) is a proposition becoming true if there is a decrease of TSB, in any context, between 4 and 6 hours after the activation of the current plan, *self*.

4   The Jaundice Protocol in Asbru

We have used Asbru to model the AAP jaundice protocol. In the model we have tried to stay as close as possible to the algorithm in the AAP protocol. Thus, for instance, the exit messages in the flowcharts have been directly translated into Asbru Displays. Likewise the AAP protocol, the Asbru version has as main components a diagnosis plan and a treatment plan. It is made up of more than 30 subplans and has a length of 16 pages. Table 1 lists the most important subplans. Finally, the protocol makes extensive use of

Table 1. Main subplans in the Asbru version of the AAP jaundice protocol. The first subplans correspond to continuous monitoring tasks to be executed in parallel. The main components are the subplans for the diagnosis and the treatment. The grouping and numbering of the plans gives an idea of their hierarchical structure. Note that several simple plans have been omitted for simplicity.

Hierarchical number	Plan name
1	Hyperbilirubinemia
1.1	Check-for-rapid-TSB-increase
1.2	Check-for-jaundice>2-weeks
1.3	Check-for-jaundice>3-weeks
DIAGNOSTIC PLANS	
1.4	Diagnostics-hyperbilirubinemia
1.4.1	Anamnesis-abnormal-signs
1.4.2	Blood-tests
1.4.2.1	Check-blood-test-mother
1.4.2.2	Perform-blood-test-child
1.4.3	Anamnesis-hemolytic-disease
1.4.3.1	Evaluation-risk-factors-hemolytic-disease
1.4.4	Jaundice-determination
TREATMENT PLANS	
1.5	Treatment-hyperbilirubinemia
1.5.1	Regular-treatments
1.5.1.1	Feeding-alternatives
1.5.1.2	Phototherapy-intensive
1.5.1.3	Phototherapy-normal-prescription
1.5.1.4	Phototherapy-normal-recommendation
1.5.1.5	Observation
1.5.2	Exchange-transfusion

many Asbru features, in particular for the combination and interleaving of diagnosis and treatment [7].

The Regular-treatments plan in table 2 illustrates the complexity of some of the protocol plans. This plan, which is fundamental in the treatment part, tries to reduce the bilirubin levels without resorting to the application of an exchange transfusion (see table 2 for details on the procedure).

5   The Critiquing Exercise

Our critiquing exercise is based on both the AAP protocol and the Asbru version we have modeled. First, we have presented a subset of the test cases to the doctor, who was trained to solve jaundice cases in a manner similar to the AAP protocol. Second, we have used the Asbru protocol to produce a recommendation for the same cases. Finally, we have tried to establish a mapping between the expert's solution and the Asbru recommendation, and to find and explain the differences. Note that, unlike traditional critiquing work, these may turn out to be problems in either the expert's solution or the Asbru protocol. Figure 1 illustrates the approach.

Table 2. Regular-treatments plan. This plan consists of two parallel parts: the study of feeding alternatives and the different therapies. The therapies can be tried in any order, one at a time. The intentions are both avoiding toxic bilirubin levels during the execution of the plan and attaining normal (observation) ones at the end. The plan completes when the feeding alternatives and the therapies complete. The latter in turn depends on the completion of observation. It aborts when either bilirubin raises to transfusion levels or intensive phototherapy fails to reduce them sufficiently, pointing to a pathologic reason.

PLAN 1.5.1	Regular-treatments	
INTENTIONS	AVOID INTERMEDIATE STATE: bilirubin=transfusion	
	ACHIEVE OVERALL STATE: bilirubin=observation	
CONDITIONS	FILTER:	(bilirubin≠transfusion any [_,_] [0,_] [_,_] *now*)
	ABORT:	(bilirubin=transfusion any [_,_] [0,_] [_,_] *now*)
		or
		(pathologic-reason=yes any [_,_] [0,_] [_,_] *now*)
PLAN BODY	DO-ALL-TOGETHER {	
	Feeding-alternatives	
	DO-SOME-ANYORDER {	
	Retry aborted children	
	Continuation specification: (**Observation**)	
	Phototherapy-intensive	
	Phototherapy-normal-prescription	
	Phototherapy-normal-recommendation	
	Observation } }	

Acquisition of expert solutions to test cases. The critiquing exercise uses the solutions given by our expert to a series of test cases. With the aim of obtaining a varied set of cases, we have carried out a *selection of data*, i.e. we have occasionally suppressed some initial lab data so as to force the expert to perform the actions requesting for them.

Then, in order to determine whether our expert's practice was coherent with the recommendations in the protocol, and hence that the critiquing made sense, we presented the protocol to her some time before the acquisition of solutions—*priming of the expert*. This was done long beforehand so that the protocol did not influence the behaviour of the expert at the time of solving the test cases.

Finally, during the acquisition we have considered both the actions of the expert and the intentions behind them—*acquisition of actions and intentions*. However, except for few points in the solutions, we have not strictly regarded the sequencing of her actions.

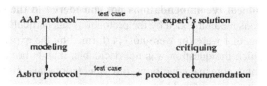

Fig. 1. Critiquing of expert solutions using the recommendations of the Asbru protocol.

Critiquing of expert solutions using the protocol. We have compared the expert's solution to a series of cases with the recommendations of the Asbru protocol to solve them. Henceforth, we will use the term action when referring to expert's actions and the terms plan or statement when making reference to elements of the Asbru protocol. First, we have studied which of her actions could be matched with (sub)plans in the protocol, and which could not. Afterwards we have studied the mismatches, i.e. the protocol recommendations which were not considered in the solution as well as the expert's actions that were not included in the protocol indications. Then, for actions that matched we have analysed their appropriateness according to conditions, time annotations and intentions as stated in the protocol. In the rest of the section we present the critiquing exercise we have carried out. For space reasons, only the critiquing of test case 1 is presented in detail.

5.1   Critiquing Test Case 1

The data provided to the expert to solve test case 1 were:

> Admission of a term icteric[4] newborn. Gestational age is 40+2 weeks. Spontaneous delivery. On day 2 after birth laboratory data show a significantly elevated total bilirubin of 17,8 mg/dl.

In addition to this, the following lab test results were available on request: blood group and rhesus factor of the mother: O positive; antibodies: negative; blood group and rhesus factor of the child: A positive; direct Coombs test: negative. Table 3 shows the actions proposed by our expert to solve the case and the intentions behind them, as she reported. Note that she did not used the Asbru terminology for expressing intentions, which implies that it has been necessary to interpret them in terms of the ACHIEVE, MAINTAIN and AVOID in Asbru.

Matching the expert's actions and the protocol. The first step is studying which of the expert's actions are included in the protocol and which are not. This matching turned out to be very difficult. The results, that also appear in table 3, show that most of times there was no direct correspondence between an action and an Asbru plan (only for action 10), but rather a variety of other situations: actions that correspond to Ask statements in an Asbru plan (e.g. action 1), or to Display statements (e.g. action 5), or even to filter conditions (action 9). Besides, it is frequent to find situations in which several actions are mapped onto the same plan (e.g. actions 5 and 6). **Conclusion.** After some difficulties, most expert's actions appear in the protocol in some form, although not always as plans in their own right.

Studying the protocol recommendations not considered in the solution. Figure 2 illustrates the actions recommended by the protocol in this particular case, with indications of the actions that were (or were not) performed by the expert. It also indicates the actions for which the question was not decidable, mainly because of unavailable data. It is important to note that conditions, time annotations and intentions of the Asbru protocol have not been considered here.

---

[4] Jaundiced.

Table 3. Solution of the expert to test case 1. This table lists the actions advised by the expert, their intentions, as she reported them, and their correspondence with elements of the Asbru protocol.

	Action	Intention	Is in protocol
1	Measurement of TSB value	(1) Determine degree of hyperbilirubinemia and (2) Determine interim therapy	in Ask of plan 1.5
2	Blood group tests: (a) mother, (b) child	Determine possibility of blood group antagonism	(a) no (b) in Ask of plan 1.4.2.2
3	Rhesus factor tests: (a) mother, (b) child	Determine possibility of rhesus conflict	(a) no (b) in Ask of plan 1.4.2.2
4	Child Coombs test	Determine (im)possibility of blood group antagonism/rhesus conflict	in Ask of plan 1.4.2.2
5	Hemoglobin test	(1) Determine presence/severity of hemolysis and (2) Determine need of blood transfusion	in Display of plan 1.4.3.1
6	Reticulocyte count	Search for clues of hemolysis	in Display of plan 1.4.3.1
7	Ratio direct/indirect bilirubin	(1) Determine first hypothesis concerning the cause of hyperbilirubinemia and (2) Determine further diagnosis/therapy	no
8	Question about geographic origin: parents, child	Determine chance of G6PD deficiency	in Ask of plan 1.4.3
9	Looking up TSB value in table	Choose correct therapy	in filter conditions of plans 1.5.1.1–5 and 1.5.2
10	Prescription of phototherapy	Prevent harmful effects of high bilirubin levels	in plan 1.5.1.3
11	New measurement of TSB value (within 6 to 12h)	(1) Determine effect of phototherapy, (2) Determine presence/severity of hyperbilirubinemia, and (3) Determine further therapy	in Ask of plan 1.5

Apart from undecidable questions, we find several points where the physician did not follow the protocol recommendations: different anamnesis questions, determination of jaundice and study of feeding alternatives. For the first two situations, we did not conclude that the expert was deviating from the protocol since we do not deem likely that she forgot to consider those aspects. For the last situation, skipping the study of feeding alternatives turned out to be a common practice in Netherlands. **Conclusion.** Summarising, except for a regional deviation of the protocol, the expert roughly followed the recommendations in the AAP protocol.

Studying the expert's actions not recommended in the protocol. Some of the expert's actions were not recommended by the protocol to solve the current case —actions 2a, 3a and 7. Even more, they are not even included in the protocol. First, the blood typing of the mother (actions 2a and 3a) is simply not considered in the protocol. When these data are not available, the diagnosis goes on with the blood typing and the Coombs test of the child. The intention of the expert, which is determining the possibility of blood group/rhesus incompatibility, causing hemolysis, is certainly relevant for the case. Since

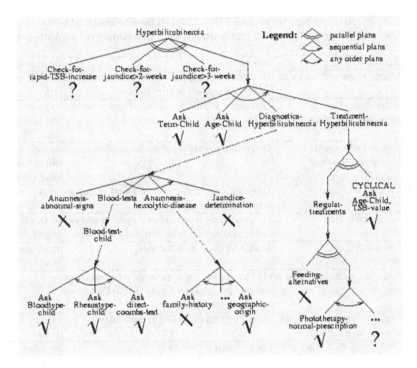

Fig. 2. Recommendations of the protocol to test case 1. Solution recommended by the protocol given the initial data of case 1, together with indications of the actions that were included in the expert's solution (signalled with $\sqrt{}$) and the ones that were not (signalled with $\times$), as well as the actions for which the question was not decidable (with **?**).

it can be fulfilled by means of a Coombs test of the child, it should be asked which is the optimal action in this case. Second, the determination of the ratio direct/indirect bilirubin is not considered either in the protocol. The intention here is to obtain additional clues concerning the cause of jaundice. This is obviously relevant to the diagnosis part of the protocol, and therefore it should be asked whether the action is optimal in the current context. According to the answers to the previous questions, the protocol can be modified to consider these alternatives. **Conclusion.** These examples show how the protocol can be improved by studying deviating actions together with their justifications.

Studying the appropriateness of expert's actions. For this analysis we grouped the actions that were mapped onto the same plan. The main reason is that intentions are in Asbru ascribed to plans rather than to individual statements of plans. Then we checked for every action group whether the conditions and time annotations of the associated plan enabled it, and whether the intentions of the plan were similar to the intentions behind the action.

   Almost all expert's actions were appropriate according to conditions and times. The only untimely actions were the two TSB measurements, which were both matched against the Ask reading a new value of plan 1.5. This was wrong for the initial measurement, but it was the only possibility given that in the protocol there is no explicit sentence for reading the initial TSB value. Regarding the second TSB measurement, which was matched correctly, it is considered untimely due to the divergence in reading intervals. **Conclusion**. These examples show how the study of actions considered untimely can also contribute to improve the protocol, in this case making explicit the initial reading of the TSB value and refining the time annotation of the second (and further) readings.

However, most expert's actions were not appropriate according to intentions. We ended up considering intentions similar in most cases, but we could only conclude this after using additional knowledge/reasoning (implicit intentions, medical knowledge or reasoning about inheritance of intentions). For instance, the intention of action 8 "determine chance of G6PD deficiency" was considered equivalent to one of plan 1.4.3 "determine possibility of hemolytic disease", because G6PD is a cause of hemolytic disease. Still, intentions are just similar, which means that only part of them match, with the possibility of subsumption. **Conclusion**. We cannot strictly rely on intentions for studying the appropriateness of expert's actions, not even in the crucial step of matching expert's actions against Asbru elements, as we would have liked to.

5.2 Critiquing Other Test Cases

We have performed similar critiquing checks with other six cases—test cases 2 through 8, except test case 7, which was discarded because the expert had problems with the terminology. Next we briefly summarise the main results of critiquing.

Matching the expert's actions and the protocol. The results of test case 1 in this regard are quite representative. In addition, there is a high number of actions corresponding to Display statements, and in some situations it is not clear whether a correspondence can be established at all. For instance, in test case 2 it was not clear whether the haptoglobin test could be considered part of the Display of plan 1.4.3.1 due to its formulation: "Perform appropriate laboratory assessment of infant including (but not limited to):...". The protocol can be improved by making this Display more explicit. Another interesting finding is that sometimes extra medical knowledge is needed for action matching. For instance, the action "determination of shape of erythrocytes" in test cases 2 and 4 was matched with the Display of plan 1.4.3.1, which includes a differential smear, because this test provides information about the shape of blood cells.

Studying the protocol recommendations not considered in the solution. In the rest of the cases the expert did not perform either of the actions she skipped in test case 1: several anamnesis questions, the determination of jaundice and the study of feeding alternatives. Our conclusion is again that these deviations from the protocol are either irrelevant or legal. Other discrepancies were found in cases 3, 5 and 8. In test case 5 the expert skipped the blood typing and Coombs test of the child. A plausible explanation is that she thinks jaundice is caused by the infant's cephalic hematoma, and that hence no other causes need to be considered. However, we cannot rely on our own interpretation of the expert's intentions to justify her actions. Discrepancies of cases 3 and 8 are different. The application of the protocol should be interrupted in both cases due to, respectively, a preterm infant and a positive Coombs test. In case 3 the expert only prescribed observation, but the actions to solve case 8 suggest a completely different approach. The latter situations are further discussed in the next paragraph.

Studying the expert's actions not recommended in the protocol. Again, some of the expert's actions were not recommended by the protocol to solve the cases, and they were not even included in the protocol. We found that the blood typing of the mother and the determination of the ratio direct/indirect bilirubin of test case 1, and the above mentioned haptoglobin test, appear as a recurrent pattern in the rest of the cases. Like in test case 1, it should be studied whether these actions are relevant to the cases and optimal in their context, in order to modify the protocol if necessary. The situations referred to in the previous paragraph are different. Here the discrepancies cannot be justified since they directly involve the applicability conditions of the whole protocol.

Studying the appropriateness of expert's actions. The results of test case 1 concerning this aspect are also representative. Again, almost all expert's actions were appropriate according to conditions and times, but not when considering intentions.

6   Results of Critiquing

Our critiquing exercise, in spite of the difficulties we have encountered, shows the utility of critiquing for quality improvement of medical protocols. The results of this exercise can be summarised as follows. *First*, we can say that most expert's actions are included in the protocol.

Second, we consider that the expert did not comply with the protocol in three of the cases.

Third, whenever the expert performs actions that are not recommended by the protocol, this occurs throughout all the cases, which means that the expert relies on a pattern of actions not considered in the protocol, therefore suggesting a gap. This impression is strengthened by the fact that these actions do not appear anywhere in the protocol, i.e. not even in subplans that are used in the particular case. We have seen that a study of the relevance and optimality of these actions can help to determine if the protocol should be modified to include them as valid alternatives.

Last, most expert's actions are appropriate according to conditions and times, but not according to intentions. The reason of this general mismatch is that the intentions we modelled in the protocol and the ones acquired from the expert when giving a solution are quite different. Since intentions are not explicitly stated in the protocol, they are very hard to model. As a result, they vary considerably in the amount of details, the level of abstraction, etc, which precludes their use even for the matching of expert's actions with Asbru plans.

7   Conclusions

Critiquing, even manually, is a difficult task. It is hard to match expert's actions with parts of the Asbru protocol. The actions do not always appear in the protocol as plans, and therefore there is no 1:1 correspondence (sometimes there is not even a correspondence) between expert's actions and protocol plans, but rather a variety of relationships. For this purpose we can think of using the intentions of both actions and plans, but, as we have already pointed out, this is also difficult. In fact, the direct use of intentions for critiquing, either for matching of actions or for studying their appropriateness, is not possible due to the difficulties inherent to their modelling/acquisition. The intentions of the protocol are not stated explicitly, which makes them very hard to model, and the intentions reported by our expert almost always differ. It is not only a problem of vocabulary, but also a matter of differences in the degree of detail, abstraction level, etc. This problem can be partly solved by using additional knowledge to fill in the gaps. Lastly, critiquing needs a lot of specific knowledge. Not only medical knowledge and vocabularies to fill the gaps between intentions, but also knowledge about the actions requiring a critique and about regional policies, for an effective critiquing.

All the above implies that the automation of critiquing will be very hard, at least in the way we have approached it. Many of the previous problems have been avoided in the critiquing literature by using *ad-hoc* solutions, basically forcing the expert to use a series of predefined actions and intentions—the ones in the system. We believe that this is not a good way of solving the natural differences that exist between the protocol and the individual practices. Besides, it assumes that the protocol constitutes the golden standard, whilst our study has shown that even a high quality protocol might have to be adjusted after systematic exposure to analysis based on test cases.

Acknowledgements. We want to thank Frea Kruizinga, the pediatrics expert without whom the critiquing exercise would not have been possible, and Andreas Seyfang and Robert Kosara, for their support in using Asbru and their feedback on this work.

References

1. American Academy of Pediatrics, Provisional Committee for Quality Improvement and Subcommittee on Hyperbilirubinemia. Practice parameter: management of hyperbilirubinemia in the healthy term newborn. *Pediatrics,* 94:558–565, 1994.
2. P. Clayton and G. Hripsak. Decision support in healthcare. *Int. J. of Biomedical Computing,* 39:59–66, 1995.
3. J. Fox, N. Johns, C. Lyons, A. Rahmanzadeh, R. Thomson, and P. Wilson. PROforma: a general technology for clinical decision support systems. *Computer Methods and Programs in Biomedicine,* 54:59–67, 1997.
4. P. M. Miller. *A Critiquing Approach to Expert Computer Advice: ATTENDING.* Research Notes in Artificial Intelligence. Pitman Publishing, 1984.
5. M. Musen, J. Rohn, L. Fagan, and E. Shortliffe. Knowledge engineering for a clinical trial advice system: Uncovering errors in protocol specification. *Bulletin du Cancer,* 74:291–296, 1987.
6. L. Ohno-Machado, J. Gennari, S. Murphy, N. Jain, S. Tu, D. Oliver, E. Pattison-Gordon, R. Greenes, E. Shortliffe, and G. Octo Barnett. Guideline Interchange Format: a model for representing guidelines. *J. of the American Medical Informatics Association,* 5(4):357–372, 1998.
7. A. Seyfang, S. Miksch, and M. Marcos. Combining Diagnosis and Treatment using Asbru, 2001. Congress of the Int. Medical Informatics Association (MEDINFO-2001).
8. Y. Shahar, S. Miksch, and P. Johnson. The Asgaard project: a task-specific framework for the application and critiquing of time-oriented clinical guidelines. *Artificial Intelligence in Medicine,* 14:29–51, 1998.
9. S. Weingarten. Using Practice Guideline Compendiums To Provide Better Preventive Care. *Annals of Internal Medicine,* 130(5):454–458, 1999.

Evaluating the Impact of Clinical Practice Guidelines on Stroke Outcomes

Silvana Quaglini[1], Carla Rognoni[1], Anna Cavallini[2], and Giuseppe Micieli[2]

[1] Dipartimento di Informatica e Sistemistica, Università di Pavia, Italy
silvana.quaglini@unipv.it
[2] Stroke Unit, IRCCS Istituto Neurologico "C. Mondino" Pavia, Italy
{cavallin,micieli}@mondino.it

Abstract. A clinical practice guideline for acute ischemic stroke has been implemented in four Italian centres. Its impact in terms of applicability and effectiveness has been analysed. The evaluation methodology is based on the correlation between the compliance to the guideline and the health and economic outcomes during a six months follow-up. The paper illustrates the fundamental role that formal guideline representation, patient data model, and health care organisation model play in the evaluation task. Results show, on the clinical side, that compliance improves stroke outcomes (relative risk due to number of non-compliance 1.07, p<0.03); on the careflow process side, they highlight organisational problems, such as lack of efficient co-operation and communication. Tasks requiring external consultants are often ruled out (e.g. physiatrist visit in 61% of cases) and tasks required to be done quickly are often delayed (e.g. preliminary patient assessment in 52% of cases).

1 Introduction

Clinical practice guidelines (GLs) diffusion requires convincing potential users about applicability and effectiveness [1]. Applicability means the possibility of implementing the GL without involving dramatic changes in the clinical practice and/or unacceptable costs. Effectiveness concerns the improvement of the health outcome and/or the cost containment maintaining the quality standard. With respect to the evaluation of a new therapeutic intervention, such as a new drug, for which randomised clinical trials are the most robust assessment method, GLs present some peculiarities. In their review Grimshaw et al. [2] illustrate the difficulties in performing clinical trials for comparing GL-supported health care delivery with current clinical practice. They affirm that "... randomised trial cannot be regarded as the gold standard in behavioural research", for multiple reasons and they suggest alternative study design, such as crossover trials, balanced incomplete blocks, controlled before-after studies. We claim, in addition, that ethical reasons may impede the creation of a control group (for example if we want to assess the organisational or the economic impact of a GL for which the health benefit has been demonstrated).
In this paper, we propose a methodology for evaluating a GL impact on health, organisational, and economic outcomes starting from the retrospective study of non-compliances (i.e. activities suggested by the GL, but not executed by the physicians). We considered a GL for the acute ischemic stroke management. The rationale is that

S. Quaglini, P. Barahona, and S. Andreassen (Eds.): AIME 2001, LNAI 2101, pp. 442–452, 2001.

if good outcomes are positively correlated (after correction for known covariates) with compliance, there are reasons for trusting in the GL effectiveness and then compliance should be fostered. On the other hand, to foster compliance, it is necessary to analyse current reasons for non-compliance. Therefore, first we investigated if there is any clinical impact related to GL compliance and then we analysed the most common deviations from the GL. Formal representation of both the GL and the healthcare organisation model and a very accurate Electronic Patient Record (EPR) are shown to be fundamental to that purpose. In particular, the latter has been designed in order to allow the detection of non-compliances by examining data after the patient discharge. We are aware this is a weak point of our study that should be addressed in the future: physicians have been allowed to enter data about their actions some time "after" the action itself has been performed; the "reconstruction" of both what they did and the time frame in which they provided treatment may constitute a bias. However, most of the information is entered in the EPR with a time-stamp associated, and the system *forces* the user entering all the necessary data. Difficulties in performing real-time check will be discussed.

2 The Clinical Application

Stroke is a serious and common illness: the death rate is approximately 30% and, at the moment, there are several million people who had a stroke yet and are still alive, with varying degrees of disability. Early stroke course is commonly divided into two phases: the acute phase is defined as the first six hours from the symptom onset, while the subacute phase is the time interval from six hours to seven days. We decided to adopt and evaluate, in four Italian hospitals, the American Heart Association (AHA) GLs for acute ischemic stroke [3], to be used for patients admitted during the acute phase, and the diagnostic procedures and recommendations for risk factors assessment and treatment [4], to be used for all survived patients. We studied 386 consecutive subjects (110 admitted in the acute phase). A follow-up of at least 6 months was planned.

3 The GL Representation and the EPR: GL Evaluation Issues

GLs have been computerised: first of all they have been represented as a flowchart through the GUIDE graphical editor [5]. GUIDE represents tasks, decision steps, monitoring steps, and allows links to decision-analytic models, to software procedures and to the EPR. Users, i.e. physicians and nurses, may browse the flowchart for both educational purposes and for obtaining real-time suggestions, since we integrated GLs with EPR. The latter, implemented with a relational database management system, was shared by the study centres and stored the data concerning the past medical history of the patient, the hospital admission modality, all the interventions carried out for each patient (including drug dosage and administration time), diagnostic test results, assessment scales' scores, complications, and follow-up information. Physicians accessed the system from fixed terminals on the wards, both for data entry and for GL browsing, being the two functionality fully integrated. Next sections illustrate the GUIDE features most related to the GL impact evaluation.

3.1 Representation of the GL Intention

A clear definition of the GL intention [6] and outcomes expected to be affected by the GL is the pre-requisite for an evaluation study. GL intention is represented through the description of one or more goals, together with the time at which goals achievement must be measured. In our case, the goals are survival improvement, disability degree reduction (quality of life improvement), and cost containment, and the evaluation time window is six months from the diagnosis. Each of these goals requires complex calculations on more than one attribute of the EPR. Thus, at the GL representation level, we decided to associate to each of them the name of a procedure that, by querying the database, produces one or more tables of data, ready for further statistical elaboration (Figure 1). For example, to estimate the quality of life pattern, it is necessary to elaborate the results of the SF36 questionnaire, administered to patients at different times. According to Apolone [7], the procedure computes two "synthetic indices", indicated as IFS and IMS in Figure 1, for the physical and mental status, respectively, that will be correlated with the GL compliance.

Similarly, other procedures pre-elaborate data for survival and cost analysis.

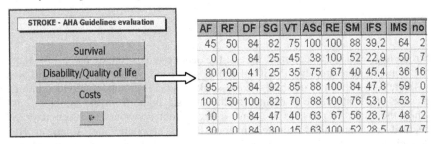

STROKE - AHA Guidelines evaluation		AF	RF	DF	SG	VT	ASc	RE	SM	IFS	IMS	no
Survival		45	50	84	82	75	100	100	88	39,2	64	2
		0	0	84	25	45	38	100	52	22,9	50	7
Disability/Quality of life		80	100	41	25	35	75	67	40	45,4	36	16
		95	25	84	92	85	88	100	84	47,8	59	0
Costs		100	50	100	82	70	88	100	76	53,0	53	7
		10	0	84	47	40	63	67	56	28,7	48	2
		30	0	84	30	15	63	100	52	28,5	47	7

Fig. 1. Left) procedures for querying the database about information related to the guideline goals; right) the table produced for analysing correlation between compliance and life quality

3.2 Compliance

As already mentioned, we want to study the correlation between outcomes and GL compliance. In this section, issues related to the *compliance* concept are discussed.

Representation of the Level of Evidence of a Task

A non-compliance to a GL task may be less or more severe, depending on the level of scientific evidence supporting that task. A well-agreed-on classification of these levels is the following[8]:

level I-   Data from randomised trials with *low* false-positive (alpha) and false-negative (beta) errors

level II- Data from randomised trials with *high* alpha and beta errors

level III- Data form non randomised cohort studies

level IV- Data from non randomised cohort studies with historical controls

level V- Data from expert experience

GUIDE allows using the five levels or any combination of them. Bullets with different colours appear at the left-top corner of each rectangle (i.e. a task/activity), indicating the degree of scientific evidence associated to that GL suggestion. For example, in our GL, three aggregated levels are used, as reported in Figure 2, that illustrates one of the 15 pages composing the whole GL, and shows some tasks with coloured bullets.

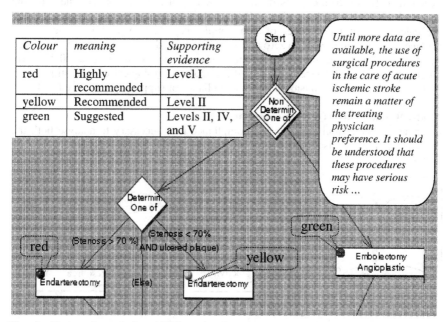

Colour	meaning	Supporting evidence
red	Highly recommended	Level I
yellow	Recommended	Level II
green	Suggested	Levels II, IV, and V

Start

Non Determin One of

Until more data are available, the use of surgical procedures in the care of acute ischemic stroke remain a matter of the treating physician preference. It should be understood that these procedures may have serious risk ...

Determin One of

(Stenosis > 70 %)   (Stenosis < 70% AND ulcered plaque)

red

(Else)

Endarterectomy

green

Embolectomy
Angioplastic

yellow

Endarterectomy

Fig. 2. The portion of the guideline showing the recommendation concerning surgical treatment. The common (if any) about a decision task may be obtained by clicking the icon.

Detection of Non-compliance

As mentioned, GUIDE implements the connection of the GL with the EPR. The GL inference engine runs in background during data input, in a "silent" modality: this means that if the performed activities are compliant with the GL, the GL presence is not perceived by the user. Only when a non-compliance is detected, looking at the information stored into the EPR, the GL reacts and shows its recommendation. However, the user can access the GL in any moment, and check both for the tasks already executed on a certain patient and the next task to execute, together with explanation about them. The GL inference engine "imposes" a sequence for data input, corresponding to the priority for actions fixed in the GL. Other types of non-compliance are very difficult to be detected in real time. For example, if there is no electronic connection between the ward and the haematho-chemical laboratories, the GL inference engine cannot be aware about which tests have been ordered until the test results are stored in the EPR. Again, some GL recommendations concern activity constraints, such as the maximum execution time: when data input is not performed in real time, and this is often the case, it is obviously impossible to detect non-compliance. For tackling these situations, we add some attributes in the EPR, explicitly representing constraints, such as " time spent for objective examination". In addition, the system embeds a specific form for writing reasons for non-compliance, but physician's resistance in writing justifications must be considered. For these reasons, a complete detection of all the non compliances is only possible "a posteriori", in our case at the discharge time, when it is assumed that the EPR has been filled accurately, including a careful inspection of the paper-based clinical chart. When the patient record is "closed", a set of SQL queries is activated to check for the "correct" treatment of that patient. The very detailed EPR allowed, for each patient, the calculation of the number of non-compliances (NC) occurred during his/her treatment: NC is initially set to zero and it is incremented by 1 for each task suggested by the GL, but not executed. NC may range between 0 and 47 (acute phase 0-17, early clinical phase 0-23, management of medical and/or neurological complications 0-7). At present, we only are considering non-compliance of supporting evidence level I.

Model-Based Analysis of Non-compliance
To understand the motivation of non-compliance it is necessary to analyse both the medical and the organisational aspects involved in the GL-based activities.

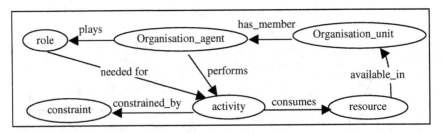

Fig. 3. The portion of the organisation ontology used for the analysis of non compliance

Table Ia. SNOMED hierarchy of activities

CODE_ CHILD	CODE_ FATHER	DESCRIPTION
C0024485	C0202565	MR-magnetic resonance
C0202565	C0202564	General radiol.Procedures
C0203887	C0203882	Physiatrist initial examination, evaluation, ..
C0203882	C0203881	GENERAL PROCED.
C0203382	C0203351	Carotid imaging

Table Ib. Roles able to perform each activity

ACT_SNOMED _CODE	ROLE_SNOMED _name
C0203887	Physiatrist
C0024485	Radiologist
C0024485	Neurologist
C0024485	Medical X-ray technician

Table Ic. Technological resources needed for each activity

Activity SNOMED CODE	Needed INSTRUMENT
C0024485	MRI scanner
C0203382	Doppler Echograph
C0202652	TC SCANNER

Table Id. View of the roles and belonging organisations for human agents

PERSON CODE	ORGANISATION UNIT	ROLE
P1	Mondino S.U.	Neurologist
P2	S.Matteo Cardiology	Cardiologist
P3	Mondino Rehabil.	Physiatrist
P4	Mondino Rad.Unit	Radiologist

An ontological approach is useful to this aim. Figure 3 illustrates a scratch of the devised organisation ontology [9], an adaptation from the TOVE project [10]. Let us focus on the characterisation of each activity in terms of technical resources needed, and roles suitable for its accomplishment. To illustrate how this information is represented within our system, let us consider the GL tasks *perform the Magnetic Resonance Imaging (MRI)* and *perform a physiatrist visit.*

Tables Ia-d are a portion of the instantiation of the ontology, showing some rows related to the above tasks. As a matter of fact, we obtain an ontology computational instance by populating a relational database, whose structure is automatically derived from the ontology itself. As described in [11] each activity is drawn from the SNOMED medical terminology server, and this allows not only to give a "standard" name to the activity, but also to put it within a hierarchy of "activity types". This is useful for the presentation of statistical results. Using this structured information we can infer possible causes of non-compliance. To this aim, the system embeds a set of rules. Let :

- "OU" be the clinical setting (Organisation Unit) where the GL is implemented;
- "External_OU" be some clinical settings collaborating with "OU"
- P% be a threshold for the percent of non compliance, that must be considered as an "alarm" (this parameter will be set by the evaluator)
- ACTno be an activity that is ruled out more than P% of times, while ACTyes an activity that is normally (ruled out less than P%) performed;
- ACTyes_C be a temporal constraint on ACTyes.

Some of the rules are:

R1. If ACTno requires instrumentation and instrumentation is present in the OU then the cause probably is: instrumentation often out of order

R2. If ACTno requires more than a role and the roles are present in the OU then the cause probably is: lack of internal co-ordination

R3. If ACTno requires roles and the roles are not present in the OU and the roles are present in External_OU then the cause probably is: failures in communication between organisations

R4. If ACTyes _C is not satisfied and ACTyes require resources and resources are present in the OU then the cause probably is: bad resource allocation or scarcity of resources

R5. If ACTyes_C is not satisfied and ACTyes require roles and roles are not present in the OU and roles are present in External_OU then the cause probably is: chronic delay in communication between organisations

....

Of course, for an activity there may be multiple causes of non compliance (more than one rule satisfied), and the "disagreement with the GL suggestions" can never be excluded. The above rules must be interpreted as a mean for devising alternative (or additional) causes of non-compliance. Since they do not involve uncertainty and they have a simple structure, rules have been implemented with SQL, exploiting the relationships derived from the organisation ontology. Results are shown in section 5.

4 Statistical Analysis

The main purpose of the statistical analysis was to investigate the relationship between outcomes and compliance to the GL.

- For the outcome *Survival* , the cumulative survival curves were derived by the Kaplan-Meier method, and the difference between two or more survival curves was assessed by the log-rank or Mantel-Haenszel test. The influence of prognostic factors (among which the number of non compliances) on survival was investigated by the Cox proportional hazard regression model. Both uni- and multivariate analyses were performed. The multivariate analysis was done by including in the model the covariates that were significant at the previous univariate analysis. Relative risks and their 95% confidence interval have been derived, after fitting the Cox model, as the antilogarithm of the coefficient estimated for each covariate included in the model itself.

- For the outcome *Disability/Quality of life* , a correlation analysis (Pearson's linear correlation coefficient) was performed between the number of non-compliances and the difference between the Barthel and SF36 scores at the admission and those measured during the follow-up.

- For the outcome *Economical cost*, we took into account both the hospitalisation phase and the costs for stroke-related visits and re-hospitalisations during the follow-up. The point of view was that of the health care organisation: only its direct costs were considered (personnel, drugs and other therapeutic interventions, diagnostic tests), while production loss and patient/family sustained costs were not taken into account. Correlation analysis was then performed between costs and number of non-compliances.

5 Results

The median number of non-compliances during the acute phase was 5 (range: 3–13), while for the early clinical/subacute phase was 3 (range: 2-15).

5.1 Motivations for Non-compliance

Table II illustrates the inferences obtained by the rules partially reported in section 3.2.3, for a threshold value P%=30%. Here non-compliances about the acute phase are considered. Interpretation of these results requires context knowledge. For example, it is very hard that an MRI scanner is out of order for a significant amount of time in a hospital with a Stroke Unit, thus more confidence will be put on the "lack of co-ordination" or "disagreement" hypothesis. Physicians involved in the study were not surprised that most of non-compliances are due do lack of co-ordination or communication, both within the same hospital, and among hospitals. This was their feeling, to which the above table provides a useful quantification: even if the collaborating organisations are in the same town it is very difficult to guarantee the intervention of an external consultant within one-two hours from the first call, and this is a major problem when "time is brain". Also the communication among

Table II - The percentage of non-compliance and the inferred motivations in the acute phase

activity	times_to_do	times_ not done	%	Possible motivation (in addition to disagreement)
Early physiotherapy	110	100	90	lack of internal co-ordination
MRI for POCS	19	17	89	Instrumentation out of order Lack of internal co-ordination
Protocol enrolment	110	97	88	lack of resource (drug)
Vital signs monitor	109	88	80	lack of resource (instrumentation)
Physiatrist visit	109	67	61	failed communication among organisations
Preliminary assessment time <=15 minutes	110	58	52	bad co-ordination or bad human resource allocation or scarcity of human resources
Chest RX	109	42	38	Instrumentation out of order Lack of internal co-ordination

different divisions of the same hospital is often difficult, because each division is self-organising, without taking into account co-ordination with the other divisions.

5.2 Compliance and Outcomes

As mentioned in the introduction, our study relies in the assumption that, if a multivariate analysis shows a good correlation between compliance and outcomes, there are reasons to think that GL performs well. Thus, we investigated this correlation.

Survival
At the univariate analysis, the Cox proportional-hazards model identified the following prognostic factors: age, type of stroke, number of non-compliance, atrial fibrillation, cardiac insufficiency and Barthel index at the admittance. Including all these variables into a multivariate model, only age, number of non-compliances and Barthel index at admission were still significant predictors.
The model is the following:

Variable:	*Relative Risk (95% CI)*
Age	$1.03 \ (1.01\text{-}1.15)$, $p<0.03$
Number of non-compliances	$1.07 \ (1.01\text{-}1.06)$, $p<0.03$
Barthel index at admission	$1.10 \ (1.05\text{-}1.16)$, $p<0.001$

Note that for continuous variables, such as age, the Barhel score, and the number of non compliance, the RR is referred to a unit change in the variable itself. This result puts the number of non-compliances among "risk factors" for early death, independently from age and the severity of the patient's initial conditions. This number has been used as a continuous variable in the regression, but for purposes of illustration Figure 4 shows the two groups of patients with more/less-equal than 5 non-compliances.

Disability/Quality of Life
As described in Figure 1, we analysed data from the SF36 questionnaire, that measures the quality of life, and from the Barthel scale, that mainly measures physical functionality. Again, encouraging results have been obtained. In particular, the SF36 physical synthetic index is inversely correlated with the number of non-

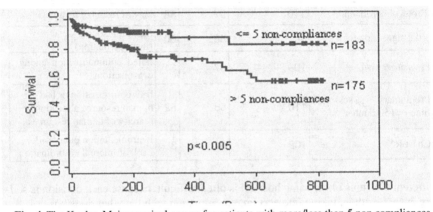

Fig. 4. The Kaplan-Meier survival curves for patients with more/less than 5 non compliances

compliances (r=-0.2, p<0.005), that also is correlated with six months residual disability in less severe patients (Barthel index: r=0.12 Pearson's correlation p<0.01)

Costs
Direct costs from the hospital point of view have been considered at the moment. Total cost (acute phase + rehabilitation) was about 10000 Euros for patients with NC>5, and about 7500 Euros for those with NC<=5. For lack of space, among several statistics performed, we only report here a very interesting result about the analysis of a particular non-compliance, i.e. lack of "vital signs monitoring", including ECG, blood pressure, pulse oxymetry. We exploit a functionality of our system that allows obtaining tables of paired cases, i.e. pairs of patients very similar for the most important variables (age, sex, severity, etc.). Pairing the patients allows analysing the effect of a particular treatment, avoiding the confounding effects of covariates. The procedure paired each patient undergoing vital signs monitoring with another one who did not. Analysing the obtained sample (about 60 + 60 patients) the Wilcoxon test showed significant difference on the duration of the hospitalisation: median 8 days (InterQuartile range: 5-12) for monitored patients versus 14 days (IQ: 11-22.5); also the number of visits during the follow-up, for problems related to the stroke, is lower in the monitored group (0.149 vs 0.857 visits/month). This can be explained by the larger number of complications detected very early in the monitored patients, allowing a better treatment and a better recovery. Considering that the overall monitoring cost for the six beds of our Stroke Unit is about 5-10 Euros/day for the instrumentation (amortisation-based estimate) it is clear that this intervention is cost-beneficial.

6 Conclusion and Future Developments

This study has pointed out that adherence to GLs improves stroke outcome and emphasises the need to develop personnel and well co-ordinated structures devoted to stroke care because an evidence-based clinical practice can significantly reduce the risk of death and improve the other outcomes.

We plan to continue analysis of collected data, refining results to take into account: non-compliance of degree II and III; the society point of view in the cost model, considering loss of productivity due to hospitalisation and residual disability, and the family involvement in these patients management; the possibility of using the SF36 scores to derive a single index [12], in order to transform survival years into QALYs (Quality Adjusted Life Years) and thus perform a cost/utility economic evaluation.

Acknowledgements. The authors thank the other components of the GLADIS study group (G.P. Anzola, L. Frattola, A. Mamoli, M. Stefanelli) for data collection and helpful discussion. This work has been partially funded by the Italian Ministry of Health.

References

1. Zielstorff R.D. Online practice guidelines: Issues, obstacles and future prospects, J Am Med Inform Assoc 1998; 5(3) 227-236.
2. Grimshaw J.M., Russel I.T. Effect of clinical guidelines on medical practice: a systematic review of rigorous evaluation. Lancet 1993; 342: 1317-1322
3. Adams H.P., Brott T.G., Crowell R.M., Furln A.J., Gomez C.R., Grotta J., Helgason C.M., Marler J.R., Woolson R.F., Zivin J.A., Feinberg W., Mayberg, M. Guidelines for the management of patients with acute ischemic stroke. Special Report. Stroke 1994;25, 9 , 1901-1911
4. Feinberg WM, Albers GW, Barnett HJM, Biller J, Caplan LR, Carter LP, Hart RG, Hobson RW, Kronmal RA, Moore WS, Robertson JT, Adams Jr HP, Mayberg M. Guidelines for the management of transient ischemic attacks. Stroke 1994;25(6):1321-1335
5. Quaglini S, Dazzi L, Gatti L, Stefanelli M, Fassino C, Tondini C. Supporting tools for guideline development and dissemination, Artificial Intelligence in Medicine 1998; 14:119-137
6. Miksch S, Shahar Y, Johnson P. ASBRU: A task-specific, intention-based, and time-oriented language for representing skeletal plans. In: E Motta, FV Harmelen, C Pierret Golbreich, I Filby, N Wijngaards (eds). Proc. Of the 7th Workshop on Knowledge Engineering:Methods and Languages. The Open University, Milton Keynes, 1997; 9.1-9.20
7. Apolone G., Mosconi P, Ware J.E. Questionario sullo stato di salute SF-36 – Manuale d'uso e guida all'interpretazione dei risultati, 1997, Guerini e Associati Ed.
8. Cook D.J., Guyatt G.H., Laupacis A., Sackett D.L. Rules of evidence and clinical recommendations on the use of antithrombotic agents. Chest. 1992; 102 (suppl. 4):305S-311S
9. Marchetti D., Lanzola G., Stefanelli M. An AI-based Approach to the Communication Problem in Health Care Organizations, ibidem

10. Fox M.S., Barbuceanu M. and Gruninger M. An organization ontology for enterprise modeling: preliminary concepts for linking structure and behaviour. Computers in Industry 1995; vol 29, pp 123-134.
11. Quaglini S, Stefanelli M, Cavallini A, Micieli G, Fassino C, Mossa C. Guideline-based Careflow Systems, Artificial Intelligence in Medicine 2000, 20(1) 5-22.
12. Brazier J., Usherwood T., Harper R., Thomas K. Deriving a Preference-Based Index from the UK SF-36 Health Survey. J. Clin. Epidemiol. 1998, 51;11;1115-11

Challenges in Evaluating Complex Decision Support Systems: Lessons from Design-a-Trial

Henry W.W. Potts[1], Jeremy C. Wyatt[1], and Douglas G. Altman[2]

[1] School of Public Policy, University College London, 29/30 Tavistock Square,
London WC1H 9QU, UK
{h.potts, jeremy.wyatt}@ucl.ac.uk
[2] Centre for Statistics in Medicine, Institute of Health Sciences, Old Road,
Oxford OX3 7LF, UK
d.altman@icrf.icnet.uk

Abstract. Decision support system developers and users agree on the need for rigorous evaluations of performance and impact. Evaluating simple reminder systems is relatively easy because there is usually a gold standard of decision quality. However, when a system generates complex output (such as a critique or graphical report), it is much less obvious how to evaluate it. We discuss some generic problems and how one might resolve them, using as a case study Design-a-Trial, a DSS to help clinicians write a lengthy trial protocol.

Keywords. Decision support, evaluation, Design-a-Trial, randomised controlled trial.

1 Introduction

It is important to evaluate decision support systems (DSSs), but most published evaluations concern DSSs producing very simple output, such as one-word advice. We are currently developing a DSS with a more complex operation: Design-a-Trial (DaT) [1, 2] aids clinicians less experienced with randomised controlled trials (RCTs) to write a high quality trial protocol (http://www.design-a-trial.net). DaT uses an interface with multiple adaptive forms, in which the user enters information about their planned research (*e.g.* target disease, study intervention), to guide the user through the process of designing a trial. Using natural language generation routines, the software produces feedback, in the form of critiques commenting on the statistical rigour and feasibility of the design, and assembles the information entered into a draft protocol.

There are many other examples of clinical DSSs with complex output, *e.g.* systems generating graphical output such as a practice guideline [3]. Several difficulties have arisen in our plans to evaluate DaT and we have identified some generic problems facing anyone evaluating a DSS with a complex output.

S. Quaglini, P. Barahona, and S. Andreassen (Eds.): AIME 2001, LNAI 2101, pp. 453–456, 2001.

2 Problems in Evaluating Complex Decision Support Systems

Table 1 outlines a number of challenges arising in evaluation studies. We will discuss these within the context of our plans to evaluate DaT. One could evaluate DaT in many different ways. One could assess user satisfaction, but the target audience, those inexperienced with RCTs, may be the least suited to judging whether DaT's advice is of use, may not recognise good advice and may dislike being corrected by a computer system. A user assessment of the DSS is an important part of the evaluation of the software, but so is a more objective assessment of the output.

Table 1. Evaluating output quality

Options	Implications
User satisfaction	Users may have poor introspection
Reference to standard guidelines; consistency of solutions	Important measure (*e.g.* risk management); standards may not exist
Exact match with DSS knowledge base	Circularity; lack of generality; tests animation of rules, not their quality
Match with a quality checklist chosen by DSS developers	Circularity; bias in choice of checklist
Get external expert(s) to choose a checklist	Which checklist to choose; duplication of effort
Use expert judges (without specified checklist)	Criteria used unclear
External measure of quality	Logistic challenges; influenced by other factors

DaT produces a complex output, a protocol of over 1000 words describing a planned RCT, the result of guided user input and natural language generation. This output should be of high quality in two respects: the design of the underlying trial should be statistically and methodologically valid; and the protocol should be an apt, concise and precise description of that trial. Assessing the quality of protocols is clearly central to evaluating DaT. In general, evaluators should check to see if there is already a scale for measuring the outcome of interest [4]. None exists in this case, but assessing protocol quality appears straightforward. One use of a protocol is for submission to bodies who make decisions about the trial described: whether to fund it, permit it on ethical grounds and so on. Bodies making these decisions routinely assess protocols in some manner. However, in considering how to formulise the assessment of protocols explicitly, we became aware of some inherent obstacles.

A complex output normally necessitates a composite measure of quality [4]. While we are unaware of any formal scales for assessing RCT protocols, there is a very considerable number of scales for assessing published reports of RCTs [5]. The issues in assessing published RCT reports are very similar to those for RCT protocols. Both have dual notions of quality: the quality of the underlying trial and of the description of the trial. It seems simple to adapt one of the many scales for RCT reports to RCT protocols. However, Jüni *et al.* [5] have shown that using different scales for assessing RCT report quality can lead to different conclusions in meta-analyses. The different scales put differing weights on the various aspects of report and design quality. For example, some concentrate on issues of internal validity, some on external validity. There is no inherent right answer to these relative weights. This problem must generalise to a potential scoring system for RCT protocols. Moreover, we suggest that it will also generalise to most composite measures of quality in a manner similar to Arrow's Theorem on the theoretical limits of group decision making [6].

If the conclusions drawn using a composite measure of quality depend on the weighting of issues within that measure, that raises certain problems. How can one ensure that the choice or design of such a measure is not biased in favour of the DSS being evaluated? Even if the measure can be chosen in an objective fashion, there is still the potential for the DSS designers to concentrate their efforts on those issues the chosen scoring system weights highest. Such problems are perhaps soluble. Decisions about assessment can be made independently from the design team. Expert judges could be set the task of choosing or designing the composite measure while blind to the details of the DSS, while the developers produce their software blind to the details of the assessment tool. However, this may be a perverse way of duplicating labour. The developers of the DSS and the judges are both concerned with quality: the former with producing it, the latter with assessing it. If the expert judges have useful insights into quality, sharing those insights could lead to a better DSS.

There is, we suggest, a generic problem: circular definitions of quality. A measure of quality defines what quality means, but the DSS in its operation may also define what quality means. We could construct a checklist for assessing RCT protocol quality, but that checklist and the DaT rule base then exist as parallel definitions of quality. As both involve arbitrary decisions, as will be the case with most complex DSSs and composite scoring scales, does it makes sense to compare one (DSS) against another (assessment tool)? The latter is no more a gold standard than the former.

An alternative approach is to ask expert judges to rate quality directly without reference to an explicit scoring system. However, this is only a superficial way of avoiding the problems raised. Judges will still use implicit quality criteria and, without a specified scoring method, we do not know what criteria they have used. Another solution is to use a pragmatic measure, one that is readily measured and an indirect result of quality. This could be seen as a test of predictive validity. In the context of RCT protocols, this might be the acceptance rate by some decision-making body, for example on funding decisions. If dealing with a prescribing system, it may be unclear what constitutes "good prescribing", but it is usually clear if patients survive longer or have higher quality of life. Although such external measures are attractive, they can pose logistic difficulties and again may fail to make quality criteria explicit.

Many of these problems arise from composite quality scores. The best way forward may be to use multiple dimensions of quality instead, although this may make it harder to draw clear conclusions from an evaluation study.

3   Conclusions

It is important to evaluate DSSs. Doing so is often not difficult, but complex DSSs present extra problems. We have underestimated these challenges in our own project and hope this paper serves to forewarn other researchers. Complex outputs may not have a gold standard. Assessment of such outputs may rely on composite scales, but there are potential biases in designing or choosing such scales. Moreover, there is a circular argument if both the operation of the DSS and the scoring system are trying to define high quality. Still other issues which we have not touched on include the choice of control and problems in ensuring blinding in comparative trials when the DSS has a distinctive output. We believe similar issues also apply to evaluations of other types of decision support, such as text checklists or websites.

However, while some compromises may be needed, work on evaluating DaT is moving ahead. Applying some ingenuity and the insights discussed here, we hope it is not too hard to perform rigorous evaluations of complex DSSs.

Acknowledgements. Peter Hammond & Sanjay Modgil; EPSRC; BUPA Foundation.

References

1. Wyatt, J., Altman, D., Heathfield, H., Pantin, C.: Development of Design-a-Trial, a Knowledge-based Critiquing System for Authors of Clinical Trial Protocols. Comp. Meth. Prog. Biomed. 43 (1994) 283-291
2. Modgil, S., Hammond, P., Wyatt, J.C., Potts, H.: The Design-a-Trial Project: Developing a Knowledge-based Tool for Authoring Clinical Trial Protocols. In: 1st European Workshop on Computer-based Support for Clinical Guidelines and Protocols (EWGLP-2000). IOS Press, Amsterdam (*in press*)
3. Fox, J., Johns, N., Rahmanzadeh, A., Thompson, R.: ProForma: A General Technology for Clinical Decision Support Systems. Comp. Meth. Prog. Biomed. 54 (1997) 59-67
4. Friedman, C., Wyatt, J.: Evaluation Methods in Medical Informatics. Springer Verlag, New York (1997)
5. Moher, D., Jadad, A. R., Nichol, G., Penman, M., Tugwell, P., Walsh, S.: Assessing the Quality of Randomized Controlled Trials. Control. Clin. Trials 16 (1995) 62-73
6. Bose, D. K., Heathfield, H. A., Andrew, M.: Collective Decision Problems in Medicine – A Basic Approach Looking for Cross-Fertilization in Clinical Surgery. Theoretical Surg. 7 (1992) 186-193

On the Evaluation of Probabilistic Networks

Linda C. van der Gaag and Silja Renooij

Institute of Information and Computing Sciences, Utrecht University,
P.O. Box 80.089, 3508 TB Utrecht, The Netherlands
{linda,silja}@cs.uu.nl

Abstract. As more and more probabilistic networks are being developed for medical applications, the question arises as to their value for clinical practice. Often the clinical value of a network is expressed as the percentage correct of predicted overall outcome, based upon an evaluation study using real-life patient data. In this paper, we propose another method of evaluation that focuses on intermediate outcomes of interest. We illustrate this method for a real-life probabilistic network for the staging of oesophageal cancer and show that it can provide valuable information in addition to a percentage correct.

1 Introduction

In various fields of clinical medicine, probabilistic networks are being developed to support physicians in the difficult tasks of diagnosis and prognostication. A probabilistic network basically is a statistical model comprised of a graphical structure and an associated set of probability distributions [1]. The graphical structure models the statistical variables that are relevant in the field of application, along with the influential relationships between them; the strengths of the relationships are captured by conditional probabilities.

To establish the value of a probabilistic network for clinical practice, it generally is subjected to an evaluation study using real-life patient data. For each patient, the available data are entered into the network whereupon the network computes the most likely diagnosis, or another outcome of interest; the computed outcome is then compared against a given standard of validity. The results of the study are often summarised in the *percentage correct*, or *accuracy*, of predicted outcome, that is, in the percentage of patients for whom the outcome is correct.

An evaluation study as described above typically focuses on a single *overall outcome*. In this paper we investigate another, more elaborate, method of evaluation that focuses on *intermediate outcomes* of interest. We illustrate this method of evaluation for a real-life probabilistic network for the staging of oesophageal cancer and show that it can provide valuable additional information for assessing the clinical value of a network. In Sect. 2, we briefly describe the oesophagus network and available patient data. We present our evaluation method in Sect. 3. The paper ends with some concluding observations in Sect. 4.

S. Quaglini, P. Barahona, and S. Andreassen (Eds.): AIME 2001, LNAI 2101, pp. 457–461, 2001.

2   The Oesophagus Network and the Patient Data

With the help of two experts in gastrointestinal oncology, we developed a probabilistic network that captures the state-of-the-art knowledge about oesophageal cancer [2]. The network describes the characteristics of an oesophageal tumour and the pathophysiological processes of invasion and metastasis. The depth of invasion and extent of metastasis are summarised in the tumour's *stage*, which is either I, IIA, IIB, III, IVA, or IVB, in the order of advanced disease. The network includes 42 variables, of which 25 are observable, and almost 1000 probabilities.

For investigating the clinical value of the oesophagus network, we have available the medical records of 156 patients diagnosed with oesophageal cancer. For each patient, various observations, for example obtained from diagnostic tests, are recorded. In addition, the tumour's stage and the values of various intermediate, unobservable variables are stated; these values basically are conjectures of the attending physician. The three most important intermediate variables pertain to the presence or absence of haematogenous metastases (the variable *Haema-metas*), to the extent of lymph node metastases (*Lymph-metas*, with the values N0, N1, and M1), and to the depth of invasion of the tumour into the oesophageal wall (*Invasion-wall*, with the values T1, T2, T3, and T4).

3   Evaluation of Intermediate Outcomes

The method of evaluation that is commonly employed for establishing the clinical value of a probabilistic network, amounts to entering patient data into the network, computing the most likely outcome, and comparing it against a given standard of validity. Such an evaluation typically focuses on a single predicted outcome. Another method of evaluation is to subsequently enter all possible outcomes, compute the expected distributions for the observable variables, and compare these against the patient data [3]. For probabilistic networks that model a large number of observable variables for which relatively few data are available, such an evaluation is infeasible. The basic idea of this evaluation method, however, can be used not just for observable variables, but also for crucial intermediate variables. We illustrate this observation for the oesophagus network.

The stage of an oesophageal tumour is defined by the values of the intermediate variables *Haema-metas*, *Lymph-metas* and *Invasion-wall*. The ability of the oesophagus network to distinguish between the various stages thus depends on how much the probability distributions for the three intermediate variables differ per stage. Fig. 1 shows the prior distributions for these variables for the six different stages. We observe, for example, that the probability distributions for *Invasion-wall* are rather similar for the stages IVA and IVB.

In the field of statistics, various measures have been developed for expressing the difference, or *distance*, between two probability distributions. An example of such a measure is the *Kullback-Leibler information divergence* [4]. For a statistical variable with m values, we consider two different distributions p and p', with probabilities p_j and p'_j, $j = 1, \ldots, m$, respectively. The Kullback-Leibler information divergence $I(p, p')$ of p from p' is defined as

	Haema-metas		Lymph-metas			Invasion-wall			
	no	yes	N0	N1	M1	T1	T2	T3	T4
stage I	1	0	1	0	0	1	0	0	0
stage IIA	1	0	1	0	0	0	0.4267	0.5733	0
stage IIB	1	0	0	1	0	0.1108	0.8892	0	0
stage III	1	0	0.0345	0.9655	0	0	0	0.8665	0.1335
stage IVA	1	0	0	0	1	0.0231	0.1234	0.6395	0.2141
stage IVB	0	1	0.4480	0.3929	0.1591	0.0089	0.2166	0.6734	0.1011

Fig. 1. The probability distributions for the three intermediate variables per stage.

$$I(p, p') = \sum_{j=1}^{m} p_j \cdot \ln \frac{p_j}{p'_j}$$

where $0 \cdot \ln \frac{0}{x} = 0$ for all values of x. The divergence $I(p, p')$ equals infinity whenever $p'_j = 0$ and $p_j > 0$; the measure is therefore not symmetric in its arguments. We illustrate the Kullback-Leibler divergence for the variable *Invasion-wall*. Writing p_i for the distributions for stage i, we find from Fig. 1 that, for example, $I(p_{IVA}, p_{IVB}) = 0.0802$, $I(p_{IVB}, p_{IVA}) = 0.0723$, $I(p_I, p_{IVB}) = 4.7217$, and $I(p_{IVB}, p_I) = \infty$. We note that the probability distributions for the stages I and IVB diverge much more than those for IVA and IVB. The network is therefore more likely to confuse the stages IVA and IVB than it is to confuse I and IVB.

Using the Kullback-Leibler divergence, we can compare the probability distributions for the three intermediate variables per stage, with the same distributions given a patient's data. As an example, Fig. 2 shows the distributions for a specific patient. Based upon these distributions, the network concludes that stage III is the most likely stage for the patient's tumour. The medical record, however, states stage IVA, which is the second most likely in the network's prediction. Upon comparing the probability distributions p_i for stage i from Fig. 1 with the distributions p for the patient, we find the Kullback-Leibler divergences shown in Fig. 3. From these divergences, we note that the probability distribution computed for the patient for the variable *Lymph-metas* points to the stages IIB and III, whereas the distribution for *Invasion-wall* favours the stages IIA, III, and IVB. The divergences for the variable *Haema-metas* reveal stage IVB to be rather unlikely. The distributions computed for the patient, therefore, do not unambiguously point to a single specific stage. The network's confusion, however, is not taken into consideration in establishing the percentage correct.

The prior divergences between the probability distributions of the intermediate variables per stage will change when a patient's data are entered into the network. The distance between the distributions for two different stages can become smaller, or the distributions can become more divergent. For example, without taking patient data into consideration, we find for the variable *Invasion-wall* that the divergence of the distribution given stage III from the distribution given stage IVA equals 0.2002. After the data of the patient described above have been entered, this divergence reduces to 0.1454: the network has become

Haema-metas		Lymph-metas			Invasion-wall			
no	yes	N0	N1	M1	T1	T2	T3	T4
0.9071	0.0929	0.0334	0.6432	0.3234	0.0088	0.1285	0.8590	0.0037

Fig. 2. The probability distributions for the three variables given a patient's data.

$I_{Haema}(p_I, p) = 0.0975$ $I_{Lymph}(p_I, p) = 3.3992$ $I_{Invasion}(p_I, p) = 4.7330$

$I_{Haema}(p_{IIA}, p) = 0.0975$ $I_{Lymph}(p_{IIA}, p) = 3.3992$ $I_{Invasion}(p_{IIA}, p) = 0.2803$

$I_{Haema}(p_{IIB}, p) = 0.0975$ $I_{Lymph}(p_{IIB}, p) = 0.4413$ $I_{Invasion}(p_{IIB}, p) = 2.0007$

$I_{Haema}(p_{III}, p) = 0.0975$ $I_{Lymph}(p_{III}, p) = 0.3933$ $I_{Invasion}(p_{III}, p) = 0.4862$

$I_{Haema}(p_{IVA}, p) = 0.0975$ $I_{Lymph}(p_{IVA}, p) = 1.1289$ $I_{Invasion}(p_{IVA}, p) = 0.6974$

$I_{Haema}(p_{IVB}, p) = 2.3762$ $I_{Lymph}(p_{IVB}, p) = 0.8566$ $I_{Invasion}(p_{IVB}, p) = 0.2837$

Fig. 3. The Kullback-Leibler divergences for the various stages, given a patient's data.

even more likely to confuse the stages III and IVA. We have found similar results for most patients for whom the network yields an incorrect stage.

4   Conclusions

To establish the value of a probabilistic network for clinical practice, it is generally subjected to an evaluation study that amounts to computing the most likely outcome for a patient from the network and comparing it against a given standard of validity. We discussed another method of evaluation that serves to gain insight in the probability distributions that are computed for crucial intermediate variables. We suggested the use of the Kullback-Leibler information divergence to investigate the distances between distributions. As it uncovers a network's degree of confusion, we feel that this method of evaluation provides valuable information in addition to a percentage correct.

Acknowledgements. This research has been (partly) supported by the Netherlands Computer Science Research Foundation with financial support from the Netherlands Organisation for Scientific Research. We are grateful to Babs Taal and Berthe Aleman from the Netherlands Cancer Institute, Antoni van Leeuwenhoekhuis, who spent much effort in the construction of the oesophagus network.

References

1. F.V. Jensen (1996). *An Introduction to Bayesian Networks*. UCL Press, London.
2. L.C. van der Gaag, S. Renooij, C.L.M. Witteman, B.M.P. Aleman, B.G. Taal (2001). Probabilities for a probabilistic network: A case-study in oesophageal carcinoma, submitted for publication.

3. S. Andreassen, F.V. Jensen, K.G. Olesen (1991). Medical expert systems based on causal probabilistic networks. *International Journal on Biomedical Computing*, vol. 28, pp. 1 – 30.
4. S. Kullback, R.A. Leibler (1951). On information and sufficiency. *Annals of Mathematical Statistics*, vol. 22, pp. 79 – 86.

Evaluation of a Case-Based Antibiotics Therapy Adviser

Rainer Schmidt, Dagmar Steffen, and Lothar Gierl

Institut für Medizinische Informatik und Biometrie, Universität Rostock
Universität Rostock, D-18055 Rostock,
Germany

Abstract. Some years ago we have developed a case-based antibiotics therapy adviser within the ICONS project. In this paper, we present steps and results of medical evaluations concerning the quality of the recommended therapies, the user friendliness of the system, and the interpretation of laboratory results. Furthermore, we have compared retrieval times of two appropriate Case-based Reasoning retrieval algorithms.

1 Introduction

Severe bacterial infections still are a life threatening complication in intensive care medicine correlated with a high mortality [1, 2]. Identification of bacterial pathogens is often difficult. It normally requires at least 24 hours to identify the pathogen that is responsible for an infection and at least another 24 hours to find out which antibiotics have therapeutic effects against the identified pathogen. To not endanger the patient, physicians often have to start an antimicrobial therapy before the responsible pathogen and its sensitivities are determined. This sort of therapy is called "calculated" in contrast to a "selective" therapy, which is used when microbiological results are already available.

The main task of ICONS is to present suitable calculated antibiotics therapy advice for intensive care patients, who have developed a bacterial infection as an additional complication. As for such critical patients physicians cannot wait for the laboratory results, we use an expected pathogen spectrum based on medical background knowledge. This spectrum should be completely covered by each advisable therapy. Furthermore, as advice is needed very quickly we speed-up the process of computing advisable therapies by using Case-based Reasoning methods [3]. We search for similar previous patients and transfer the suggested therapies made for their situations to the current patient. These previous suggestions are adapted to be applicable to the new medical situation of the current patient.

1.1 Strategy for Selecting Advisable Antibiotic Therapies

Since ICONS is not a diagnostic system, we do not attempt to deduce evidence for diagnoses based on symptoms, frequencies or probabilities, but instead pursue a strategy that can be characterised as follows: Find all possible solutions and reduce them using the patient's contraindications and the complete coverage of the calculated pathogen spectrum (establish-refine strategy).

S. Quaglini, P. Barahona, and S. Andreassen (Eds.): AIME 2001, LNAI 2101, pp. 462–466, 2001.
© Springer-Verlag Berlin Heidelberg 2001

First, we distinguish among different groups of patients (infection acquired in- or outside the ward resp. the hospital, immuncompromised patients). A first list of antibiotics is generated by a susceptibility relation, which for each group of pathogens provides all antibiotics that usually have therapeutic effects. This list contains all those antibiotics that can control at least a part of the potential pathogen spectrum. We obtain a second list of antibiotics by reducing the first one by applying two constraints: The patient's contraindications and the desired sphere of activity. Using the antibiotics of this second list, we try to find antibiotics that under consideration of the expected susceptibility cover the whole pathogen spectrum individually.

Except for some community-acquired infections, monotherapies have to be combined with synergistic or additive effecting antibiotics. If no adequate single therapy can be found, we use combination rules to generate combinations of antibiotics. Each possible combination must be tested for the ability to cover the expected spectrum completely.

2 Medical Evaluation of ICONS

ICONS was originally developed for an intensive care unit of the University clinic in Munich within a project, which was also named ICONS. Since we moved to Rostock, the evaluation of ICONS remained unfinished in Munich. In Rostock we changed those parts in ICONS which depend on the local environment. Subsequently, we evaluated ICONS in Rostock. Here we present first results. At present a second evaluation in Rostock is still in progress.

2.1 Evaluation in Munich

A first evaluation dealt with the interpretation of microbiological findings to adapt general information from literature to the local situation [4]. We interpreted about 14800 microbiological findings to test parts of our initial medical knowledge base (calculated pathogen spectra, known resistances). The laboratory data mainly corresponded with the data from literature, which we had used to build up an initial knowledge base. A few pathogens had developed resistances against specific antibiotics and some calculated pathogen spectra had to be widened.

Secondly, we asked experienced physicians to assess our adviser. Since no golden standard exists about antibiotics therapy, we developed a questionnaire to evaluate the user friendliness, the men-machine-interaction, and especially the correctness and the quality of the recommended therapies. Experienced physicians of intensive care units filled in the questionnaire, which contained typical clinical case descriptions. They were asked to recommend antibiotic therapies for these cases. We asked them to do the same task with ICONS again. The results of this evaluation by questionnaire can be summarised as follows [4]:

- The general idea of ICONS, namely to determine calculated pathogen spectra concerning the infected organ systems and the groups of patients and subsequently to attempt to cover the current patient's spectrum, was approved by all physicians.

- Concerning the correctness and the quality of ICONS's recommendations the opinions of the physicians deviated from each other. Though most physicians rated

ICONS's recommendations as correct, suitable and useful, few of them said that specific therapies should not be recommended.

- The comments on the user-friendliness and on the interface of ICONS were positive. However, some physicians made suggestions and we enriched some menus by additional explanations.

2.2 Evaluation in Rostock

After moving to Rostock we wanted to establish ICONS here. However, many parts of the adviser had to be updated. First, partly different antibiotics are available on the wards. So we had to remove a few antibiotics from the knowledge base and had to put in a few others instead. And the rules, which contain information about which antibiotics should be combined with each other, also had to be modified. Furthermore, an antibiotics therapy adviser has to consider local characteristics; e.g. the resistance situation is mainly general, but has to be adapted to local characteristics.

Because of the high variability between the physicians concerning the assessment of ICONS's recommendations (see section 2.1), we now chose a different strategy. After all necessary updates were finished, we started with an examination of more than 50 cases of three intensive care units (internal medicine, surgery, and one for children). In a first step we have checked if the therapies introduced by the physicians were recommended by the updated ICONS too. Fig.1. shows that about 70% of the introduced therapies were also recommended by ICONS, about 12% were used as single therapies while ICONS recommended them in combination with antibiotics that have additive or synergistic effects, and for nearly 18% of the cases the physicians prescribed therapies that were not recommended by ICONS. The 12% combinations instead of single therapies are no a problem, because ICONS simply prefers to be on the safer side. For those therapies ICONS did not recommend at all, it was difficult to decide if they were suitable or not, because we did not have any information about the quality of the prescribed therapies. We tried to discuss with the physicians who prescribed these therapies about their reasoning. One problem with the retrospective cases was that the physicians sometimes had difficulties to remember all details. Another problem was to assess the justifications of the explanations given by the physicians. So, as a result we have modified the combination rules only slightly.

Very recently we have started another evaluation in Rostock. We use a questionnaire again, this time we ask only about the quality of ICONS's recommendations and we do not ask physicians, but experts working in the microbiological laboratory (biologists, chemists), who not only provide antibiograms, but who additionally make suggestions which antibiotics should be used.

3   Applying Case-Based Reasoning

In this application, the main argument for using CBR methods is to speed-up the process of finding adequate therapies. We shorten the above described strategy (see paragraph 1.1) of selecting advisable antibiotic therapies by searching for a similar case, retrieving its suggested therapies and by adapting them to the situation of the current patient.

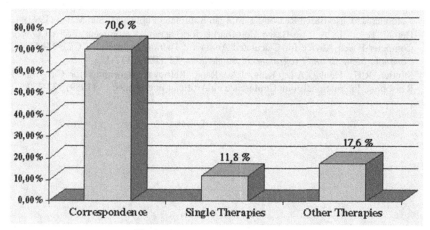

Fig.1. First evaluation results in Rostock

Retrieval. Since the attributes in ICONS are nominal valued, we have originally applied the Hash-Tree-Retrieval algorithm of Stottler, Henke, and King [5], which has been developed for large case bases containing cases with nominal valued attributes. We compared retrieval times of the Hash-Tree-Retrieval algorithm with those of "simple indexing" [3]. Tree-Hash retrieval is very fast when the number of attributes is low (up to about ten). Its retrieval time does not increase with the number of cases if a hashing scheme is used, because in a pre-processing step a tree is constructed, which consists of nodes for every possible combination of the attributes. From these nodes corresponding cases can be hashed.

Since simple indexing does not construct a Hash-Tree, but hashes directly, the results of comparing both algorithms are no surprise. Simple indexing works much faster, but the retrieval time increases with the number of stored cases, while Hash-Tree retrieval does not depend on the number of stored cases. So, in our application both algorithms have equal retrieval times, when the case base contains about 3.000 cases. With even more cases Hash-Tree retrieval is faster than simple indexing. As a result of comparing retrieval times we have replaced Hash-Tree retrieval by simple indexing, because ICONS contains just a few hundreds of cases.

Adaptations. In ICONS three sorts of adaptations occur: A CBR adaptation to obtain sets of calculated advisable therapies for current patients, an adaptation of chosen therapies to laboratory findings, and a periodical update of laboratory information used by the system.

References

1. Bueno-Cavanillas, A. et al.: Influence of nosocomial infection on mortality rate in an intensive care unit. *Crit Care Med 22* (1994) 55-60
2. Daschner, F.D. et al.: Nosocomial infections in intensive care wards: a multicenter prospective study. *Intensive Care Med 8* (1982) 5-9

3. Kolodner, J.: Case-Based Reasoning. Morgan Kaufmann Publishers, San Mateo (1993)
4. Heindl ,B. et al.: A Case-Based Consiliarius for Therapy Recommendation (ICONS): Computer-Based Advice for Calculated Antibiotic Therapy in Intensive Care Medicine. *Computer Methods and Programms in Biomedicine 52* (1997) 117-127
5. Stottler, R.H., Henke, A.L., King, J.A.: Rapid Retrieval Algorithms for Case-Based Reasoning. International Joint Conference on Artificial Intelligence 11 (1989) 233-237

Author Index

Lecture Notes in Artificial Intelligence (LNAI)

Lecture Notes in Computer Science